ESSAYS IN BIOCHEMISTRY

ESSAYS IN BIOCHEMISTRY

volume 56 2014

Amyloids in Health and Disease

Edited by Sarah Perrett

portlandpress**limited**
publishing innovation

Essays in Biochemistry is published by Portland Press Limited on behalf of the Biochemical Society

Portland Press Limited
Third Floor, Charles Darwin House
12 Roger Street
London WC1N 2JU
U.K.
Tel: +44 (0)20 7685 2410
Fax: +44 (0)20 7685 2469
email: editorial@portlandpress.com
www.portlandpress.com

British Library Cataloguing-in-Publication Data
A catalogue record for this book is available from the British Library
ISBN   978-1-85578-192-4
ISSN (print)   0071 1365
ISSN (online)   1744 1358

Typeset by Techset Composition Ltd, Salisbury, U.K.
Printed in Great Britain by Berforts Information Press, Eynsham, U.K.

CONTENTS

4   Protein folding, misfolding and quality control: the role of molecular chaperones 53

Katharina Papsdorf and Klaus Richter

5   Insights into amyloid disease from fly models 69

Ko-Fan Chen and Damian C. Crowther

6   Yeast models for amyloid disease 85

Barry Panaretou and Gary W. Jones

7 Amyloid β-peptide and Alzheimer's disease 99

David Allsop and Jennifer Mayes

8 The physiology and pathology of microtubule-associated protein tau 111

Jian-Zhi Wang, Xinya Gao and Zhi-Hao Wang

9 Role of α-synuclein in neurodegeneration: implications for the pathogenesis of Parkinson's disease 125

Shun Yu and Piu Chan

10 Oligomers of α-synuclein: picking the culprit in the line-up 137

Nikolai Lorenzen and Daniel E. Otzen

11 Many roads lead to Rome? Multiple modes of Cu,Zn superoxide dismutase destabilization, misfolding and aggregation in amyotrophic lateral sclerosis 149

Helen R. Broom, Jessica A.O. Rumfeldt and Elizabeth M. Meiering

12 Spontaneous self-assembly of pathogenic huntingtin exon 1 protein into amyloid structures 167

Philipp Trepte, Nadine Strempel and Erich E. Wanker

13 Prion disease and the 'protein-only hypothesis' 181

Jiyan Ma and Fei Wang

14 Amyloid diseases of yeast: prions are proteins acting as genes 193

Reed B. Wickner, Herman K. Edskes, David A. Bateman,
Amy C. Kelly, Anton Gorkovskiy, Yaron Dayani and Albert Zhou

15 Functional amyloid: widespread in Nature, diverse in purpose 207

Chi L.L. Pham, Ann H. Kwan and Margaret Sunde

PREFACE

Misfolding and aggregation of proteins to form amyloid deposits is a characteristic of a number of human diseases, including Alzheimer's, Parkinson's, amyotrophic lateral sclerosis, polyglutamine diseases such as Huntington's, and the prion diseases. Although genetically inherited factors play a role in each of these diseases to a greater or lesser extent, age is also a risk factor, as the manifestation of these diseases reflects a breakdown in the cellular quality control mechanisms that usually ensure that proteins attain and maintain their correctly folded conformations. Understanding the protective mechanisms of the cell, as well as the pathological mechanisms of each of these diseases, is of increasing concern and importance for an aging world population. Interestingly, amyloid aggregates are also found in functional roles in a range of organisms, such as formation of fimbriae (or curli) in bacteria and epigenetic prion-like factors in fungi. Understanding how bacteria, fungi and even mammalian cells can control and utilize protein 'misfolding' to provide biological functions is not only a fascinating biological question, but may also shed light on the pathological mechanisms of amyloid diseases.

Protein folding, misfolding and amyloid formation is no longer considered a specialist subject, of interest only to those carrying out research in this area, but is now a core part of any advanced undergraduate or graduate biochemistry course. It is also a rapidly developing field, with a broad range of approaches being applied, ranging from *in silico* theoretical modelling; via biophysical, biochemical and cellular characterization of molecular mechanisms; to whole organism and systems biology approaches. Importantly, these wide-ranging approaches and techniques are being used in combination to great effect, meaning that research in this area has become truly multi-disciplinary. It is hoped that this volume will provide an accessible overview, highlighting recent progress in this field.

In Chapter 1, Louise Serpell sets the scene by providing an introduction to amyloid structure. The biophysical theme continues in Chapter 2, by Alex Buell, Chris Dobson and Tuomas Knowles, which provides a comprehensive overview of the thermodynamics and kinetics of amyloid fibril formation; and Chapter 3, by Greet De Baets, Joost Schymkowitz and Frederic Rousseau discusses prediction of aggregation prone sequences in proteins. Chapter 4, by Katharina Papsdorf and Klaus Richter, addresses the roles of the protein quality control machinery, particularly molecular chaperones, in health and disease. Chapter 5, by Ko-Fan Chen and Damian Crowther, describes the application of fly models to study amyloid diseases; and Chapter 6, by Barry Panaretou and Gary Jones, discusses yeast models for amyloid disease. Chapters 7–13 provide an overview of research on specific amyloid diseases and the role of key protein players: Chapter 7, by David Allsop and Jennifer Mayes, is focused on amyloid β-peptide in Alzheimer's disease; Chapter 8, by Jian-Zhi Wang and colleagues, focuses on the physiology and pathology of microtubule-associated tau; Chapter 9, by Shun Yu and Piu Chan, addresses the role of α-synuclein in neurodegeneration in the context of Parkinson's disease; Chapter 10, by Nikolai Lorenzen and Daniel Otzen, continues discussion of α-synuclein from the viewpoint of its biophysical properties and cytotoxicity; Chapter 11, by Elizabeth Meiering and colleagues discusses the role of Cu,Zn superoxide dismutase in amyotrophic lateral sclerosis; Chapter 12, by Erich Wanker and colleagues, addresses polyglutamine disease and aggregation of the protein fragment, Huntingtin exon 1; and Chapter 13, by Jiyan Ma and Fei Wang, discusses prion disease and the 'protein-only hypothesis'. Chapter 14, by Reed Wickner and colleagues, is focused on yeast prions. Finally, in Chapter 15, Margaret Sunde and colleagues give an overview of the many functional roles of amyloids found in Nature.

I would like to thank each author who has contributed to this fascinating collection of articles. I would also like to thank the *Essays in Biochemistry* Editorial Advisory Panel as well as the staff at Portland Press, particularly Clare Curtis, for their guidance and assistance at all stages of this project. Finally, I would like to thank Chris Dobson and Tuomas Knowles for facilitating a 6-month sabbatical in Cambridge, coinciding with the main period of work on this volume.

Sarah Perrett is a Professor at the Institute of Biophysics (IBP), Chinese Academy of Sciences, where she has been a group leader since 2003. She obtained her undergraduate and Ph.D. degrees from the University of Cambridge, where she then held a Sidney Sussex College Research Fellowship. After a year of full-time Chinese language study at the National University of Singapore, she moved to IBP in 2000, initially supported by fellowships from the Royal Society and the Royal Commission for the Exhibition of 1851. Her current research is supported by the National Natural Science Foundation of China, the Ministry of Science and Technology of China and the Chinese Academy of Sciences. She has returned to Cambridge as a visiting scientist in 2005, 2009 and 2014. Her laboratory is studying the structure and assembly of functional amyloids, and the structure and function of molecular chaperones, using a variety of biochemical and biophysical techniques.

Louise Serpell is a Professor of Biochemistry at the University of Sussex, where she has run a research group looking at the structure of amyloid fibrils since 2003. Previously, she worked at the University of Cambridge and Medical Research Council Laboratory of Molecular Biology in Cambridge where she did much of her early work to visualize the β-sheet structure of amyloid fibrils. She spent 18 months as a postdoctoral researcher at the University of Toronto after completing her D.Phil. in the laboratory of Dr Colin Blake at the University of Oxford, where she worked on the generic structure of the amyloid fibril.

Alexander Buell studied Chemistry and Biochemistry at the University of Tübingen from 2002 to 2004. He was then awarded a 'Sélection Internationale' scholarship to continue his studies at Ecole Normale Supérieure, Paris and the University Paris VI. He graduated in 2007 with a Master's degree in Physical and Theoretical Chemistry. He then did his Ph.D. studies with Professor Sir Mark Welland and Professor Christopher M. Dobson on the kinetics of protein aggregation into amyloid fibrils. In 2011, he was awarded a Thomas Nevile research fellowship from Magdalene College, Cambridge and in 2013, a Leverhulme Trust Early Career Fellowship, both to be held in the Department of Chemistry in Cambridge in order to continue and extend his research on the physical principles and mechanisms underlying amyloid fibril formation.

Christopher Dobson studied Chemistry at the University of Oxford, where he also carried out his Ph.D. work under Robert J.P. Williams on structural characterizations of proteins by the then emerging technique of NMR spectroscopy. He held research fellowships at Merton and Linacre colleges, Oxford and then an Assistant Professorship at Harvard University, before being appointed to a Lectureship in Oxford in 1980, followed by a Readership and Professorship. Until his move to Cambridge in 2001 to take up the John Humphrey Plummer Professorship in Chemical and Structural Biology, his research was mainly directed towards the understanding of protein folding mechanisms, to which he made seminal contributions. Towards the end of the 1990s, he became interested in the link between protein folding and misfolding that can lead to aggregation into amyloid fibrils. His research has contributed groundbreaking fundamental understanding about the causes of protein aggregation and its link with human disorders, such as Alzheimer's disease. Professor Dobson has published more than 700 scientific articles and has been awarded numerous prizes for his work, most recently, the Heineken prize for Biochemistry and Biophysics.

Tuomas Knowles studied Biology at the University of Geneva and Physics at ETH Zurich. He obtained his Ph.D. in Physics from the University of Cambridge, working at the Cavendish laboratory and Nanoscience Centre with Professor Christopher Dobson, Professor Sir Mark Welland and Professor Cait MacPhee. He then spent time as a St John's College Research Fellow at Cambridge and Harvard University and joined the Department of Chemistry in Cambridge in 2010. His research is focused on the development and application of both theoretical and experimental methods to the study of biological macromolecules, work that has been recognized through a number of prizes, including the British Biophysical Society Medal, Young Investigator Prize and the Royal Society of Chemistry Harrison Meldola Award.

Greet De Baets obtained her Ph.D. in 2013 in the Switch Laboratory (VIB, University of Leuven). She combines computational modelling and cell biological experimentation to investigate the mechanisms of protein aggregation.

Joost Schymkowitz obtained his Ph.D. in 2001 from the University of Cambridge in Professor Sir Alan Fersht's laboratory under the supervision of Laura Itzhaki. He completed his postdoctoral research at the European Molecular Biology Laboratory in Luis Serrano's laboratory. He is now one half of a group leader duo running the Switch Laboratory at the VIB and University of Leuven. The research of the Switch Laboratory combines computational modelling and biophysical and cell biological experimentation to investigate the mechanisms of protein misfolding and aggregation. Specifically, Switch investigates how sequence composition determines the structure of protein aggregates as well as their specificity, their mode of interaction with molecular chaperones and their toxicity to cells.

Frederic Rousseau obtained his Ph.D. in 2001 from the University of Cambridge in Professor Sir Alan Fersht's laboratory under the supervision of Laura Itzhaki. He completed his postdoctoral research at the European Molecular Biology Laboratory in Luis Serrano's laboratory. He is now one half of a group leader duo running the Switch Laboratory at the VIB and University of Leuven. The research of the Switch Laboratory investigates the mechanisms of protein misfolding and aggregation. In order to relate the sequence specificity of aggregation to aggregation-related disease mechanisms, Switch has built an integrated research platform that combines bioinformatics, biophysics, cell biology and now, also increasingly, animal models.

Katharina Papsdorf is a Ph.D. student in Klaus Richter's group. She works on the Hsc70 chaperone system in *Caenorhabditis elegans* and polyglutamine aggregation models in *Saccharomyces cerevisiae*.

Klaus Richter is a group leader at the Technische Universität München. He works on *Saccharomyces cerevisiae* and *Caenorhabditis elegans* model systems to study the function of molecular chaperones and protein misfolding diseases. He is particularly interested in understanding the molecular mechanisms of the chaperones Hsp90 and Hsc70 during their cellular functions. Klaus Richter earned his Ph.D. in the laboratory of Johannes Buchner and completed his postdoctoral studies at Rick Morimoto's Laboratory at Northwestern University.

Ko-Fan Chen is a postdoctoral scientist with a particular interest in using *Drosophila melanogaster* to study neurodegenerative disease and aging, and their impact on circadian biology. His Ph.D. was awarded by Queen Mary University of London where he worked in Ralf Stanewsky's circadian group.

Damian Crowther has a background in clinical neurology and has been working on *in vitro* and *Drosophila*-based models of neurodegenerative diseases for over a decade. He is currently interested in understanding prion-like mechanisms in disorders such as Alzheimer's disease.

Barry Panaretou is a Senior Lecturer within the Institute of Pharmaceutical Science, King's College London (KCL). His primary research interests focus on the function of the Hsp90 chaperone, using yeast as a model organism. Prior to establishing the Yeast Genetics Laboratory at KCL in 2000, he held postdoctoral positions at University College London and the Chester Beatty Laboratory, Cancer Research UK. He obtained his Ph.D. in Biochemistry in 1993 from University College London.

Gary Jones is a Senior Lecturer within the Department of Biology, National University of Ireland Maynooth (NUIM). His primary research interests focus on the influence of chaperone proteins on amyloid formation, using yeast as a model organism. Prior to establishing the Yeast Genetics Laboratory at NUIM in 2004, he held postdoctoral positions at the National Institutes of Health, University College London and University of Wales Swansea. He obtained his Ph.D. in Molecular Biology in 1996 from the University of Liverpool.

David Allsop is a Professor of Neuroscience in the Faculty of Health and Medicine at University of Lancaster. He has more than 30 years of research experience working on the role of β-amyloid in Alzheimer's disease. He was the first person to isolate senile plaque amyloid from frozen post-mortem brain tissue and was one of the founders of the 'amyloid cascade' hypothesis. His current research is focused on the development of biomarkers for neurodegenerative diseases, and on the development of inhibitors of protein aggregation.

Jennifer Mayes is a Research Associate and Senior Teaching Associate in the Faculty of Health and Medicine, University of Lancaster. She has worked with clinicians and patients to set up studies to investigate measures of inhibitory control and working memory as an aid to diagnosis of Alzheimer's disease and other dementias. She now focuses her research on the redox processes associated with β-amyloid aggregation and on the development of inhibitors to target these processes.

Jian-Zhi Wang is a Professor and Director of the Pathophysiology Department, Key Laboratory of Ministry of Education of China for Neurological Disorders, and Deputy Director of the Faculty of Basic Medicine and Research Institutes for Medical Science. Her laboratory is involved in exploring the mechanisms underlying Alzheimer's neurodegeneration, especially the role of the microtubule-associated protein tau. In the search for new strategies to arrest disease progression, the laboratory develops methods, and cell and animal models to measure abnormal tau proteins, and cellular or systemic effects of tau proteins.

Xinya Gao is a student in the laboratory of Jian-Zhi Wang working on exploring the mechanisms underlying Alzheimer's neurodegeneration.

Zhi-Hao Wang is a student in the laboratory of Jian-Zhi Wang working on exploring the mechanisms underlying Alzheimer's neurodegeneration.

Shun Yu obtained his Ph.D. in 1998 from Shiga University of Medical Science in Japan. After a 2 year postdoctoral position in the Academy of Military Medical Sciences of China, he moved to the Department of Neurobiology, Beijing Institute of Geriatric Medical and Research Center, Xuanwu Hospital, Capital Medical University. Since then, he has focused on the study of Parkinson's disease, especially the pathogenic mechanism and diagnostic biomarkers.

Piu Chan graduated from Hunan Medical College in 1983 followed by clinical postgraduate training at the First Affiliated Hospital (Xiangya Hospital). He received his Ph.D. in Neuroscience from Sun Yat-Sen University of Medical Science in 1990, followed by a 2 year postdoctoral position at the Parkinson's Institute in California. Dr Chan was then the Director of the Molecular Genetics Laboratory at the Parkinson's Institute until he returned to China in 2000. Since then, he has been Professor of Neurology, Geriatrics and Neurobiology at the Beijing Institute of Geriatric Medical and Research Center and Xuanwu Hospital of Capital Medical University in Beijing. He has focused on studies of Parkinson's and related diseases, especially epidemiology, genetics, biomarkers and animal models.

Nikolai Lorenzen obtained his B.Sc. degree in Civil Engineering (Biotechnology) from Aalborg University in 2008. He was then enrolled as an M.Sc. student in Peptide and Protein Chemistry at Stockholm University for 1 year until he was enrolled as a Ph.D. student under the supervision of Daniel Otzen. He finished his Ph.D. in November 2013, working on the topic of α-synuclein aggregation and the use of small-molecule drugs to inhibit this process. He now works as a Research Scientist in protein biophysics at Novo Nordisk.

Daniel Otzen is Professor of Nanobiotechnology at the Interdisciplinary Nanoscience Center (iNANO) at Aarhus University. He obtained his Ph.D. at Aarhus University in 1995 after protein folding studies in Professor Sir Alan Fersht's laboratory at the University of Cambridge. He has also worked as a staff scientist at Novozymes within the field of stability and folding of industrial enzymes. His interests include pathological and functional amyloid formation, the structures and properties of pre-fibrillar species, approaches to prevent aggregation and oligomer formation and also the folding and stability of membrane proteins. He is a member of the Danish Royal Society of Sciences and Letters.

Helen Broom is a Ph.D. candidate at the University of Waterloo, working under the supervision of Elizabeth Meiering. She began her graduate studies in 2008, after completing a B.Sc. in Biochemistry and Biotechnology at the University of Waterloo. Her graduate research is on characterizing folding, misfolding and aggregation of metal-free forms of SOD1.

Jessica Rumfeldt obtained her Ph.D. on stability and folding mechanisms of SOD1 in 2006 from the University of Waterloo under the supervision of Elizabeth Meiering. She was a postdoctoral research fellow at the University of Waterloo and then the University of California San Diego under the supervision of Dr James R. Halpert and Dr Dimitri R. Davydov, investigating substrate binding co-operativity in cytochrome P450s. She is now a Research Associate studying various proteins including SOD1 in the Meiering group.

Elizabeth Meiering completed her Ph.D. on the folding and function of barnase with Professor Sir Alan Fersht at the University of Cambridge in 1992. Her postdoctoral research used NMR to analyse the roles of mutations and hydration on dihydrofolate reductase, with Professor Gerhard Wagner at Harvard Medical School. Since joining the University of Waterloo in 1996, her group's research has focused on the folding, misfolding and design of numerous proteins of fundamental, medical or biotechnological interest. She has held a John Charles Polanyi Award and University Research Chair, and has served on the ALS Society of Canada Scientific Advisory Board, as Associate Dean of Graduate Studies, and on the Editorial Board for Protein Engineering Design and Selection.

Philipp Trepte is currently doing his Ph.D. in the laboratory of Erich Wanker, working on the systematic generation and characterization of a protein interaction map of synaptic proteins. During his Master's degree in Cell Biology at the University of Osnabrück, he visited the laboratory of Douglas Cyr at the University of North Carolina School of Medicine, before he joined the Philipp Khaitovich's laboratory at the Partner Institute for Computational Biology for his Master's thesis. His research interests focus on protein–protein interactions, neurodegenerative diseases and synapse biology.

Nadine Strempel is working towards her Ph.D. in Erich Wanker's laboratory with a focus on the molecular mechanisms of huntingtin aggregation and its modulation by small molecules. Before coming to the Max Delbrück Center, she completed a diploma degree with a thesis in Molecular Biology and Virology at the Department of Applied Tumor Virology of the German Cancer Research Center. To deepen her knowledge in Immunology and Biochemistry, she studied one semester abroad at the University of Copenhagen.

Erich Wanker is Chair of Molecular Medicine at Charité University Medicine Berlin and heads the Neuroproteomics research group at the Max Delbrück Center for Molecular Medicine Berlin-Buch. He graduated in Chemical Engineering and Biochemistry from the University of Technology Graz, where he also completed his Ph.D. in 1992. After a postdoctoral fellowship at the University of California, Los Angeles he became a group leader at the Max-Planck-Institute for Molecular Genetics and was appointed to his present positions in 2001. His research interests are in protein misfolding and neurodegeneration, molecular mechanisms of protein–protein and protein–drug interactions and on high-throughput network biology.

Jiyan Ma received training in Medicine and studied leukaemia viruses at the Shanghai Medical University. He received his Ph.D. degree in 1997 from the University of Illinois. Dr Ma started to study prion disease when he was a postdoctoral fellow in Dr Susan Lindquist's laboratory at the University of Chicago. Ma started his group at Ohio State University in 2002 and continued to study the pathogenic mechanism of prion disease. Currently, he is a Professor at the Center for Neurodegenerative Science and Head of the laboratory of prion mechanisms in neurodegeneration at the Van Andel Research Institute.

Fei Wang received his B.Sc. degree from Nankai University. He joined Dr Jiyan Ma's laboratory and started his Ph.D. thesis research on prion disease in 2003. Dr Wang's graduate work focused on the biochemical characterization of interactions between recombinant PrP and lipids. Dr Wang's current research interests lie in molecular mechanisms of prion infectivity. Dr Wang has co-authored 14 peer-reviewed articles on prion research, including one invited methodology paper and one invited review article, and he is the recipient of the Alberta Prion Research Institute International Young Researcher Prize.

Reed Wickner majored in Mathematics at Cornell University and obtained his MD from Georgetown University. After studying yeast RNA viruses, he discovered, in 1994, that the non-chromosomal genes [URE3] and [PSI+] are yeast prions of Ure2p and Sup35p. He is currently interested in expanding knowledge of the in-register parallel β-sheet prion amyloid structure, the mechanisms by which prions cause disease in yeast, the means by which Btn2p and Cur1p cure the [URE3] prion, and the mutability of the prion cloud.

Herman Edskes obtained his Ph.D. at the University of Kentucky studying plant pararetroviruses with Professor Robert Shepherd. He carried out postdoctoral work with Dr Reed Wickner at the National Institutes of Health investigating viruses and prions of the yeast *Saccharomyces cerevisiae*. Currently, he is a staff scientist at the National Institute of Diabetes, Digestive and Kidney Diseases in the Laboratory of Biochemistry and Genetics and focuses on yeast prions.

David Bateman obtained his Ph.D. from the University of Toronto in the department of Medical Biophysics. He is currently investigating the cloud of prion variants, using yeast as a model system.

Amy Kelly is currently a postdoctoral fellow in the Wickner laboratory at the National Institutes of Health. She acquired her Ph.D. from the University of Illinois, Urbana-Champaign in the laboratory of Dr Jan Novakofski, where she studied population genetics of mammalian prion diseases. Her current research focuses on elucidating the molecular ecology of yeast prions.

Anton Gorkovskiy is a visiting fellow in the Laboratory of Biochemistry and Genetics, National Institute of Diabetes and Digestive and Kidney Diseases, National Institutes of Health. Dr Gorkovskiy obtained his Ph.D. in Biochemistry in 2009 from the Institute of Biochemistry and Physiology of Microorganisms, Russian Academy of Sciences. Working in Dr Tatyana Kalebina's group, Dr Gorkovskiy was investigating *Saccharomyces cerevisiae* cell wall proteins possessing amyloid properties. Currently, he is studying metastable and toxic *S. cerevisiae* prion variants and working on determining the fine structure of amyloid fibrils formed by one of the prion-forming proteins, Sup35.

Yaron Dayani is currently a postdoctoral fellow in the Wickner laboratory at the National Institute of Diabetes and Digestive and Kidney Diseases. He completed his Ph.D. studies at the Faculty of Life Sciences, The Hebrew University of Jerusalem, in collaboration with Dr Simchen and the Lichten laboratory at the National Cancer Institute, where he studied activities responsible for the resolution of double Holliday junctions. Before that, he completed his undergraduate and Master's studies in Genetics with a focus on aging using nematode models in the Gruenbaum laboratory. His present research focuses on prion propagation using yeast as a model.

Albert Zhou graduated with a B.Sc. in Biochemistry and Molecular Biology from the University of Maryland, Baltimore County and is currently a post-baccalaureate fellow working with Dr Reed Wickner. Zhou is investigating the prion-forming ability of various proteins.

Chi Pham joined Professor Roberto Cappai's laboratory in the Department of Pathology at The University of Melbourne, working on amyloid diseases associated with neurodegeneration, specifically on Alzheimer's disease and Parkinson's disease following the completion of her Ph.D. Currently located in the Discipline of Pharmacology at The University of Sydney, her research focus is now on the role of amyloid-forming fungal hydrophobin proteins in rice blast infections.

Ann Kwan received her Ph.D. in Biochemistry from the University of Sydney. After working as an Australian postdoctoral fellow, she took up the position of NMR Facility Manager at the School of Molecular Bioscience, University of Sydney. She is currently a research fellow at the School as well as being responsible for the NMR facility. Her research focuses on investigations of protein structures and functions, and protein assemblies including functional amyloids. Ann has received Young Investigator Awards from the East Coast Protein Meeting, Lorne Protein Conference, ISMAR and AMZMAG societies.

Margaret Sunde received her Ph.D. in Biochemistry from the University of Cambridge. Her interest in amyloid was sparked during her postdoctoral work with Colin Blake and Chris Dobson in Oxford, where she focused on structural and biophysical studies of disease-associated amyloid fibrils and the role of protein misfolding in amyloid formation. Now a senior lecturer at the University of Sydney, Sunde's research efforts have turned to the study of functional amyloid, particularly the formation and biological application of amyloid formed by the fungal hydrophobin proteins.

ABBREVIATIONS

AA	arachidonic acid
AAA ATPases	ATPases associated with various cellular activities
ACE	angiotensin-converting enzyme
AD	Alzheimer's disease
ADAM	a disintegrin and metalloproteinase
ADDL	amyloid β-derived diffusible ligand
ADF	*Araneusdiadematus* fibroin
aDrs	anionic dermaseptin
AD-tau	abnormally hyperphosphorylated tau from AD brain
AFM	atomic force microscopy
AGE	advanced glycation end product
ALS	amyotrophic lateral sclerosis
ANS	8-anilinonaphthalene-1-sulfonic acid
APH-1	anterior pharynx defective 1
APOE	apolipoprotein E
apoSH	metal-free disulfide-reduced monomer
apoSS	metal-free disulfide-intact dimer
APP	amyloid precursor protein
APR	aggregation-prone region
Aβ	amyloid β-peptide
Aβ42	amyloid β-peptide 42-residue fragment
BACE1	β-site amyloid precursor protein cleaving enzyme 1
BBB	blood–brain barrier
BSE	bovine spongiform encephalopathy
CaMKII	Ca^{2+}/calmodulin-dependent protein kinase II
CASA	chaperone-assisted selective autophagy
CCS	copper chaperone for SOD-1
CCT	chaperone-containing T-complex protein
CDK	cyclin-dependent kinase
CFTR	cystic fibrosis transmembrane conductance regulator
CHIP	C-terminus of the heat-shock cognate 70-interacting protein
CK1	casein kinase 1
CMA	chaperone-mediated autophagy
CNS	central nervous system
CPEB	cytoplasmic polyadenylation element-binding protein
CSPα	cysteine string protein α
Cu,Zn-SOD1	copper/zinc superoxide dismutase 1
CWD	chronic wasting disease
DA	dopamine
DAT	dopamine transporter

DIC	dynein intermediate chain
DISC	death-inducing signalling complex
DLS	dynamic light scattering
DSC	differential scanning calorimetry
dSTORM	direct stochastic optical reconstruction microscopy
DYRK1A	dual-specificity tyrosine-phosphorylation-regulated kinase 1A
ECE	endothelin-converting enzyme
EGCG	(−)-epigallocatechin gallate
EM	electron microscopy
ER	endoplasmic reticulum
ERK	extracellular-signal-regulated kinase
fAD	familial Alzheimer's disease
fALS	familial amyotrophic lateral sclerosis
FAP	familial amyloid polyneuropathy
FRET	Förster resonance energy transfer
FTDP-17	frontotemporal dementia with Parkinsonism-linked to chromosome-17
FTLD	frontotemporal dementia lobar degeneration
FUS	fused-in-sarcoma
GA	geldanamycin
GFP	green fluorescent protein
GndHCl	guanidine hydrochloride
GndSCN	guanidinium thiocyanate
GPI	glycosylphosphatidylinositol
GPx	glutathione peroxidase
GSK-3	glycogen synthase kinase 3
GWAS	genome-wide association study
HD	Huntington's disease
HDAC6	histone deacetylase 6
3-HK	3-hydroxykynurenine
holoSS	mature, fully metallated and disulfide-intact dimer
Hsc70	heat-shock cognate 70 stress protein
Hsp	heat-shock protein
HSPB1	heat-shock 27 kDa protein 1
5-HT	serotonin
HTT	huntingtin
HTTex1	huntingtin exon 1
IAPP	islet amyloid polypeptide
IB	inclusion body
IDE	insulin-degrading enzyme
IDP	intrinsically disordered polypeptide
iLBD	incidental Lewy body disease
IPOD	insoluble protein deposit
iPS	induced pluripotent stem

ITC	isothermal titration calorimetry
JNK	c-Jun N-terminal kinase
KLC	kinesin light chain
KMO	kynurenine 3-monooxygenase
KPI	kunitz-type protease inhibitor
LB	Lewy body
LN	Lewy neurite
LRP	low-density lipoprotein receptor-related protein
M	folded monomer
β2M	β_2-microglobulin
MAPK	mitogen-activated protein kinase
MARK	microtubule affinity-regulating kinase
MASS	Mutant Aggregation and Stability Spectrum
MAT	monoamine transporter
MBD	microtubule-binding domain
MCI	mild cognitive impairment
mHTT	mutant HTT
NAC	nascent chain-associated complex or non-amyloid β-peptide component
NBD	N-terminal ATP-binding domain
NCC	nucleated conformational conversion
NCP	10-[4′-(N-diethylamino)butyl]-2-chlorophenoxazine
NE	norepinephrine
NEF	nucleotide exchange factor
NET	norepinephrine transporter
NFT	neurofibrillary tangle
NMDA	*N*-methyl-D-aspartate
NMDAR	*N*-methyl-D-aspartate receptor
OPTN	optineurin
PAR1	partitioning defective 1
PASTA	Prediction of Amyloid STructure Aggregation
PD	Parkinson's disease
PDPK	proline-directed protein kinase
PE	phosphatidylethanolamine
PEN-2	presenilin enhancer 2
PFD	prion-forming domain
PHF	paired helical filament
PICALM	phosphatidylinositol-binding clathrin assembly protein
PiD	Pick's disease
PIMA	Peptide Interaction Matrix Analyzer
Pin1	peptidylprolyl *cis–trans* isomerase NIMA-interacting 1
PI-PLC	phosphoinositide-specific phospholipase C
PK	proteinase K
PMCA	protein misfolding cyclic amplification

polyQ	polyglutamine
POPG	1-palmitoyl-2-oleoyl-*sn*-glycero-3-phospho-(10-rac-glycerol)
PP2A	protein phosphatase 2A
PrP	prion protein
PrP^C	normal cellular prion protein
PrP^{Sc}	disease-specific conformation of prion protein
PSP	progressive supranuclear palsy
PSSM	position-specific scoring matrix
QCM	quartz crystal microbalance
QUIN	quinolinic acid
RAC	ribosome-associated complex
RAGE	receptor for advanced glycation end products
recPrP	recombinant PrP
RHIM	RIP homotypic interaction motif
RIP	receptor-interacting protein
ROS	reactive oxygen species
sALS	sporadic amyotrophic lateral sclerosis
SALSA	Simple ALgorithm for Sliding Averages
SAXS	small-angle X-ray scattering
SBD	substrate-binding domain
SEC	size-exclusion chromatography
SERT	serotonin transporter
SH3	Src homology 3
sHsp	small heat-shock protein
SNAP-25	25 kDa synaptosome-associated protein
SNARE	soluble *N*-ethylmaleimide-sensitive fusion protein-attachment protein receptor
SOD1	superoxide dismutase 1
SR	sepiapterin reductase
SSA	senile systemic amyloidosis
SSP	secretion signal peptide
SUMO1	small ubiquitin-like modifier protein 1
αsyn	α-synuclein
TBP	TATA-binding protein
TCP	T-complex protein
TDP-43	transactive response DNA binding protein 43
TG	transglutaminase
TH	tyrosine hydroxylase
ThT	thioflavin-T
TIRF	total internal reflection fluorescence microscopy
TMAO	trimethylamine N-oxide
TriC	TCP1-containing ring complex
TPR domain	tetratricopeptide domain
TREM2	triggering receptor expressed on myeloid cells 2

TSE	transmissible spongiform encephalopathy
TTR	transthyretin
UPR	unfolded protein response
UPS	ubiquitin–proteasome system
vCJD	variant Creutzfeldt–Jacob disease
VMAT2	vesicular monoamine transporter 2
WT	wild-type

© The Authors Journal compilation © 2014 Biochemical Society
Essays Biochem. (2014) 56, 1–10: doi: 10.1042/BSE0560001

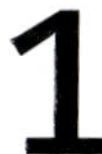

Amyloid structure

Louise Serpell[1]

School of Life Sciences, University of Sussex, Falmer BN1 9QG, U.K.

Abstract

Amyloid fibrils are formed by numerous proteins and peptides that share little sequence homology. The structures formed are highly ordered and extremely stable, being composed of β-sheet structure and stabilized along their length by hydrogen bonding. The fibrils are formed by several protofilaments that wind around one another in rope-like structures, lending further strength and stability to the resulting fibres. The fact that so many proteins and peptides form amyloid structures under suitable conditions, seems to suggest that the sequence of the precursor is unimportant. However, it is now clear that side chains play a central role in forming interactions between several β-sheets to further stabilize and regulate the structures. The primary sequence plays a central role in determining the rate of fibril formation, the stability of the resulting structure to degradation and the final morphology of the fibrils. The side chains regulate the elongation and growth, and also the lateral association of the protofilament and fibrils, having a significant impact on the final architecture.

Keywords:

amyloid, cross-β, protofilament, β-sheet, templated aggregation.

Introduction

Amyloid fibrils formed in disease are renowned for their resistance to degradation and clearance [1]. This is probably due to their extreme stability provided by their highly repetitive and ordered molecular architecture. This has been likened to the structure of silk, which is known to have a very high tensile strength [2]. The finding that amyloid fibrils deposit in diseases as diverse as Alzheimer's disease, Type 2 diabetes and multiple myeloma has meant that the

[1]To whom correspondence should be addressed (email l.c.serpell@sussex.ac.uk).

structure of these fibres is of particular interest. Importantly, the elucidation of the structure is thought to be helpful to provide a rational basis for drug design to prevent or reverse aggregation of the precursor protein. Each disease is characterized by the deposition of a different precursor protein and the native structures of these precursors vary enormously, from the all α-helical apolipoprotein A to the α-β structure of lysozyme and the mostly β structure of transthyretin. Despite these enormous differences, the fibrillar structures formed are indistinguishable, leading to the belief that the precursor proteins unfold and then refold to form the β-sheet-rich amyloid fibril.

Although the central role for amyloid fibrils in disease places them as a focus for research, the observation that they are utilized in Nature by a range of organisms makes them all the more fascinating. Amyloid fibrils are found to decorate bacteria and provide host defence [3]. They also form a protective coat on melanosomes [4] and they are involved in another level of genetic control in yeast [5]. Details of these roles are given in other chapters, but it is important to point out that it is the highly organized stable structure and self-propagating nature of the amyloid fibrils that means they are useful in these roles.

Techniques to examine amyloid structure

Amyloid fibrils may be observed using negative stain electron microscopy whereby the structures are enhanced by the use of a heavy metal stain that surrounds the protein (Figure 1). The magnification of ×20000–80000 allows observation of the size of the filaments as well as any details within them, such as the association of narrower protofilaments (Table 1). Cryo-electron microscopy has also been used and the advantage is that the fibre is hydrated and encased in ice resulting in a more physiologically preserved sample. It is also possible to

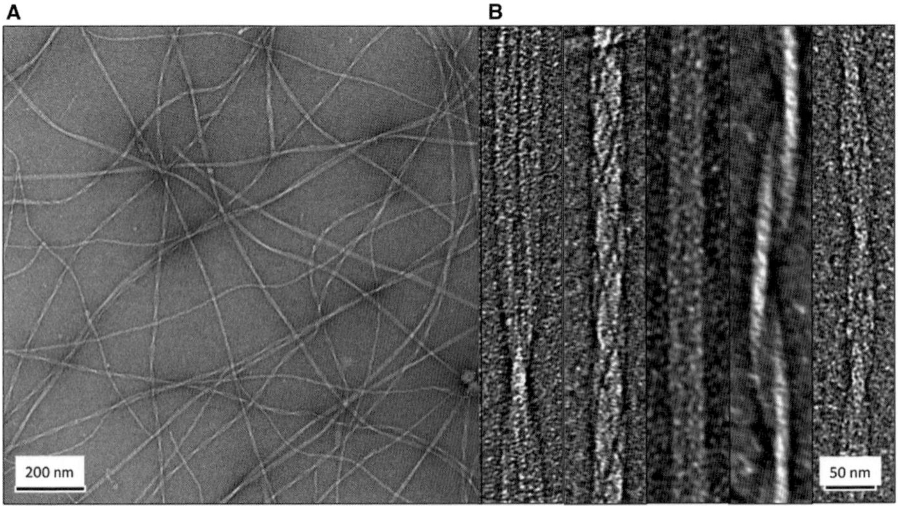

Figure 1. Electron micrographs of negatively stained amyloid fibrils
(**A**) Amyloid fibrils formed by the islet amyloid polypeptide associated with Type 2 diabetes.
(**B**) Alternative morphologies that can be formed by amyloidogenic peptides such as twisted ribbons, tubes, tapes and ropes.

Table 1. Nomenclature for amyloid terms

Term	Description	Conformation
Oligomer	Small and generally spherical structures formed by several monomers of the precursor molecule	Some β-sheet content
Protofibril	Elongated 'curvy linear', but relatively short assemblies of the precursor molecule	β-sheet
Protofilament	Narrow filamentous structure that associates further to form the amyloid fibril (~2.5–50 nm in diameter, indeterminate length).	Cross-β
Amyloid fibril	Straight unbranched fibres composed of several protofilaments (7–12 nm in diameter, indeterminate length). Sheets can laterally associate further to form ribbons	Cross-β with lateral association

directly image the protein rather than the stain and so this technique can provide much more structural information at a higher resolution (as we will see in the section below) [6,7].

Fibrous molecules are difficult to study by conventional structural techniques such as X-ray crystallography and solution-state NMR. These fibres are large, insoluble and heterogeneous. These qualities make them quite unsuitable for crystallization or solution-state techniques. However, they do contain crystalline structure and this means they can be studied using X-ray fibre diffraction (Figure 2). X-ray fibre diffraction is a technique made famous by the discovery of the structure of DNA by Watson and Crick [8] and relies on the diffraction from the repetitive features along the fibre axis. Amyloid fibrils consistently give a cross-β

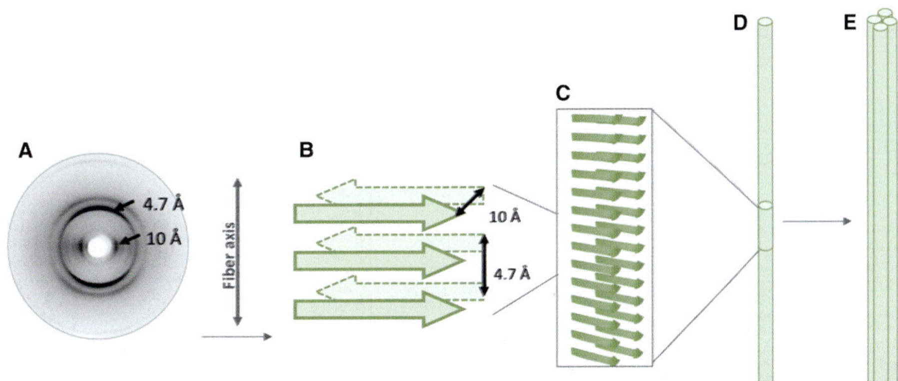

Figure 2. X-ray fibre diffraction gives information about the repetitive structure within the amyloid protofilament
(**A**) The cross-β diffraction pattern obtained from amyloid fibrils which arises from the (**B**) cross-β structural core of the protofilament shown in (**C**). The protofilaments shown in (**D**) self-associate to form the mature amyloid fibril (**E**).

diffraction pattern [9] similar to that first observed for cross-β silk [10]. This arises from the β-strands that run perpendicular to the fibre axis and the association of the β-sheets (see Figure 3 and more detail below). The diffraction patterns give a strong reflection at 4.7 Å (1 Å = 0.1 nm) on the vertical meridional axis of the pattern and a more diffuse reflection at 10 Å on the horizontal equatorial axis. This pattern was observed from many amyloid fibrils formed by different precursor molecules [11] (Figure 2).

Solid-state NMR [12] has been developed for the elucidation of amyloid structure, yielding a number of high resolution structures for the fibres and revealing that many amyloid-ogenic peptides form parallel, in register arrangements whereby the side chains stack up along the fibre axis. These structures again reinforce the importance of sequence composition. Solid-state NMR requires the use of spin-labelled peptides and allows information to be drawn regarding the distances between the spin labels, resulting in a model structure [13].

Biophysical techniques have been used extensively to examine the conformation of the protein backbone, particularly as the precursor protein assembles to form the fibrils (Figure 3). These techniques include circular dichroism, Fourier transform infrared spectroscopy and fluorescence that can inform regarding the secondary structural content of the sample and the environment of chromophores (such as side chains of tryptophan, tyrosine and

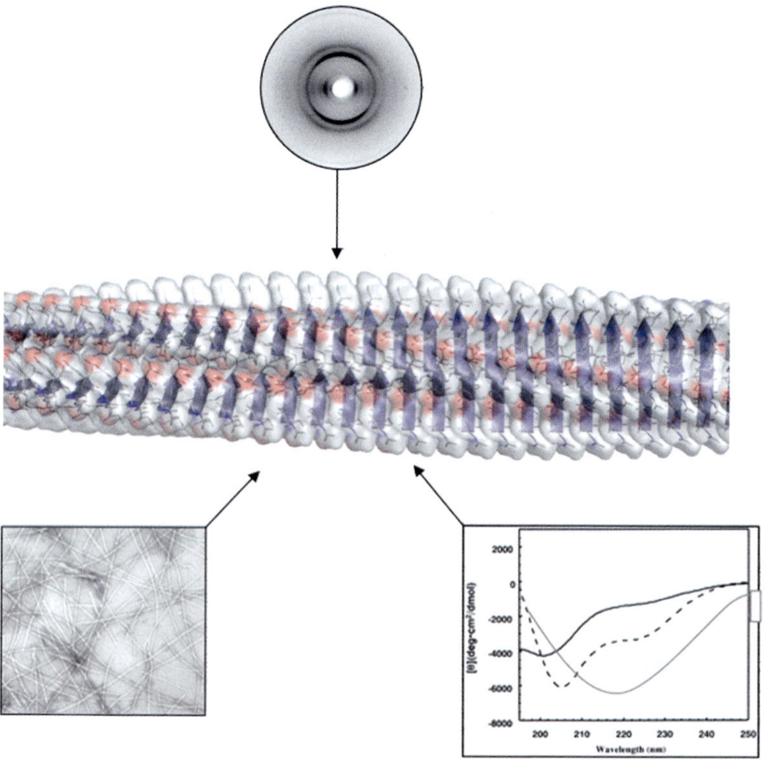

Figure 3. Structural methods can be combined to elucidate models for the amyloid structure
The diagram shows the contribution of X-ray fibre diffraction, electron microscopy and circular dichroism that can be combined to produce a structural model for the amyloid fibril [32].

phenylalanine), that change as the protein assembles. Circular dichroism can reveal a conformational change from the native structure of the precursor protein to the β-sheet-rich structure of the fibrils [14].

Structure of the fibril

The mature amyloid fibrils formed by the range of precursor molecules can vary depending on the assembly conditions. Fibrils can be ribbons, tubes and laterally associated sheets, composed of the narrow subunit filaments known as protofilaments (Figures 2D and 2E). Early work showed that amyloid fibrils purified from tissue were composed of several protofilaments (four to six) [15] and more recently, a number of cryo-electron microscopy studies have revealed more information about the interaction and association of the protofilaments to make up the final fibre [6,7]. The variability of the numbers of protofilaments has been studied in detail by Goldsbury et al. [16] who showed that individual protofilaments can be observed and that the morphology of the final fibre can vary. In later studies, the protofilament structure of fibrils and their variability were shown by processing of cryo-electron micrographs from amyloid fibrils formed by insulin [6], Aβ (amyloid β-peptide) [17] and β2 microglobulin [18]. Interestingly, fibrils formed by the same protein even under the same conditions can vary in the number of protofilaments that associate to form the mature fibril. Studies on both Aβ [17] and insulin [6] have revealed significant polymorphisms in the arrangement of the protofilaments from pairs of twisted protofilaments to association of six or more protofilaments (Figure 4).

Structure of the protofilaments

Each individual protofilament is made up of β-sheet-rich structure in which the β-strands run perpendicular to the fibre axis (Figure 2C). The hydrogen bonding along their length strengthens the β-sheets. Several β-sheets are then associated via side chain interactions. The importance of these interactions has been highlighted by work using X-ray crystallography of short amyloidogenic peptides, which show a 'steric zipper' structure whereby the side chains complement one another across the sheet–sheet interface [19]. It is clear that these interactions can have higher-order implications and that each peptide may associate in several different ways leading to changes in the macromolecular structure of the mature fibril. The protofilaments themselves associate via the side chains that radiate from the protofilaments and so the organization can be influenced by changes in assembly conditions such as pH and ionic strength [20].

The elucidation of the structures for amyloid protofilaments has often required the contribution of many different structural methods including electron microscopy, X-ray fibre diffraction and solid-state NMR. A good example is the recent structure of a short fragment of the transthyretin protein that forms amyloid fibrils *in vitro*. This structure was elucidated using many complementary techniques [21].

Solid-state NMR has revealed that many fibrils are composed of peptides arranged in a parallel and in-register arrangement [22]. Very recent work provided a structure for the amyloid fibrils found in brains of patients with Alzheimer's disease composed of Aβ(1–40) that shows a cross-β architecture in a triangular arrangement. Each molecule forms a β-bend structure that then associates with two others [23] (Figure 5). The β-bends then stack up so that

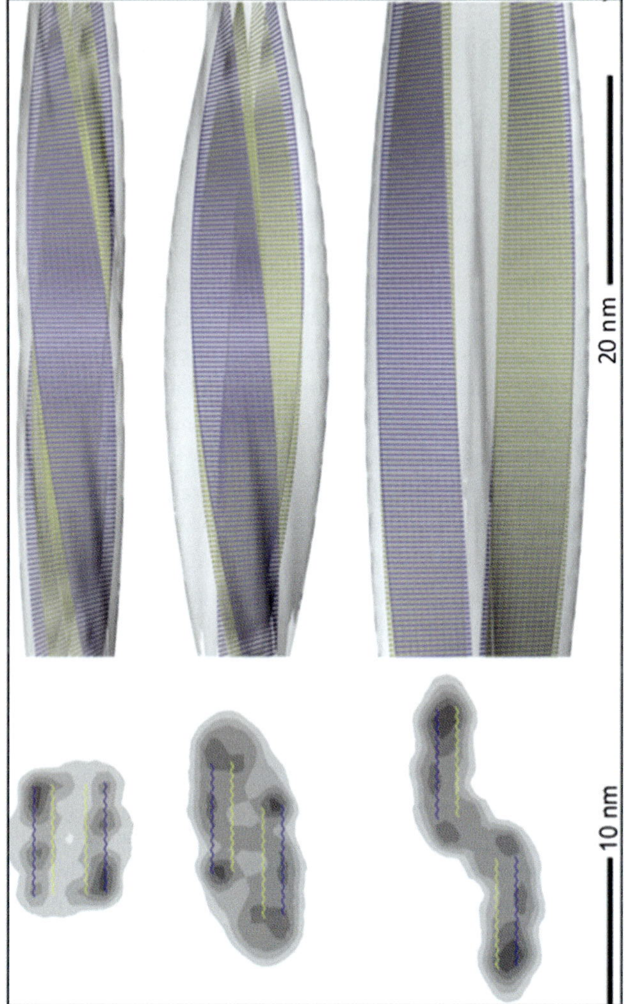

Figure 4. Cryo-electron microscopy analysis from amyloid fibrils formed by Aβ(1–40)
The figure shows alternative morphologies formed in which the protofilament number differs as well as the organization of the protofilament in the fibre. Reprinted from [33]; J. Mol. Biol. **386**, Meinhardt, J., Sachse, C., Hortschansky, P., Grigorieff, N. and Fandrich, M., Aβ(1–40) fibril polymorphism implies diverse interaction patterns in amyloid fibrils, 869–877, Copyright (2009), with permission from Elsevier.

identical side chains from one molecule stack on the same side chain of the next. Thus this structure results in three essentially flat surfaces of the protofilament lined with rows of identical amino acid side chains (Figure 5).

The role of side chains and the importance of precursor sequence

As already described, many proteins and peptides have the ability to assemble to form amyloid fibrils under particular conditions. In some cases, the protein must unfold in order to

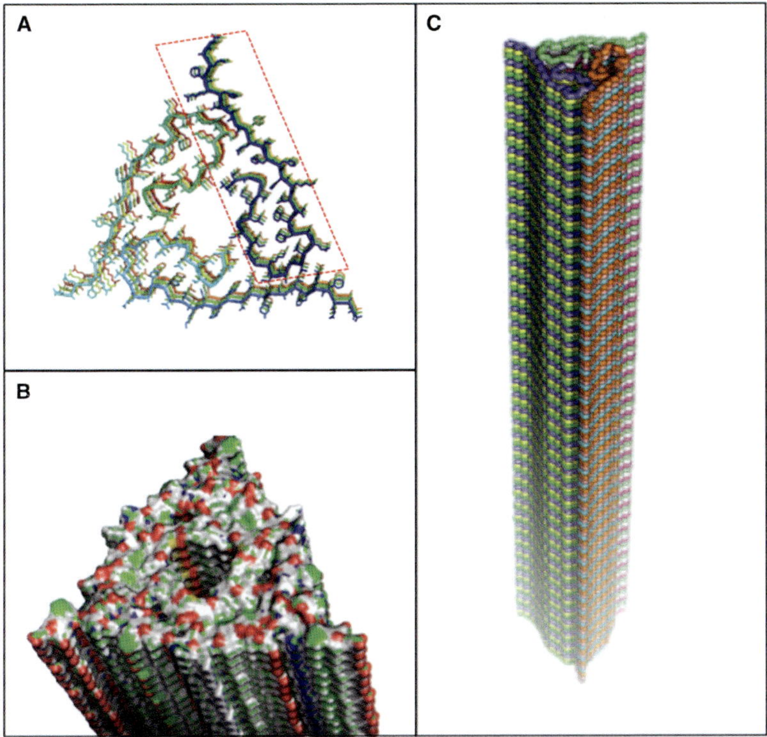

Figure 5. The structure of the Aβ(1–40) amyloid fibril (2M4J.ent) elucidated using solid-state NMR [23]
(**A**) The view down the axis of the fibre showing the side chains. A single Aβ(1–40) molecule is highlighted and the molecules are coloured according to chain identifier. (**B**) A surface representation showing the fibre coloured according to atom type and revealing the nature of the stacking along the fibre axis. (**C**) The full fibre is generated from the PDB code 2M4J by using PyMOL (http://www.pymol.org), coloured by chain and represented as ribbons.

assemble. For example, for insulin to assemble *in vitro*, it is necessary to incubate the native protein at pH 2 and 60°C to induce amyloid assembly. Therefore these proteins must unfold and then refold. Many of the short amyloidogenic peptides are natively unstructured and therefore their propensity to aggregate can be more simply correlated with their primary sequence. The importance of sequence has been extensively examined using algorithms designed to correlate the primary sequence to the propensity to form amyloid fibrils [24–26]. These algorithms incorporate analysis of the β-sheet propensity of the sequence as well as hydrophobicity and amino acid size. In later studies, the algorithms were developed by taking into account structural information from a training set of amyloidogenic sequences [26,27], resulting in increasingly accurate prediction of amyloid propensity.

Stability of the fibrils

The highly regular repeating structure of the amyloid fibril, which is held together by extensive hydrogen bonding and side chain interactions across and along the β-sheets, provides a structure with significant strength [28]. It is interesting to note that amyloid structures share many structural characteristics with insect and spider silk, and silk has long been highlighted for its very high tensile strength [29]. It is also interesting that the amyloid structure has been 'used' extensively by organisms as a functional material providing protection and support [4] due to these properties.

Infectivity and seeded aggregation

Prion diseases such as bovine spongiform encephalopathy and Creutzfeldt–Jakob disease are a very specific class of amyloid diseases that are infectious. In these conditions, a small amyloid 'seed' can be inoculated into an organism to lead to disease and it is thought that the basis of this is templated aggregation. In this scheme, the β-sheet-rich structure of the seed somehow acts as a template that can convert the non-β-sheet native structure of the PrP^C (normal cellular prion protein) into the infectious, β-sheet form. Recent studies have suggested that, although the other amyloid diseases are not infectious between organisms, similar mechanisms may exist in propagation of the amyloid structure between cells leading to 'spreading' of the pathology [30]. Prion diseases have also highlighted the importance of 'strains' whereby a particular 'strain' of infective agent can propagate a particular structure which has a particular resulting phenotype (i.e. time of infection, rate of progression of disease, site of deposition and pattern of spread). It has been suggested that differences at the structural level are responsible for the differences in these strains [31]. This is an intriguing question and one that structural studies promise to contribute to answering in the coming years.

Conclusions

Amyloid fibrils represent a very special class of protein fold, one of high strength lent by the presence of hydrogen bonded β-strands in β-sheet ribbons that associate to form amyloid protofilaments and further into the mature amyloid fibril. As research progresses from *in vitro* structures to those coming from *in vivo* sources, we are gaining more insight into the structure of the amyloid fibrils found in tissue in disease and beginning to understand the basis of templated aggregation and strains.

Summary

- Many unrelated peptides can form amyloid.
- Amyloid can be pathological or functional.
- Amyloid fibrils are extremely ordered and stable.
- Amyloid fibrils are composed of several protofilaments.
- The protofilaments are composed of cross-β structure.

I am very grateful to Kyle Morris for providing help with the Figures and to Alexander Barret for reading the chapter before submission. I have received support from ARUK (Alzheimer's Research UK) and MRC (Medical Research Council).

References

1. Marshall, K.E. and Serpell, L.C. (2009) Structural integrity of β-sheet assembly. Biochem. Soc. Trans. **37**, 671–676
2. Heim, M., Keerl, D. and Scheibel, T. (2009) Spider silk: from soluble protein to extraordinary fiber. Angew. Chem. Int. Ed. Engl. **48**, 3584–3596
3. Sawyer, E.B., Claessen, D., Haas, M., Hurgobin, B. and Gras, S.L. (2011) The assembly of individual chaplin peptides from *Streptomyces coelicolor* into functional amyloid fibrils. PLoS ONE **6**, e18839
4. Fowler, D.M., Koulov, A.V., Balch, W.E. and Kelly, J.W. (2007) Functional amyloid: from bacteria to humans. Trends Biochem. Sci. **32**, 217–224
5. Lindquist, S., DebBurman, S.K., Glover, J.R., Kowal, A.S., Liu, J.J., Schirmer, E.C. and Serio, T.R. (1998) Amyloid fibres of Sup35 support a prion-like mechanism of inheritance in yeast. Biochem. Soc. Trans. **26**, 486–490
6. Jimenez, J.L., Nettleton, E.J., Bouchard, M., Robinson, C.V., Dobson, C.M. and Saibil, H.R. (2002) The protofilament structure of insulin amyloid fibrils. Proc. Natl. Acad. Sci. U.S.A. **99**, 9196–9201
7. Stromer, T. and Serpell, L.C. (2005) Structure and morphology of the Alzheimer's amyloid fibril. Microsc. Res. Tech. **67**, 210–217
8. Watson, J.D. and Crick, F.H. (1953) Molecular structure of nucleic acids; a structure for deoxyribose nucleic acid. Nature **171**, 737–738
9. Morris, K.L. and Serpell, L.C. (2012) X-ray fibre diffraction studies of amyloid fibrils. Methods Mol. Biol. **849**, 121–135
10. Geddes, A.J., Parker, K.D., Atkins, E.D. and Beighton, E. (1968) "Cross-beta" conformation in proteins. J. Mol. Biol. **32**, 343–358
11. Jahn, T.R., Makin, O.S., Morris, K.L., Marshall, K.E., Tian, P., Sikorski, P. and Serpell, L.C. (2010) The common architecture of cross-β amyloid. J. Mol. Biol. **395**, 717–727
12. Tycko, R. (2011) Solid-state NMR studies of amyloid fibril structure. Annu. Rev. Phys. Chem. **62**, 279–299
13. Wasmer, C., Schutz, A., Loquet, A., Buhtz, C., Greenwald, J., Riek, R., Bockmann, A. and Meier, B.H. (2009) The molecular organization of the fungal prion HET-s in its amyloid form. J. Mol. Biol. **394**, 119–127
14. Serpell, L.C., Berriman, J., Jakes, R., Goedert, M. and Crowther, R.A. (2000) Fiber diffraction of synthetic alpha-synuclein filaments shows amyloid-like cross-beta conformation. Proc. Natl. Acad. Sci. U.S.A. **97**, 4897–4902
15 Serpell, L., Sunde, M., Benson, M., Tennent, G., Pepys, M. and Fraser, P. (2000) The protofilament substructure of amyloid fibrils. J. Mol. Biol. **300**, 1033–1039
16. Goldsbury, C., Goldie, K., Pellaud, J., Seelig, J., Frey, P., Muller, S., Kistler, J., Cooper, G. and Aebi, U. (2000) Amyloid fibril formation from full-length and fragments of amylin. J. Struct. Biol. **130**, 352–362
17. Sachse, C., Fandrich, M. and Grigorieff, N. (2008) Paired β-sheet structure of an Aβ(1–40) amyloid fibril revealed by electron microscopy. Proc. Natl. Acad. Sci. U.S.A. **105**, 7462–7466
18. White, H.E., Hodgkinson, J.L., Jahn, T.R., Cohen-Krausz, S., Gosal, W.S., Muller, S., Orlova, E.V., Radford, S.E. and Saibil, H.R. (2009) Globular tetramers of β$_2$-microglobulin assemble into elaborate amyloid fibrils. J. Mol. Biol. **389**, 48–57
19. Nelson, R. and Eisenberg, D. (2006) Recent atomic models of amyloid fibril structure. Curr. Opin. Struct. Biol. **16**, 260–265
20. Morris, K. and Serpell, L. (2010) From natural to designer self-assembling biopolymers, the structural characterisation of fibrous proteins and peptides using fibre diffraction. Chem. Soc. Rev. **39**, 3445–3453
21. Fitzpatrick, A.W., Debelouchina, G.T., Bayro, M.J., Clare, D.K., Caporini, M.A., Bajaj, V.S., Jaroniec, C.P., Wang, L., Ladizhansky, V., Muller, S.A. et al. (2013) Atomic structure and hierarchical assembly of a cross-β amyloid fibril. Proc. Natl. Acad. Sci. U.S.A. **110**, 5468–5473

22. Petkova, A.T., Yau, W.M. and Tycko, R. (2006) Experimental constraints on quaternary structure in Alzheimer's β-amyloid fibrils. Biochemistry **45**, 498–512

23. Lu, J.X., Qiang, W., Yau, W.M., Schwieters, C.D., Meredith, S.C. and Tycko, R. (2013) Molecular structure of β-amyloid fibrils in Alzheimer's disease brain tissue. Cell **154**, 1257–1268

24. Pawar, A.P., Dubay, K.F., Zurdo, J., Chiti, F., Vendruscolo, M. and Dobson, C.M. (2005) Prediction of "aggregation-prone" and "aggregation-susceptible" regions in proteins associated with neurodegenerative disease. J. Mol. Biol. **350**, 379–392

25. Rousseau, F., Schymkowitz, J. and Serrano, L. (2006) Protein aggregation and amyloidosis: confusion of the kinds? Curr. Opin. Struct. Biol. **16**, 118–126

26. Thompson, M.J., Sievers, S.A., Karanicolas, J., Ivanova, M.I., Baker, D. and Eisenberg, D. (2006) The 3D profile method for identifying fibril-forming segments of proteins. Proc. Natl. Acad. Sci. U.S.A. **103**, 4074–4078

27. Maurer-Stroh, S., Debulpaep, M., Kuemmerer, N., de la Paz, M.L., Martins, I.C., Reumers, J., Morris, K.L., Copland, A., Serpell, L., Serrano, L. et al. (2010) Exploring the sequence determinants of amyloid structure using position-specific scoring matrices. Nat. Methods **7**, 237–242

28. Knowles, T.P. and Buehler, M.J. (2011) Nanomechanics of functional and pathological amyloid materials. Nat. Nanotechnol. **6**, 469–479

29. Romer, L. and Scheibel, T. (2008) The elaborate structure of spider silk: structure and function of a natural high performance fiber. Prion **2**, 1–8

30. Jucker, M. and Walker, L.C. (2013) Self-propagation of pathogenic protein aggregates in neurodegenerative diseases. Nature **501**, 45–51

31. Paravastu, A.K., Leapman, R.D., Yau, W.M. and Tycko, R. (2008) Molecular structural basis for polymorphism in Alzheimer's β-amyloid fibrils. Proc. Natl. Acad. Sci. U.S.A. **105**, 18349–18354

32. Morris, K.L., Rodger, A., Hicks, M.R., Debulpaep, M., Schymkowitz, J., Rousseau, F. and Serpell, L.C. (2013) Exploring the sequence–structure relationship for amyloid peptides. Biochem. J. **450**, 275–283

33. Meinhardt, J., Sachse, C., Hortschansky, P., Grigorieff, N. and Fandrich, M. (2009). Aβ(1–40) fibril polymorphism implies diverse interaction patterns in amyloid fibrils. J. Mol. Biol. **386**, 869–877

Essays Biochem. (2014) 56, 11–39: doi: 10.1042/BSE0560011

2

The physical chemistry of the amyloid phenomenon: thermodynamics and kinetics of filamentous protein aggregation

Alexander K. Buell[1], Christopher M. Dobson and Tuomas P.J. Knowles

Department of Chemistry, University of Cambridge, Lensfield Road, Cambridge CB2 1EW, U.K.

Abstract

In this chapter, we present an overview of the kinetics and thermodynamics of protein aggregation into amyloid fibrils. The perspective we adopt is largely experimental, but we also discuss recent developments in data analysis and we show that only a combination of well-designed experiments with appropriate theoretical modelling is able to provide detailed mechanistic insight into the complex pathways of amyloid formation. In the first part of the chapter, we describe measurements of the thermodynamic stability of the amyloid state with respect to the soluble state of proteins, as well as the magnitude and origin of this stability. In the second part, we discuss in detail the kinetics of the individual molecular steps in the overall mechanism of the conversion of soluble protein into amyloid fibrils. Finally, we highlight the effects of external factors, such as salt type and concentration, chemical denaturants and molecular chaperones on the kinetics of aggregation.

Keywords:

activation energy, electrostatics, fragmentation, energy landscape, kinetics, linear polymerization, nucleation, thermodynamics.

[1]*To whom correspondence should be addressed (email ab761@cam.ac.uk).*

Introduction

Protein molecules can adopt a variety of conformations in their soluble forms, ranging from compact natively structured states to the random coils of completely denatured states, with a multitude of species in between these two extremes [1]. Likewise, the insoluble forms of proteins have many guises, ranging from three-dimensional crystals to amorphous species, again with a multitude of intermediate states of varying nature and size [1]. Some forms of aggregates may be small enough to form stable colloidal suspensions under commonly encountered solution conditions, therefore bridging the gap between soluble and insoluble forms of a given protein.

Amorphous aggregates are characterized by the absence of translational symmetry and conventional highly ordered crystals exhibit three-dimensional translational symmetry. Amyloid fibrils are a particularly interesting state and are often described as one-dimensional crystals, linear assemblies of proteins with translational symmetry along the long axis. Although this simplified description has been shown to allow a detailed analysis of the kinetics and thermodynamics of amyloid formation (see sections below), detailed structural information that is available shows that amyloid fibrils can have three-dimensional order as they can often be composed of several individual protofilaments that wrap around each other, and that exhibit a twist that breaks translational symmetry [2,3].

The discovery in the late 1990s that amyloid fibrils can be formed in the laboratory by proteins entirely unrelated to well-established amyloid diseases led to the hypothesis that the fibrillar state represents a generic state that polypeptides can adopt, which can be the thermodynamically most stable state under some conditions [1,4]. This hypothesis was supported by the discovery that even archetypal folded proteins with mostly α-helical secondary structure, such as myoglobin, readily form amyloid fibrils under appropriate conditions [5], as indeed do homopolymeric polypeptides, such as polythreonine and polylysine [6]. In the case of globular proteins, a combination of conditions that are known to destabilize the native state, such as extremes of pH [7], high temperature and co-solvents, often induces amyloid formation.

In the present chapter, we discuss the current state of understanding of the thermodynamics of amyloid fibrils, as well as the factors that determine the kinetics of interconversion between the various soluble, intermediate and aggregated states that a polypeptide can adopt.

Before we embark on this journey through the energy landscapes of proteins, we would like to clarify the meaning of a range of terms that we will be using frequently. When we speak of soluble peptides or proteins, we mean the native functional form, in most cases monomeric, of folded (e.g. lysozyme) or intrinsically disordered (e.g. α-synuclein) proteins or the monomeric proteolytic fragments of proteins {e.g. Aβ(1–42) [amyloid β-peptide (1–42)]}. The term aggregate comprises both ordered (e.g. amyloid fibrils) and disordered (e.g. amorphous) multimeric forms of proteins. An insoluble aggregate is defined as a structure that does not form a stable colloidal suspension at 1 g gravitational acceleration. In between these two extremes are situated what we refer to as oligomers. These aggregates are small enough to form a colloidal suspension at 1 g, but can be separated from soluble protein at elevated forces in a centrifuge. A protein is amyloidogenic if conditions have been identified under which the formation of protofilaments and/or amyloid fibrils can be readily observed. A protofilament is a linear assembly of individual peptide or protein molecules, which form a continuous β-sheet. An amyloid fibril is usually composed of two or more protofilaments that are helically entwined. We often speak of amyloid fibrils as templates for further conversion of monomeric protein molecules, as these soluble molecules will adopt the structure of the monomers in the fibril upon attachment to the end of the fibril (see below).

Thermodynamics of amyloid formation

The classical analysis of the thermodynamics of protein folding usually focuses on the two-state (or sometimes multistate) transition between a folded and an unfolded state. Here, the thermodynamics are determined through the competition between interactions of the protein with the solvent and intramolecular interactions. However, above a certain critical concentration, the presence of aggregates, stabilized by intermolecular interactions, will become thermodynamically favourable. In order to be able to analyse the thermodynamics of a system of aggregating protein molecules, the polydisperse nature of the aggregates has to be taken into consideration, rendering the use of a two-state folding model inappropriate.

A linear polymerization model of amyloid formation

The simplest possible model for the formation of a series of linear multimers is an infinite number of equilibria with identical equilibrium constants K [8]:

$$M + M \underset{}{\overset{K}{\rightleftharpoons}} M_2$$

$$M_2 + M \underset{}{\overset{K}{\rightleftharpoons}} M_3$$

$$\ldots$$

$$M_n + M \underset{}{\overset{K}{\rightleftharpoons}} M_{n+1}$$

In this framework,

$$K = \frac{[M_i][M]_0}{[M_{i-1}][M]}$$

and $[M] = [M_1]$ is the concentration of the soluble building block, in most cases a monomer, and $[M]_0$ is a standard concentration to make K unitless. The total quantity of protein in this system can be written as:

$$M_{tot} = \sum_{i=1}^{\infty} i[M_i] = \sum_{i=1}^{\infty} i \left(\frac{K}{[M]_0} \right)^{i-1} [M]^i = \frac{[M]}{\left(1 - \frac{K}{[M]_0}[M] \right)^2} \tag{1}$$

which leads to:

$$K = \frac{[M]_0}{[M]} - \sqrt{\frac{[M]_0^2}{M_{tot}[M]}} \tag{2}$$

For high enough M_{tot}, we obtain:

$$K = \frac{[M]_0}{[M]} = e^{-\frac{\Delta G^0}{RT}}$$

where ΔG^0 is the free energy difference between a monomer in solution and as part of an aggregate. We can therefore estimate the free energy difference between the insoluble and the soluble states of the protein from measurements of the concentration of soluble protein at equilibrium. However, the equilibrium concentration of soluble protein is usually low (in the µM to nM range [9,10]) and therefore not straightforward to measure. Also, it is not always easy to determine whether an aggregated protein sample has truly reached equilibrium, due to processes such as gelation, which can slow down the equilibration process considerably [11].

A way around these experimental problems is to measure an equilibrium dissociation curve similar to the denaturation of soluble protein with a chaotrope like urea or GndHCl (guanidine hydrochloride). The free energy difference between the monomeric and aggregated states depends on the concentration of the denaturant, in the simplest model in a linear manner: $\Delta G = \Delta G^0 + m[D]$, where $[D]$ is the concentration of denaturant and m is a proportionality constant. The fraction of soluble protein, assumed to consist exclusively of the (monomeric) building block, as a function of denaturant concentration can then be fitted to obtain ΔG^0 and m as fitting parameters (see Figure 1A). This method has been shown to be applicable to amyloid fibrils [12] and recently it has been applied to a large number of amyloidogenic proteins [10]. This latter analysis has yielded an interesting scaling relationship between the sequence length of amyloidogenic proteins and the free energy per residue. Amyloid fibrils of short peptides were found to be much more stable per residue (soluble compared with insoluble) than folded proteins (folded compared with unfolded), whereas longer sequences form fibrils that have similar stabilities per residue to folded proteins (Figure 1B). Indeed, short amino acid sequences (<50 residues) do not usually fold into globular structures, whereas many such short sequences have been found to form amyloid fibrils [13]. These results provide support for the hypothesis that the amyloid state represents, for many polypeptides, and particularly for those with less than approximately 150 residues, the lowest energy state at concentrations above the threshold for aggregation even under physiological concentrations. Many polypeptides exist *in vivo* at concentrations above this critical concentration [10], stimulating questions about the exact nature of the forces that favour intermolecular interactions with respect to intramolecular and peptide–solvent interactions.

It has to be noted here that the linear polymerization model is an incomplete description of amyloid formation, as it neglects the experimental finding that the nucleation of amyloid fibrils is a process with different kinetics and thermodynamics compared with the growth of an amyloid fibril through addition of a monomer. In addition, this model neglects other processes that can change the number and size of aggregates, such as fragmentation [14] and secondary nucleation [15]. For these reasons, the linear polymerization model in most cases predicts incorrect length distributions for amyloid fibrils at equilibrium. Nevertheless, the model is useful for the thermodynamic analysis described above as it is largely independent of the length distribution at high enough total protein concentrations.

Calorimetric experiments of amyloid growth and dissociation

It is interesting to explore the molecular origins of the high thermodynamic stability of amyloid fibrils. A decomposition of the free energies measured in equilibrium experiments into enthalpic and entropic contributions can be useful in this context, although, as in the case of globular proteins, this analysis is far from straightforward [16]. We know, for example, that

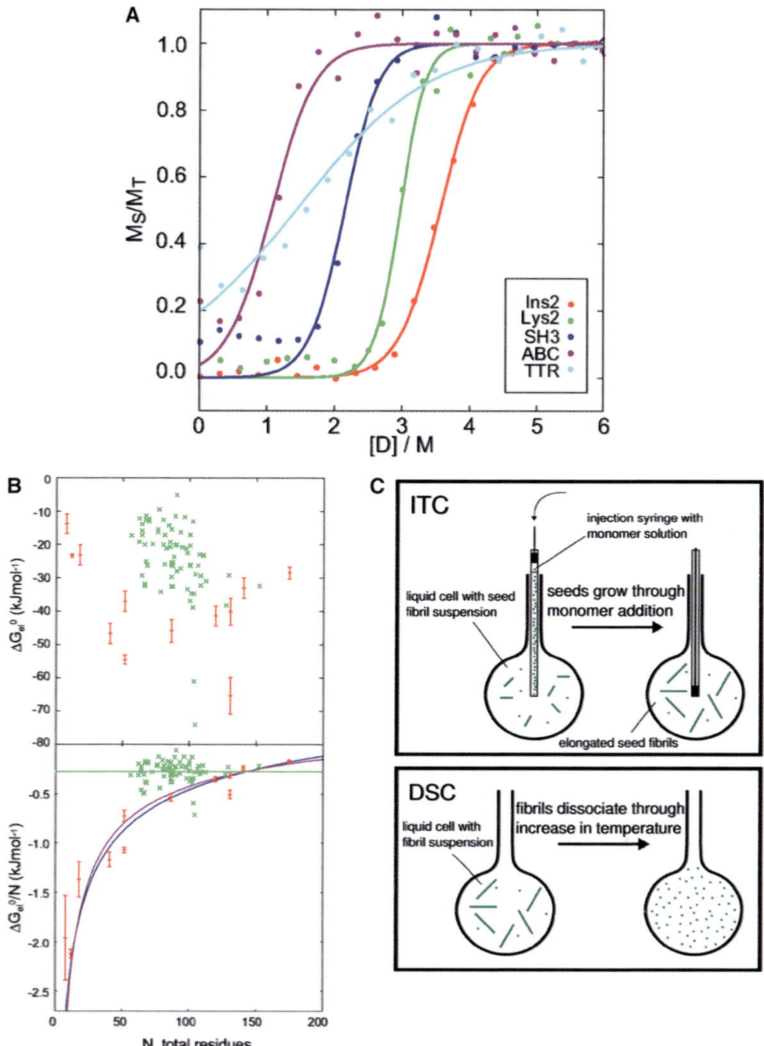

Figure 1. Thermodynamics of amyloid fibril formation

(**A**) Equilibrium denaturation curves of amyloid fibrils formed from a range of different peptides and proteins. (**B**) Measurements such as the ones shown in (**A**) allow the determination of the free energy of fibril formation ΔG^0. The top panel shows ΔG^0 as a function of the number of amino acid residues (N). The red data points are for amyloid fibrils, and the green data points are for globular proteins (in the latter case comparing the stabilities of folded and unfolded states). The bottom panel shows $\Delta G^0/N$ as a function of N. It can be seen that short peptides form amyloid fibrils that are more stable per residue, compared with the average stability of a folded protein; however, the longer the sequence, the more the stability per residue of the amyloid state approaches the stability per residue of the globular state. (**C**) Illustrations of calorimetric experiments to probe the enthalpic signature of amyloid formation. The top panel shows ITC, where the enthalpy released or consumed during fibril growth is measured. The bottom panel shows DSC, where the thermal dissociation ('melting') of fibrils is measured. (**A**) and (**B**) are reprinted (adapted) with permission from [10]; Baldwin, A.J., Knowles, T.P.J., Tartaglia, G.G., Fitzpatrick, A.W., Devlin, G.L., Shammas, S.L., Waudby, C.A., Mossuto, M.F., Meehan, S., Gras, S.L. et al., 2011, Metastability of native proteins and the phenomenon of amyloid formation, J. Am. Chem. Soc., vol. 133, pp. 14160–14163. Copyright (2011) American Chemical Society.

hydrogen bonding and van der Waals interactions are enthalpic in nature, whereas hydrophobic interactions (in a certain range of temperatures and length scales [17]) and the conformational freedom of the peptide backbone contribute to the entropy of the system.

Calorimetry is the most obvious choice of experimental technique to explore the enthalpic nature of the process of amyloid formation. Indeed, it has been applied to the study of amyloid fibril formation in the form of both DSC (differential scanning calorimetry) [18], where the change in heat capacity as a function of temperature is monitored, as well as ITC (isothermal titration calorimetry) [19], where the heat released or absorbed upon interaction of two molecular species can be measured (see Figure 1C). The general picture that emerges from such experiments is that amyloid fibrils usually dissociate at temperatures far higher than the unfolding temperature of the soluble monomeric state (in cases where the monomeric precursor is a folded protein) [18,20] (see Note added in proof). The thermal dissociation of fibrils, however, can depend profoundly on kinetic as well as thermodynamic parameters as shown by the strong heating rate dependence of the enthalpy of fibril 'melting' [18]. Furthermore, while the thermal unfolding of a globular monomeric protein is usually reversible, the dissociation of amyloid fibrils, if quantitative, is irreversible in the framework of a DSC experiment [18]. These findings can be rationalized in light of the complex and often slow kinetics of the reverse process, i.e. fibril formation (see Kinetics of amyloid formation section).

The enthalpic signature of amyloid fibril growth at any given temperature, as measured by ITC, where soluble (monomeric) protein can be titrated into pre-formed seed fibrils, as well as seed fibrils into soluble protein, has been shown to be exothermic in most cases [19,21]. However, the temperature-induced dissociation as observed in DSC can be both exothermic [18] and endothermic [20]. Experimental results from those two techniques are, however, difficult to compare; both measurements are necessarily performed out of equilibrium and usually in very different temperature ranges. Amyloid fibril growth can only be studied under conditions where fibrils are stable, whereas the observation that amyloid fibrils can be dissociated at elevated temperatures of course indicates that above a certain temperature, the soluble monomeric form of the protein becomes the thermodynamic minimum. As expected, the melting temperature depends on the total concentration of protein in the system [18,20].

We can conclude, therefore, that the balance of the fundamental forces that stabilize amyloid fibrils is strongly temperature dependent, not only because of the general temperature dependence of the free energy, $\Delta G = \Delta H - T\Delta S$, but also because the fundamental interactions responsible for the formation of amyloid fibrils, in particular the hydrophobic effect, are temperature dependent. At this stage, no general conclusions can be drawn as to the enthalpic or entropic origin and nature of the thermodynamic stabilities of amyloid fibrils.

Electrostatic effects on the stability of amyloid fibrils

One particular type of energetic contribution to the stability of amyloid fibrils that has been studied in some detail involves electrostatic interactions. It has been shown by calorimetry that under pH conditions where the monomers are highly positively charged, the dissociation temperature of fibrils rises with increasing salt concentration [18]. This reflects the fact that the electrostatic contribution to the free energy of aggregation is unfavourable in such cases of self-assembly of highly charged species and that this repulsion can be screened by the presence of ions. Interestingly, this stabilization necessitates salt concentrations (hundreds of mM) where the Debye length, the characteristic distance over which the electrostatic potential decreases through screening, is formally less than 1 nm (this concentration regime is, of course, outside the range of validity of simple Debye–Hückel theory [22,23]), in agreement with the idea of very closely packed charges of the same sign within an amyloid fibril. In such a situation, the salt ions can only exert screening if they are in very close proximity to the charges on the fibrils. In addition, it has been shown that a change in pH that leads to a change in sign and an increase in magnitude of the net charge of the protein can destabilize amyloid fibrils [24]. Therefore, as expected for a homopolymer, electrostatic interactions are generally unfavourable. However, often conditions that accelerate amyloid fibril formation are those that increase the net charge, for example extremes of pH. This paradox is easily explained by the fact that these are cases where the soluble amyloid precursor state has a stable fold and the native interactions within this folded state are more strongly destabilized by changes in charge state than those in the fibrillar state. This effect leads to a net decrease in the free energy barrier for aggregation (see below).

Fibril-crystal polymorphism

As mentioned in the Introduction, polypeptide aggregates can take many forms, in particular amorphous, fibrillar or crystalline species. For the crystalline form, we have to distinguish between crystals where the polypeptide retains its native fold, and which are for example used for structure determination at atomic resolution of folded proteins, and microcrystals, formed exclusively by short peptides. It has been demonstrated that many short peptides, in particular those derived from the sequences of highly amyloidogenic proteins, are capable of forming microcrystals, and in some cases, these crystals can coexist with amyloid fibrils [25]. The opportunity to study, via X-ray diffraction, the atomic structure of these microcrystals is an interesting route towards a detailed description of interactions akin to those in amyloid fibrils in more readily studied systems [26].

Recently, a theory has been developed that treats the fibril-crystal polymorphism and transition of short peptides analogously to a phase transition [2]. According to this description, the free energy of the fibril/crystal is a function of twist angle, with the latter adopting a finite value in the fibrils and zero in the crystal. The fundamental origin of the twist is the chiral nature of the peptide building blocks. The balance between the intersheet interactions and the elastic energy of torsion determines the coexistence [25], or not, of twisted fibrillar and constrained crystalline phases of a given peptide.

Kinetics of amyloid formation

Having established above that the aggregated state of many proteins represents the free energy minimum at finite ($>\mu$M) concentrations, close to those found in living systems, we can now ask what prevents many proteins from aggregating *in vivo*. A phenomenological answer has been proposed as the 'life on the edge' hypothesis [27]. According to this idea, proteins are expressed at concentrations which are, generally speaking, inversely related to their kinetics of aggregation. Just enough protein is expressed for it to be functional, but not more, in order to minimize the risk of deleterious aggregation. It is crucial in this context that the proteins are prevented from aggregation through kinetic, rather than thermodynamic factors. Many attempts have been made to identify the physico-chemical and sequence determinants of the so-called 'aggregation propensity' [28] and to use this insight to predict the tendency of given sequences to aggregate [29,30]. In the framework of an energy landscape perspective on protein aggregation [31] (Figure 2A), the heights of the energy barriers that separate the soluble from the amyloid states are responsible for the kinetic (meta-)stability of soluble proteins [32].

At the beginning of a detailed description of the kinetics of amyloid formation is the realization that protein aggregation cannot be described as a one-step reaction, but consists of a range of molecular processes (Figure 2B). The observation that amyloid formation from soluble protein molecules usually displays a lag time, which can be shortened or even abolished when pre-formed aggregates are added, suggested that nucleation, as well as growth processes have to be considered. The pre-formed ('seed') fibrils act as templates for the addition of further monomers and the rates of addition to these templates are faster than the *de novo* formation of fibrils through nucleation, thereby accelerating the aggregation. Primary nucleation and growth of fibrils alone are, however, in most cases not able to explain the observed kinetic behaviour, including cases where the aggregating samples are subjected to strong mechanical action. Such conditions can induce the fragmentation of fibrils, which can strongly accelerate the aggregation reaction due to an exponential increase in growth-competent fibril ends [14]. Even under quiescent conditions, however, fragmentation of fibrils can be important; it has been shown, for example that the chaperone Hsp104 (heat-shock protein 104) can fragment yeast prion amyloid fibrils [33]. Finally, some proteins display a mechanism of proliferation of fibrils that depends on both the concentration of already fibrillar protein, as well as of monomeric species in solution, a process described as 'secondary nucleation' (Figure 2B).

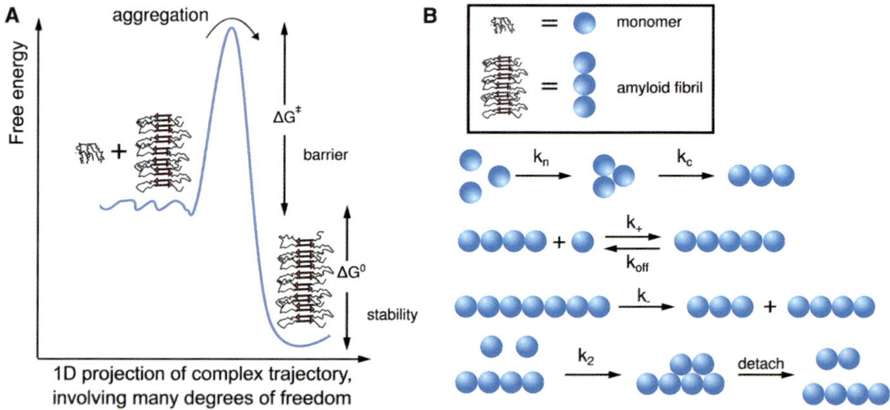

Figure 2. The mechanism of amyloid formation

(**A**) Highly simplified free energy landscape for protein aggregation, in this particular case of amyloid fibril growth. The amyloid fibril is thermodynamically more stable than the monomeric state. However, the latter is metastable due to a free energy barrier that separates the two states. (**B**) The elementary processes involved in the conversion of soluble protein molecules into amyloid fibrils: nucleation of an aggregate (k_n), that may be followed by conversion steps (k_c) in order to form an amyloid fibril of minimal size. Also shown are fibril growth by addition of a soluble building block (k_+) and the reverse process, dissociation (k_{off}). Secondary processes are processes which lead to an increase in the number of amyloid fibrils, and the rates of which depend on the concentration of existing fibrils. Examples are fibril fragmentation (k_-) and monomer-dependent secondary nucleation (k_2), where the newly formed nucleus may detach from the nucleation site. All molecular processes are described in detail in the text. Reprinted with permission from [15]; Cohen, S.I.A., Vendruscolo, M., Welland, M.E., Dobson, C.M., Terentjev, E.M. and Knowles, T.P.J., 2011, Nucleated polymerization with secondary pathways. I. time evolution of the principal moments, J. Chem. Phys. Vol. 135, p65105, Copyright 2011, AIP Publishing LLC.

All of those processes can operate in parallel as well as in series and render the theoretical description of the reaction highly complex. In the following sections we discuss both experimental and theoretical approaches to exploring and analysing the kinetics of amyloid formation.

Experimental methods to measure the kinetics of aggregation

Measuring quantitatively the kinetics of supramolecular protein aggregation into amyloid fibrils, as well as gaining useful insights from such measurements is challenging. The fundamental difficulty lies in the fact that a transition from a soluble to an insoluble form needs to be studied. Experimental techniques that are powerful for the investigation of the soluble states of proteins (such as NMR spectroscopy) are often not easily applicable to insoluble states of proteins.

Kinetic measurements of protein aggregation can be made in bulk solution or on surfaces, and measurements are possible for single particles, as well as for multimolecular ensembles. In the latter cases, the average evolution of a large number of molecules and aggregates is monitored. All of those experiments can be performed starting either from pure soluble protein or in the presence of pre-formed (seed) aggregates. When the concentration (by number) of seed fibrils is high enough, the growth of those seeds is the dominant process and the data analysis differs considerably from that where nucleation is rate-limiting [11]. As a general strategy, the variation of the concentrations of the reaction partners, as well as of the external conditions allows, in combination with kinetic analysis, extraction of the kinetic parameters of the individual molecular processes [34].

The kinetics of amyloid formation were initially studied almost exclusively in bulk solution, using light as a probe, either through light scattering [35] (Figure 3B) or through the change in fluorescence intensity and spectral properties of small fluorescent molecules upon binding to amyloid fibrils, in particular ThT (Thioflavin T) [36] (Figure 3A). Both methods have provided useful insight into the bulk kinetics of aggregation, although it is not always easy to relate the observed signal to a specific molecular process. Light scattering suffers from the highly non-linear scaling of the scattering intensity with particle size, which makes it challenging to follow the time evolution of the populations of monomers and small- and medium-sized aggregates. In addition, the scattering from large non-spherical particles is difficult to treat [37]. ThT fluorescence has yielded useful data in hundreds of studies, but it is essential to ensure that it is not influenced by various external factors, in particular other small molecules that can compete for binding sites on the fibrils and/or quench the fluorescence [38]. In addition, protein aggregation in the bulk solution of a test tube is rather different to the processes happening within or outside living cells, where the surface-to-volume ratios are very high, and where a variety of chemically diverse soluble species and surfaces may influence the aggregation process. Table 1 shows experimental techniques that can be used to monitor the kinetics of the aggregation mechanism.

In response to these potential limitations, surface-based biosensing methodologies have been developed; the deposition of amyloid fibrils on a surface for the detailed study of their kinetics of growth explicitly takes their nature as insoluble structures into account. These experiments do not require the use of a label molecule such as ThT; the change in size of surface-bound protein aggregates is directly measured through the change in refractive index of the surface-bound layer in the SPR (surface plasmon resonance) [49] and related optical biosensing techniques, or through the change in (hydrodynamic) mass of the attached aggregates

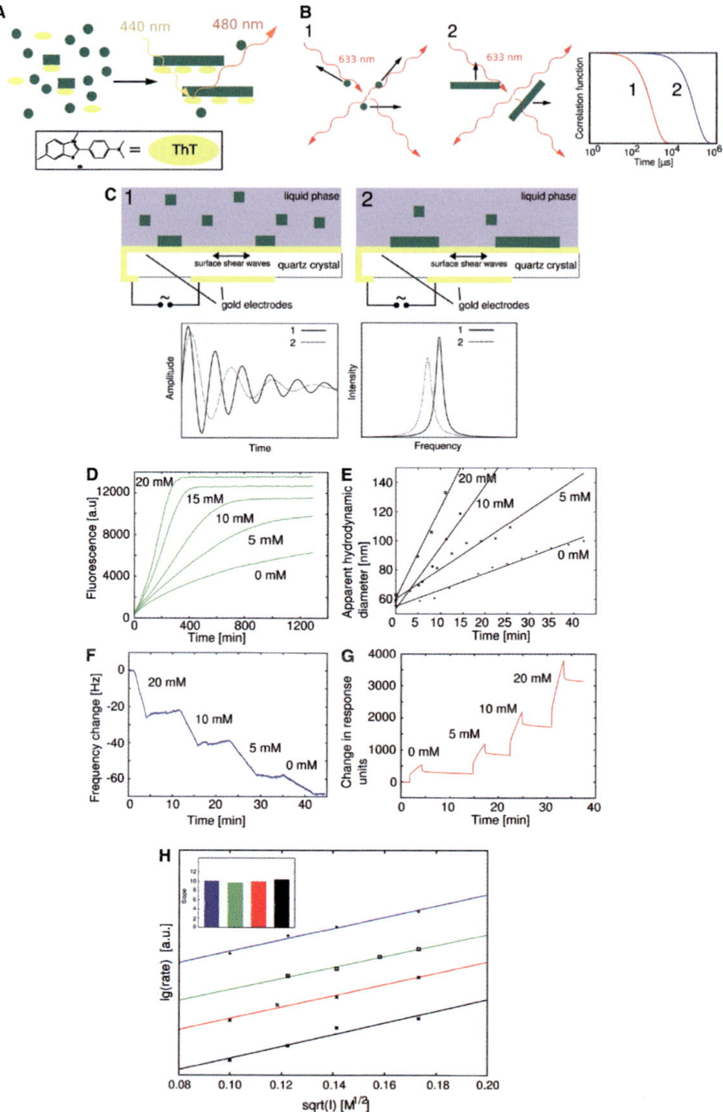

Figure 3. A comparison of important experimental methods for studying different steps of protein aggregation

(**A**) ThT binds to amyloid fibrils and this interaction induces a shift in the fluorescence frequency maximum and intensity. (**B**) Dynamic light scattering can be used to monitor a change in particle size over time. The time auto-correlation function (shown schematically as an inset) reflects the diffusive motion of the particles in solution. (**C**) A QCM allows the change in mass of growing surface-bound aggregates to be monitored very accurately. The resonant frequency of the crystal decreases upon addition of mass to the surface. (**D**)–(**G**) Experimental results on the effects of changes in NaCl concentration on the elongation kinetics of insulin amyloid fibrils at pH 2, acquired with two bulk solution and two surface-based experimental techniques. (**D**) ThT fluorescence, (**E**) dynamic light scattering, (**F**) QCM, (**G**) SPR and (**H**) summary of the results shown in (**D**)–(**G**), in the form of a Debye–Hückel plot. The inset shows a comparison of the slopes of the Debye–Hückel plots, demonstrating the equivalence of these different experimental techniques. (**D**)–(**H**) were reproduced from [52]; Buell, A.K., Hung, P., Salvatella, X., Welland, M.E., Dobson, C.M. and Knowles, T.P.J., (2013), Electrostatic effects in filamentous protein aggregation, Biophys. J., vol. 104, pp. 1116–1126.

Table 1. Summary of the most important experimental techniques that can be used to monitor the kinetics of different steps of the aggregation mechanism of soluble proteins into amyloid fibrils.

For *Ex situ* techniques, aliquots are taken from the reaction mixture and analysed after quenching the reaction (e.g. through dilution or surface deposition and drying). For *in situ* techniques, the reaction mixture is analysed during the reaction, for example through the presence of ThT in the reaction mixture or AFM imaging of growing fibrils in liquid. DLS, dynamic light scattering; SLS, static light scattering; TCCD, two-colour coincidence detection; TEM, transmission electron microscopy.

(a) Ensemble measurements

Technique	Process that can be monitored	Advantages	Disadvantages	Reference
Dye (e.g. ThT) fluorescence in bulk solution (*in situ*)	Overall aggregation time course and fibril elongation	Easy and rapid	Can be perturbed by the presence of the dye itself or by other molecules and fluorescence is often not linear with respect to total fibril mass M(t)	[34]
Ex situ aggregation time course (e.g. ThT fluorescence or measurement of soluble protein concentration)	Overall aggregation time course and fibril elongation	Dye does not interfere with aggregation and can be more quantitative than *in situ*	Time consuming	[39]
Spectroscopy in bulk solution (circular dichroism and tryptophan fluorescence)	Overall aggregation time course and fibril elongation	Label-free	Large aggregates strongly scatter UV light and can make measurement difficult	[40]
Light scattering (e.g. DLS and SLS)	Overall aggregation time course and fibril elongation	Label-free	For polydisperse samples, data analysis and interpretation are challenging and scattering by large aggregates can mask small structures	[35]
Small-angle scattering	Overall aggregation time course	Label-free	Similar challenges as DLS and SLS	[41]

(Continued)

Table 1. Summary of the most important experimental techniques that can be used to monitor the kinetics of different steps of the aggregation mechanism of soluble proteins into amyloid fibrils.   (*Continued*)

(a) Ensemble measurements

Technique	Process that can be monitored	Advantages	Disadvantages	Reference
Biosensing (e.g. QCM and SPR)	Fibril elongation	Label-free and highly quantitative due to monitoring of constant quantifiable ensemble of aggregates	Surface interactions can bias measurements, and data analysis can be challenging due to complex interactions between surface and liquid	[42]
Ex situ AFM/TEM	Nucleation and fibril elongation	Enables determination of time-resolved fibril length distribution	Time-consuming and samples can be perturbed through drying	[43]
Dye fluorescence in microdroplets	Nucleation and spatial propagation	Low sample consumption, can probe spatial propagation and can give robust statistics due to large number of droplets that can be monitored	Same potential disadvantages as bulk dye fluorescence	[44]

(b) Single molecule/particle measurements

Technique	Process that can be monitored	Advantages	Disadvantages	Reference
TIRF	Nucleation and fibril elongation	Real-time monitoring of individual aggregates	Surface interactions can bias measurements	[45]
In situ AFM	Nucleation and fibril elongation	Real-time monitoring of individual aggregates	Surface interactions can bias measurements	[46]
Single molecule fluorescence (e.g. TCCD and FRET)	Nucleation and conversion steps	Time evolution of size distribution and structural characteristics of oligomeric structures can be determined	High levels of dilutions involved can perturb measurements	[47]
Super-resolution optical microscopy (e.g. dSTORM)	Nucleation and fibril elongation	Possibility to monitor aggregation *in vivo*	Relatively slow and time courses of individual aggregates difficult due to photobleaching	[48]

in QCM (quartz crystal microbalance) experiments [42,50] or similar mechanical biosensors (Figure 3C). In the latter measurements, the sensor surface is excited to vibrate in shear mode and the growth of protein aggregates leads to a shift and broadening of the resonance. In such experiments, when irreversible surface attachment of the seed aggregates is ensured [51], the evolution of a constant ensemble of seeds is monitored, which can be successively exposed to soluble protein under varying conditions, leading to growth of the seed fibrils, and the influence of those conditions on the fibril growth rate can be very accurately measured [32,42,52]. In a systematic study of the effects of changes in solution ionic strength on the rate of amyloid fibril growth, it was established recently that the most commonly used bulk and surface-based experiments yield very similar results [52] and (Figure 3).

Both surface-based and bulk experiments performed in the ways described above measure the average behaviour of a large number of aggregates, even if only one molecular process, such as fibril elongation, is monitored. However, the complex nature of macromolecular interactions manifests itself in a large degree of stochasticity at the level of the individual molecules or aggregates. Therefore it is useful to try and follow the evolution of individual particles in an aggregating sample. Both the nucleation and the growth of amyloid fibrils have thus been studied using single particle techniques. The early stages of aggregation have been followed with single molecule fluorescence measurements where the diffusion of fluorescently labelled protein molecules through the focal volume of a laser is monitored [53]. Size and structural information about the oligomeric aggregates can be obtained from the intensity of the fluorescence signal and the FRET (Förster resonance energy transfer) efficiency of the monomers, labelled with two different dyes within the oligomeric aggregates [47].

The growth of individual fibrillar aggregates, on the other hand, has been monitored by AFM (atomic force microscopy) in liquid [46,54], TIRF (total internal reflection fluorescence microscopy) [45] and super-resolution (i.e. not diffraction-limited) microscopy techniques, such as dSTORM (direct stochastic optical reconstruction microscopy) [48]. In these experiments, it was established that the description of fibril growth by a single rate constant only captures the average behaviour and that there are extremely important variations between the behaviour of individual particles (see below).

Kinetic theories

In order to be able to obtain insightful information about the mechanism of amyloid formation from experiments such as the ones described above, an appropriate theoretical description is indispensable. Depending on the specific experimental design, a mathematical framework needs to be constructed that describes the relevant molecular processes and where fitting of the data allows the determination of the average rate constants of these individual microscopic processes. In addition, if a reaction rate theory for any given molecular process is available, such as is the case for example for fibril growth [31], detailed insight into the magnitude and composition of the relevant free energy barriers can be obtained [32].

The master equation approach

The time evolution of an aggregating protein solution can be modelled by a set of differential equations that describe the interconversion of the species that are populated, a concept similar to that of a master equation in quantum mechanics and other fields of physics. Owing to the large number of possible aggregated states, the number of differential equations that needs to be solved simultaneously is astronomical and numerical approaches usually need to be adopted [55]. However, a breakthrough has recently been made through the realization that the experimentally most easily accessible observable, namely the total mass of fibrillar aggregates as a function of time (e.g. from ThT fluorescence experiments), can be obtained by summing up the (theoretically infinitely many) differential equations, leading to a set of two coupled differential equations for the total mass and total number of aggregates [14,15]. This set of equations can be solved iteratively, leading to better analytical descriptions with each iteration. The availability of analytical expressions allows global fits to large datasets to be performed. The greatest asset of this approach is that a large dataset can only be fitted to a set of equations with a small number of unknowns (three to four rate constants) if the data are consistent with the model used to derive the equations. In addition, the fact that the analytical expressions contain the molecular rate constants as parameters allows fundamental connections to be revealed and explained, such as the one between the lag time and the maximum conversion rate [56]. Furthermore, the availability of the molecular rate constants allows predictions to be made about the kinetics of aggregation in regions of parameter space that are difficult or time-consuming to access experimentally.

Theories of primary nucleation

In the master equation formalism described above, the primary nucleation term is usually approximated as:

$$\frac{d[P]}{dt} = k_n [m]^{n_c} \tag{3}$$

where [P] and [m] denote the concentrations of nuclei (defined as the smallest multimer that can act as a seed fibril, i.e. that can grow by monomer addition) and monomers respectively, and k_n is the nucleation rate constant. However, this approach can mask more complex nucleation mechanisms than simple collisions of n_c monomers to form a nucleus. In particular for $n_c > 2$, this picture becomes non-physical owing to the small probability of simultaneous multiparticle encounters. Attempts have been made to develop theories of primary nucleation of amyloid fibrils in analogy to classical nucleation theory where the critical nucleus is the structure with the highest free energy on the reaction co-ordinate [57], which results from a competition between surface and volume effects. The resulting theory predicts the existence of concentration regimes with different scaling exponents of the nucleation rate with the monomer concentration. However, no experimental data exist to date that are appropriate to validate, or otherwise, this approach. A further complication stems from the fact that one or several conversion steps may be required in order to convert the initial nucleus into a growth competent species that can progress to a fibril. Recently, a theoretical framework was presented that allows prediction of the consequences of a cascade of conversion events [58]. In this work, it was shown that a range of different regimes exist, depending on the relative kinetics of nucleation, conversion and growth, and that only some of those regimes lead to the formation of elongated fibrils.

Mechanistic aspects of the molecular steps in amyloid formation

Despite the many remaining open questions on the mechanistic details of amyloid formation by individual proteins, enormous progress has been made in recent years towards understanding the individual molecular steps in the reaction, as well as their relative contribution towards the overall conversion process. Below, we give a summary of the most important processes. All processes are shown in Figure 2(B).

Primary nucleation

Primary nucleation, the formation of a protein multimer from monomeric protein molecules that will ultimately evolve into an amyloid fibril, is the most elusive process on the pathway from soluble to aggregated protein. As is well known from studies of related processes such as crystallization, nucleation itself cannot usually be studied experimentally by conventional means due to the very nature of the critical nucleus as a species of high(est) free energy and therefore low(est) population. Owing to the downhill energetic nature of the growth of a nucleus, the nuclei are not only usually slow to form, but also evolve very rapidly into larger aggregates. Most experimental setups are not able to detect the presence of very small numbers of aggregates, but rather have a threshold concentration above which their presence can be detected. In cases where secondary processes, such as fragmentation or secondary nucleation (see below) are important, the lag time, i.e. the time until a detectable quantity of aggregates is present, is likely to depend only weakly on the primary nucleation rate [14,15]. Therefore, in these cases, the primary nucleation rate cannot normally be determined very accurately from bulk aggregation experiments. In some studies it has been proposed that the variability of aggregation time courses, in particular at low protein concentrations, is a direct consequence of the stochastic nature of primary nucleation. Recent experimental [9] and theoretical [15] insights, however, show that this is unlikely to be the case in bulk experiments, but that the true origin of the variability in such cases is the lack of control over all experimentally relevant parameters, such as the presence of pre-formed aggregates. Indeed, in at least some cases where all possible efforts have been undertaken to remove such aggregates, in order to create a well-defined reproducible starting point of the experiment, variations in the aggregation time courses have been very small [9].

In order for the intrinsic stochasticity in primary nucleation to be able to manifest itself, nano- or pico-litre volumes are usually required. A small calculation shall serve to illustrate this point. Recently, an estimate for the primary nucleation rate constant of the $A\beta(1-42)$ peptide has been presented ($k_n \sim 3 \times 10^{-4}$ $M^{-1} \cdot s^{-1}$; $n_c = 2$ [34]), obtained from global fitting to aggregation time courses in bulk solution. This system is characterized by the presence of a monomer-dependent secondary nucleation pathway (see below) that dominates the production of new aggregates, except at the very beginning of an experiment, when only monomers are present, and where primary nucleation dominates. In a typical bulk experiment, 100 µl aliquots of solution at a concentration of 1 µM are used. The rate of production of nuclei under those conditions is $\sim 1.8 \times 10^4$ s^{-1}. This number is too large, and its associated variation, assuming the nucleation obeys Poisson statistics, is too small to be expected to generate detectable variability in macroscopic experiments, and indeed, as mentioned above, careful control of all experimentally relevant parameters results in highly reproducible data. On the other hand, in recent microdroplet experiments [44], it was shown that through the reduction in the experimental volumes to the nanolitre scale, only a single primary nucleation event per droplet is likely to occur over a time course of several hours, and hence the observed variability of the time to nucleation reflects stochasticity on the molecular level.

However, in some amyloid systems, under certain conditions, no significant secondary processes are detected, and in those cases, the aggregation time courses contain more information about the primary nucleation step than is possible in the presence of significant secondary nucleation. The most important case in this respect is the aggregation of α-synuclein, a hallmark of Parkinson's disease, at neutral pH [11]. It has been demonstrated in a range of studies that homogeneous primary nucleation in simple aqueous solution of this protein is undetectable [11], and that the formation of α-synuclein fibrils is a surface-catalysed heterogeneous process. Various interfaces, such as the air–water interface [59] or (of particular significance in biology) lipid membranes [60] are able to induce α-synuclein nucleation. In order to account for the heterogeneous nature of nucleation, the classical models of nucleation and growth [8] have to be modified, making it possible to determine nucleation rates accurately from bulk aggregation data.

Overall, many open questions remain with respect to primary nucleation, given the multitude of oligomeric species that are observed under conditions of amyloid fibril formation. There is strong evidence that some of those oligomeric structures are not nuclei to fibril formation, but rather products of alternative aggregation pathways [61]. However, in other cases, the kinetics of oligomer formation and evolution suggest that they could be structures that are direct precursors of amyloid fibrils [47]. In this case, however, it can be expected that a significant conformational conversion step is required to transform the oligomeric structures, which show some β-sheet content, into all β-sheet amyloid fibrils [58].

Fibril growth

The growth, or elongation, of amyloid fibrils is probably the best-studied molecular process on the pathway from monomeric protein to amyloid fibrils. In experiments where a sufficiently high concentration of seed fibrils is initially added to the soluble protein, fibril growth is the only relevant process that results in further aggregation. A fundamental question in this context is whether or not fibrils grow via the addition of monomeric protein or soluble oligomeric structures that are often observed to coexist with fibrils and monomers under conditions where fibrils grow; indeed, this coexistence has been advanced as a strong argument for growth by oligomer addition. However, the populations of such oligomers, if at equilibrium with monomers, can be expected to show a highly non-linear dependence on the total protein concentration. Therefore the growth rate of fibrils, if growth occurs by oligomer addition, should depend in a similar, higher than linear, manner on the total concentration of soluble protein molecules (monomers plus oligomers; Figure 4A) as the concentration of oligomers. For some proteins, experiments have been performed where the dependence of fibril elongation on the concentration of soluble protein has been measured specifically, for example in seeded growth experiments in bulk solution [11,62,63] and using biosensing [31]; it has been found in all cases that the growth rate depends linearly on the concentration of soluble protein at low concentrations, as expected if elongation occurs by monomer addition, and becomes independent of the soluble protein concentration at higher concentrations (Figure 4B). This saturable behaviour is reminiscent of Michaelis–Menten enzyme kinetics, whose origin can be found in the two-step nature of substrate conversion by an enzyme, a diffusive 'docking' step is followed by a chemical transformation or 'locking' step, which have distinct rate constants and energy barriers. However, it has been shown that in the case of amyloid fibril growth, a separation of the incorporation of a monomer into the fibril into diffusive and reactive parts is neither supported by experimental data nor by the energy landscape view of protein folding and misfolding, which treats all processes and movements that the polypeptide chain undergoes as

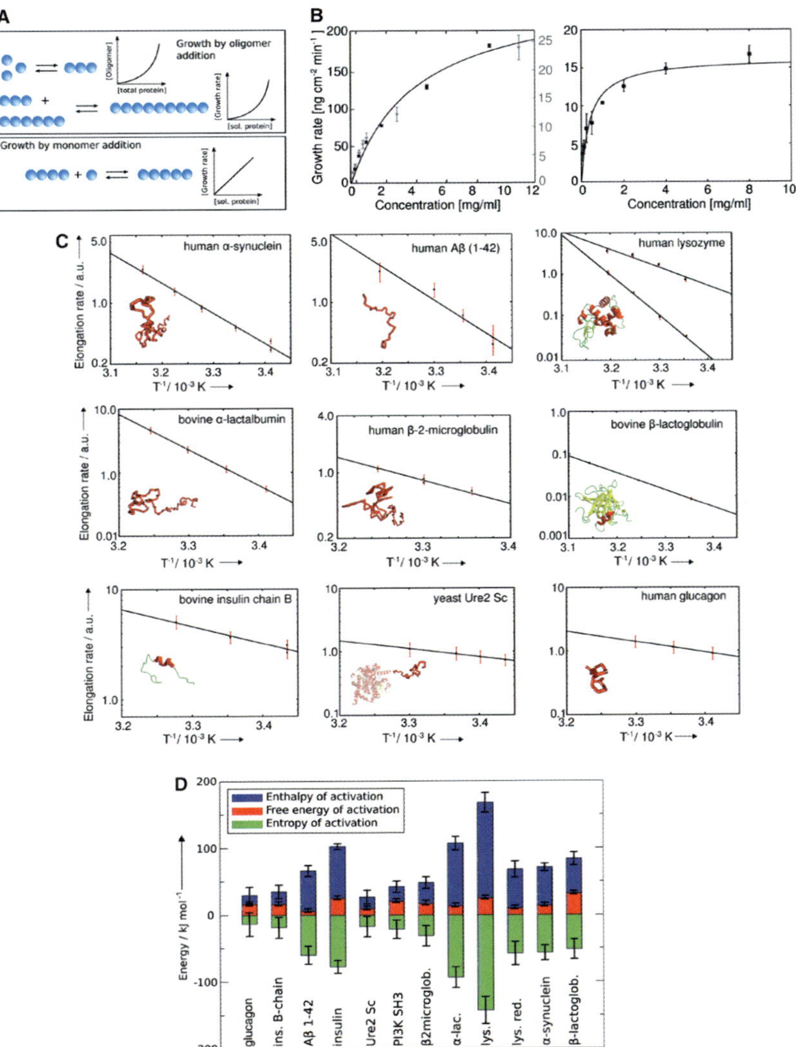

Figure 4. The energy barriers of amyloid fibril growth
(**A**) Illustration of two different models for amyloid fibril elongation. Fibrils can in principle grow via the addition of oligomeric structures or by the addition of monomeric protein molecules. These two models make different predictions about the concentration dependence of elongation (see text for details). (**B**) The elongation rate of amyloid fibrils from insulin (left panel; two different solution conditions) and α-lactalbumin (right panel) as a function of the concentration of soluble protein [31]. (**C**) Analysis of the temperature dependence of amyloid fibril elongation by a range of peptides and proteins [32], measured with a QCM. The data are shown as Arrhenius plots (**D**). The data shown in (**C**), together with estimates of the absolute rate of fibril growth and an appropriate kinetic theory [31], allow the determination of the thermodynamic parameters of activation, $\Delta H^{\ddagger}$, $\Delta G^{\ddagger}$ and $\Delta S^{\ddagger}$. This analysis shows that in general, an unfavourable enthalpy of activation, $\Delta H^{\ddagger}$, is partly compensated by a favourable entropy of activation, $\Delta S^{\ddagger}$. (**B**) was reproduced from [31]; Buell, A.K., Blundell, J.R., Dobson, C.M., Welland, M.E., Terentjev, E.M. and Knowles, T.P.J., 2010, Frequency factors in a landscape model of filamentous protein aggregation, Phys. Rev. Lett., vol 104, 228101. (**C**) and (**D**) were reproduced with permission from [32]; Buell, A.K., Dhulesia, A., White, D.A., Knowles, T.P.J., Dobson, C.M. and Welland, M.E., 2012, Detailed analysis of the energy barriers for amyloid fibril growth, vol.51, pp. 5247–5251 copyright 2012 WILEY-VCH Verlag GmbH & Co. KGaA, Weinheim.

diffusive. Therefore the elongation reaction in the context of ensemble experiments can overall be described as a diffusive crossing of a single highest free energy barrier [31]; the diffusive arrival of the protein molecule from the bulk solution at the fibril end and the incorporation are not separate processes, but form a continuous diffusive process. In this scenario, the saturation of the growth rate stems from the finite time that is on average required for a monomer to incorporate into a fibril in such a way as to act as a template for the subsequent monomer.

Overall, the kinetics of fibril elongation are determined by an expression of the form:

$$R_{el} = \Gamma e^{-\frac{\Delta G^{\ddagger}}{RT}}$$

where Γ is a diffusive pre-factor, or attempt rate, and $\Delta G^{\ddagger}$ is the free energy barrier for the process of fibril elongation (see below). If the absolute rates of fibril growth can be measured, as is possible in seeded growth experiments both in bulk solution and using biosensing, and a model for Γ is available, the magnitude of the free energy barriers $\Delta G^{\ddagger}$ can be determined. Such an analysis has been performed with a simple Smoluchowski-type pre-factor [64] and recently, an extensive analysis of the elongation kinetics of a wide variety of proteins has been presented [32], using a polymer science model for Γ [31] (Figure 4C). The principle result of this analysis is that the absolute rates of fibril growth in amyloid-forming proteins can vary over more than four orders of magnitude, owing to the different heights of the free energy barriers. In most cases, the free energy of activation was found to be composed of an unfavourable enthalpy of activation, which correlates with sequence length and residual structure of the monomer, and a favourable entropy of activation, which correlates with the hydrophobicity of the sequence (Figure 4D).

This type of ensemble analysis neglects the experimental finding of 'stop-and-go' kinetics that have been observed in a range of single particle studies on fibril growth, using *in situ* AFM [54,65] and ThT TIRF techniques [66]. These studies have found that different morphologies of amyloid fibrils formed from the same protein can exhibit different elongation rates. In addition, it has been shown that only a fraction of the fibrils being monitored grows at any one time. This intriguing finding is explained by proposing that the monomer at the end of the fibril can sometimes adopt a conformation that does not act as a template for further attachment. After dissociation or rearrangement of this monomer, the templating effect resumes. These results illustrate that ensemble experiments of fibril growth are not able to capture all the features of the elongation reaction and that the energy landscape of a monomer and a seed fibril can have local minima corresponding to partly incorporated states. It is interesting to note, however, that although the results on the elongation of single fibrils give valuable insight into the nature of this process, the observed durations of 'stop' periods do not require significant corrections to the free energy barriers extracted from ensemble experiments. Furthermore, the description in terms of an average growth rate is fully sufficient for the modelling and fitting of bulk aggregation data [11,34].

Finally, we comment on the existence of so-called fibril strains, subtle differences in the molecular structure of amyloid fibrils, formed from the same protein, which manifest themselves in different kinetics of elongation. Highly quantitative studies of this phenomenon have been carried out, for example using a fragment of the yeast prion Sup35 as a model system. It was found that a change in solution conditions, such as an increase in temperature from 4°C to 37°C, can induce the formation of a different fibril strain [67]. However, even under one set of conditions, different types of fibrils with very different growth characteristics can be formed [68] that are not straightforward to distinguish with low-resolution techniques, such as AFM. Similar results have been obtained in a recent study of the elongation kinetics of fibrils of Aβ(1–40), where two forms with distinguishable morphology were shown to have different growth and dissociation rate constants [65].

Fragmentation

The fragmentation of amyloid fibrils is an important factor in many *in vitro* experiments of amyloid formation. It is well known that mechanical action such as agitation or sonication accelerates amyloid formation, often dramatically [69], and it has been proposed that the main effect of these processes is the fragmentation of fibrils, which increases the number of growth competent fibril ends and therefore accelerates the conversion of monomeric into fibrillar protein. It has been shown that in *in vitro* experiments of amyloid formation that are dominated by fragmentation, the lagtimes scale as $[M_0]^{1/2}$, where $[M_0]$ is the initial concentration of monomer [14].

It has been proposed that the fragmentation of fibrils can also play an important role in the proliferation and transmission of aggregation *in vivo*, in particular in the case of yeast prions, where the chaperone Hsp104 is thought to fragment the amyloid fibrils, thereby increasing infectivity and transmission efficiency of the prions [33]. Similarly, for mammalian prions, the finding that the disease onset in transgenic mice scales with the expression levels with the said scaling exponent of 0.5, suggests that fragmentation plays an important role in this case [14].

The mechanical stabilities that enable individual amyloid fibrils to resist fragmentation have been probed by experiments [70], as well as simulation [71], and from these studies it can be concluded that amyloid fibrils can fragment with low rates even in the absence of mechanical action. The mechanisms and effects of fibril fragmentation under the influence of shear forces have been investigated in detail using *ex situ* single particle analysis by AFM [43]. In that study, it was demonstrated that the probability of fragmentation of any link between monomers within an amyloid fibril strongly depends on the overall length of the fibril, as well as the relative position of the link.

Monomer-dependent secondary nucleation

Secondary pathways other than fragmentation, in particular processes that create new amyloid fibrils in a manner that depends on the concentrations of both the soluble protein and the concentration of fibrillar protein already present, have been shown to play an important role in the proliferation of a range of amyloid systems. They have been suggested to contribute to the aggregation of a fragment of the IAPP (islet amyloid polypeptide) [72], and it has been shown recently that the aggregation kinetics of the Aβ42 peptide are dominated by secondary nucleation under quiescent conditions [34]. Mechanistically, it is thought that secondary nucleation is a form of surface catalysis. This hypothesis is supported by recent findings on the dependence of secondary nucleation of the intrinsically disordered protein α-synuclein on the solution conditions [11]. In particular, it has been found that the kinetics of secondary nucleation for this protein depends extremely sensitively on the pH of the solution, with an increase of more than four orders of magnitude from pH 7 to pH 5. Over this pH interval, the charge of the C-terminal residues of α-synuclein, which are not in the fibril core, changes dramatically. This change in electrostatic properties probably enables the nucleation of new amyloid fibrils on the surface of existing fibrils.

Spatial propagation of aggregation

Until very recently, the spatial propagation of a protein aggregation reaction has not generally been considered in the context of amyloid formation. The spread of aggregates is, however, of great significance in protein misfolding disorders, such as Alzheimer's and Parkinson's diseases, where the migration of aggregates through the affected organism and the infection of formerly healthy cells can take place just as it can in the prion diseases. The spatial propagation of aggregation generally proceeds through one of two distinct mechanisms, namely direct growth (gelation) or diffusion of aggregates that form through secondary processes and that then act as seeds distant from the location of their formation [73]. Under conditions where primary nucleation is slow and in the total absence of macroscopic transport processes such as convection, the spatial spread can be most readily observed and its velocity measured. Such experiments have been carried out in microdroplets for insulin amyloid formation and the results suggest that under those conditions the spatial spread is dominated by diffusion [44], which is much faster than gelation, the velocity of which is limited by the growth rate of individual fibrils. The velocity of spatial spread is hence not influenced by a change in solution condition that changes the fibril growth rate [73]. On the other hand, if the velocity of the growth of insulin spherulites (compact higher-order aggregates of amyloid fibrils) is measured, it can be shown that it is defined by the growth rates of the individual fibrils [73]. This difference in behaviour is likely to be due to the different maturation stages of the amyloid fibrils directly after nucleation and in a spherulite.

Effects of external factors on the aggregation kinetics

A very large number of studies has been published in the last decade, where the influence of a multitude of physical or chemical factors on amyloid formation of proteins has been investigated. Nevertheless, in most of these studies, it has not been possible to elucidate the effect of the specific factor under study on each of the individual molecular processes involved in amyloid formation. Such an analysis is, however, indispensable as a result of the complex nature of amyloid formation (see above) and the large variation in the relative importance of primary nucleation, growth and secondary processes for different proteins. Such a detailed description can either be achieved through global fitting of large datasets of complete aggregation time courses, or through an experimental design that specifically probes individual molecular processes. In the following section, we describe the most important results obtained in explorations of various aspects of the aggregation process.

Salt type and concentration

As outlined above, in many cases amyloid fibrils form most readily under conditions of extreme pH, where the native form of the protein is destabilized. However, under these conditions, protein molecules are often highly charged, and therefore electrostatic factors oppose aggregation (Figure 5A). It came therefore as no surprise when it was found that an increase in the ionic strength of the aggregating buffer or solution accelerates protein aggregation in many cases [74].

However, it has also been shown that a change in the concentration and the chemical nature of the dissolved ions can change the pathways of aggregation and lead to different aggregate morphologies. In particular, it has been found that, above a certain ionic strength, amorphous aggregates are formed rather than ordered fibrillar structures [74,75]. This finding suggests that a certain degree of electrostatic repulsion is required in order to favour ordered

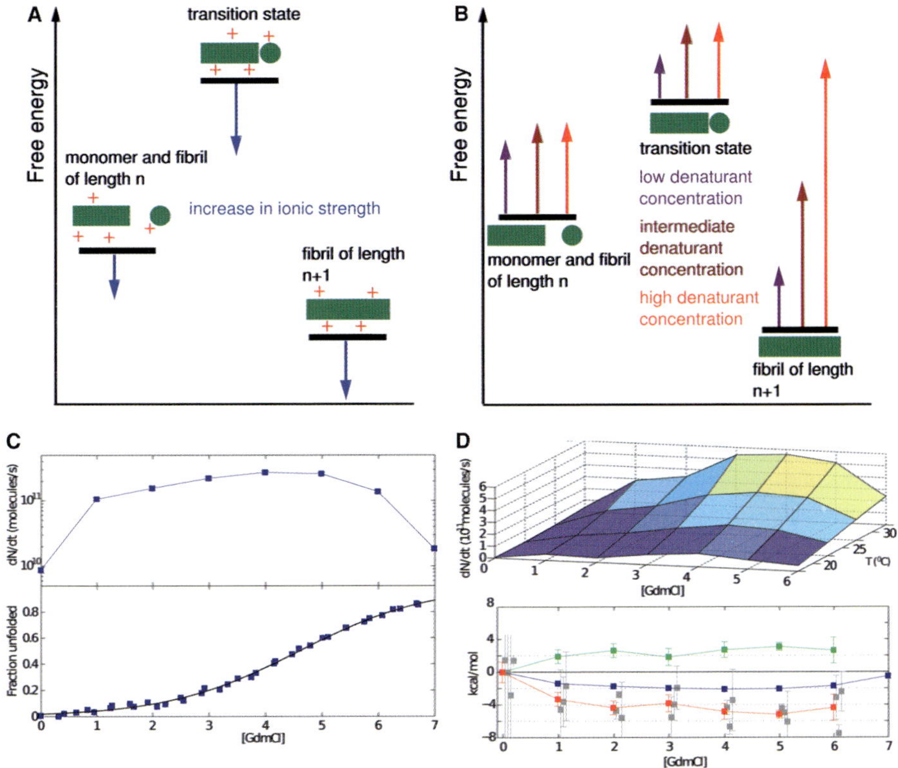

Figure 5. Modifying the energy landscape of protein aggregation
(**A**) The effect of a change in ionic strength on the self-assembly of peptides and proteins into amyloid fibrils under conditions where the proteins carry a high net charge. An increase in ionic strength stabilizes all states, but in particular the transition state for aggregation, due to the presence of ions between the two reaction partners, the monomer and the fibril end. (**B**) The effect of denaturant on the aggregation rate and process depends on the concentration. At low concentrations, the globular structure of the soluble state is most destabilized, and hence aggregation is accelerated. At intermediate concentrations, the transition state is also destabilized and hence the aggregation no longer accelerates, or even decreases. At very high concentrations, all protein–protein interactions, intra- as well as inter-molecular, are strongly destabilized and hence the (unfolded) monomer represents the free energy minimum. (**C**) Elongation rate of insulin amyloid fibrils (top panel) and fraction of unfolded insulin (bottom panel) as a function of denaturant (GndHCl) concentration. (**D**) Insulin amyloid fibril elongation rate as a function of both temperature and GndHCl concentration (top panel) and analysis of the activation parameters (bottom panel). (**C**) and (**D**) were reproduced from [42]; Knowles, T.P.J., Shu, W., Devlin, G.L., Meehan, S., Auer, S., Dobson, C.M. and Welland, M.E, 2007, Kinetics and thermodynamics of amyloid formation from direct measurements of fluctuations in fibril mass, Proc. Natl. Acad. Sci. U.S.A., vol.104, pp. 10016–10021 © 2007 by The National Academy of Sciences of the USA.

aggregation. This repulsion will prevent most of the molecular encounters in an aggregating solution from leading to permanent interactions. The interactions will persist only in those cases where the molecules meet in a configuration that enables them to gain some of the favourable free energy of aggregation early on the reactive trajectory. In the absence of electrostatic repulsion, a larger fraction of encounters will result in permanent interactions, leading to disordered aggregation. Overall, it has been found that the effects of salts on amyloid formation in general, and fibril elongation in particular, is a combination of Debye screening (for simple ions at low concentrations), (specific) ion binding and Hoffmeister-type effects, where the salt influences the protein–solvent interactions [52,76] (Figures 3D–3H).

Denaturants and osmolytes

Denaturants and osmolytes are small molecules that, at high concentrations (typically several molar), modify the stability of proteins. Denaturants such as urea, GndHCl and GndSCN (guanidinium thiocyanate) destabilize the fold of globular proteins, an effect attributable to preferential hydrogen bonding to the backbone of the polypeptide and weakening of the hydrophobic effect [77]. In contrast, osmolytes such as some amino acids and TMAO (tri-methylamine N-oxide) are excluded from the surface of folded proteins and hence stabilize the globular structure [78]. As discussed in the first part of the present chapter, despite their large thermodynamic stability, amyloid fibrils can be dissociated by high concentrations of denaturants. It has been found, however, that at moderate concentrations of denaturants, the kinetics of amyloid formation and growth can be accelerated, in particular in cases where the soluble amyloid precursor is a globular protein, such as insulin [42]. Hence, under these con-ditions, the structure of the monomeric building block is destabilized by the denaturant to a larger degree than the transition state for fibril growth, which, being intermediate in structure between the native and fibrillar states, is likely to be less structured than either of these two states and hence less destabilized by denaturants. At higher concentrations of denaturants, however, the aggregation kinetics are observed to slow down, before finally the fibril ceases to be the thermodynamic minimum energy state (see Figure 5B). The expected converse effect, the inhibition of amyloid fibril growth by a stabilizing osmolyte at moderate concentrations, has also been observed [42].

Crowding agents

In living cells, a large volume fraction (up to 40% by mass) is occupied by macromolecules [79], and an important question is the degree to which biochemical or biophysical reac-tions in such a crowded environment are affected relative to environments in which such systems are normally studied *in vitro*, e.g. a dilute regime in a test tube. In this context, a distinction needs to be made between chemically specific interactions and interactions that are independent of the chemical nature of the 'crowding agent'. An important challenge in studies of crowding effects has always been to distinguish the effects of the artificial crowd-ing agent on the properties of the solvent water, such as its viscosity or its hydrogen bond-ing structure and dynamics, from direct consequences of crowding. In the simplest case, the crowding agent only exerts excluded volume effects, i.e. it occupies some fraction of the available volume and therefore increases the effective concentration of reacting species [80]. Such excluded volume effects have been shown to influence both the folding and aggregation rates of proteins [81] due to the favouring of compact forms of the proteins. Indeed, it has been shown that crowding effects can both slow down [82] and accelerate [83,84] the formation of amyloid fibrils. In a detailed study that selectively investigated crowding effects on fibril growth, it has been shown that these apparently contradictory effects can be rationalized and depend on the structure of the monomeric amyloid precur-sor. Owing to the favouring of compact states in crowded environments, fibril elongation by natively disordered monomers is accelerated by crowding and that by monomers with a globular structure is inhibited [85].

Molecular chaperones and antibodies

A large body of literature exists that addresses the nature and consequences of the interactions between molecular chaperones and amyloid species. This interest stems from the discovery that molecular chaperones co-localize with amyloid deposits in neurodegenerative diseases [86]. In addition, the role of chaperones in assisting protein folding, which is mediated through a preferential interaction between the chaperone and partly folded intermediates [87], renders an interaction between chaperones and amyloid species and intermediates likely, given the partly unfolded nature of oligomeric precursors or even fully formed amyloid fibrils that often have large parts of the polypeptide sequence exposed rather than buried in the compact fibril core. Detailed studies have shown that chaperones can interact in a rather promiscuous and non-specific way with soluble amyloid precursors, such as monomers and oligomers [88, 89], and also bind to amyloid fibrils where they can inhibit both growth [88, 90] and nucleation processes [91]. In stark contrast with molecular chaperones, specifically raised antibodies can bind highly specifically to amyloid fibrils of a given protein and in some cases are even able to distinguish between different amyloid fibril morphologies [92].

Small molecules and peptides

The common structural feature of all amyloid fibrils, a cross-β structure, exhibits specific binding of a range of small molecules, in particular several dyes. This feature is used in the histological identification of amyloid fibrils [93], in non-invasive diagnosis of neurodegenerative diseases [94], as well as for the detection of amyloid fibrils in *in vitro* experiments [36]. These multiple potential applications are of great interest and therefore the design and the study of amyloid ligands is a very active field of research. However, in even the most well-studied molecules, the exact mode of binding, as well as the affinity and stoichiometry are not yet fully understood. The finding that some small molecules, in particular dye labels, such as ThT and Congo Red, exhibit a specific interaction with amyloid species motivates a large research effort devoted to discovering small molecule inhibitors of protein aggregation. One main challenge that these efforts face is to find small molecules whose interaction with amyloid species or precursors has comparable energetics with the highly favourable intermolecular interactions within amyloid fibrils. This feature, combined with the difficulties associated with the experimental validation of the amyloid binding and inhibitory effects of inhibitor candidates [95], has led to the fact that despite extensive efforts few convincing small molecule inhibitors have been presented.

In parallel with the search for effective small molecules, peptides and peptide analogues are also being developed as inhibitors. Already in the earliest days of *in vitro* studies on amyloid formation, it has been shown that short fragments of amyloidogenic peptides can bind to aggregates and inhibit their further growth [96]. One advantage of peptide inhibitors is the possibility of rational discovery and design strategies (through sequence complementarity), as well as energetics of interactions with the amyloidogenic polypeptide that are comparable with the self-interaction of the aggregating peptide.

We conclude this section with the remark that, depending on the exact mechanism of aggregation of a specific disease-related protein, the inhibition of the formation and growth of amyloid fibrils may, or may not, be a useful and efficient therapeutic strategy. Owing to the complex feedback mechanism enabled by secondary processes, the concentrations of toxic aggregated species can both increase and decrease if amyloid formation is inhibited.

Note added in proof (received 30 June 2014)

While this chapter was in press, it was reported that certain amyloid fibrils can also be cold-denatured, i.e. they dissolve when incubated for prolonged times at temperatures close to the freezing point of water [97].

Summary

- Amyloid fibrils are thermodynamically more stable than the soluble forms under conditions often found *in vitro* and *in vivo*. Therefore the soluble states of many proteins are only kinetically stable towards amyloid formation.

- Equilibrium dissociation and calorimetric experiments can provide insight into the origin of this thermodynamic stability, and into the relative balance of intra- and inter-molecular, as well as protein–solvent, interactions.

- Amyloid formation is a complex multistep process, including nucleation and growth processes, as well as secondary processes, that lead to the proliferation of aggregates. These processes can act in series or in parallel and lead to highly complex overall kinetic behaviour.

- In order to determine the overall mechanism of amyloid formation of a given protein, large datasets can be globally fitted to a range of models and different mechanisms can be discarded or validated based on the quality of the fit.

- A complementary strategy is to design experiments that are sensitive to only one out of the variety of different processes that contribute to amyloid formation. An example is the use of biosensing experiments to probe amyloid fibril elongation.

- The individual molecular steps in the overall amyloid formation pathway, as well as the overall aggregation process, are influenced by a variety of external factors, such as solution composition (ionic strength, denaturants and osmolytes) and the presence of small molecules, peptides or molecular chaperones.

- Understanding the mechanism of protein aggregation into amyloid fibrils in detail is the key to the rational design of potential therapeutic strategies.

Christopher Dobson and Tuomas Knowles thank the Wellcome Trust and Elan Pharmaceuticals for support. Alexander Buell thanks Magdalene College, Cambridge, and the Leverhulme Trust for their support.

References

1. Dobson, C.M. (2003) Protein folding and misfolding. Nature **426**, 884–890
2. Knowles, T.P.J., Simone, A.D., Fitzpatrick, A.W., Baldwin, A., Meehan, S., Rajah, L., Vendruscolo, M., Welland, M.E., Dobson, C.M. and Terentjev, E.M. (2012) Twisting transition between crystalline and fibrillar phases of aggregated peptides. Phys. Rev. Lett. **109**, 158101
3. Fitzpatrick, A.W.P., Debelouchina, G.T., Bayro, M.J., Clare, D.K., Caporini, M.A., Bajaj, V.S., Jaroniec, C.P., Wang, L., Ladizhansky, V., Mller, S.A. et al. (2013) Atomic structure and hierarchical assembly of a cross-β amyloid fibril. Proc. Natl. Acad. Sci. U.S.A. **110**, 5468–5473

4.   Gazit, E. (2002) The "correctly folded" state of proteins: is it a metastable state? Angew. Chem. Int. Ed. Engl. **41**, 257–259

5.   Fändrich, M., Fletcher, M.A. and Dobson, C.M. (2001) Amyloid fibrils from muscle myoglobin. Nature **410**, 165–166

6.   Fändrich, M. and Dobson, C.M. (2002) The behaviour of polyamino acids reveals an inverse side chain effect in amyloid structure formation. EMBO J. **21**, 5682–5690

7.   Guijarro, J.I., Sunde, M., Jones, J.A., Campbell, I.D. and Dobson, C.M. (1998) Amyloid fibril formation by an SH3 domain. Proc. Natl. Acad. Sci. U.S.A. **95**, 4224–4228

8.   Oosawa, F. and Kasai, M. (1962) A theory of linear and helical aggregations of macromolecules. J. Mol. Biol. **4**, 10–21

9.   Hellstrand, E., Boland, B., Walsh, D.M. and Linse, S. (2010) Amyloid β-protein aggregation produces highly reproducible kinetic data and occurs by a two-phase process. ACS Chem. Neurosci. **1**, 13–18

10. Baldwin, A.J., Knowles, T.P.J., Tartaglia, G.G., Fitzpatrick, A.W., Devlin, G.L., Shammas, S.L., Waudby, C.A., Mossuto, M.F., Meehan, S., Gras, S.L. et al. (2011) Metastability of native proteins and the phenomenon of amyloid formation. J. Am. Chem. Soc. **133**, 14160–14163

11. Buell, A.K., Galvagnion, C., Gaspar, R., Sparr, E., Vendruscolo, M., Knowles, T.P., Linse, S. and Dobson, C.M. (2014) Solution conditions determine the relative importance of nucleation and growth processes in α-synuclein aggregation. Proc. Natl. Acad. Sci. U.S.A. **111**, 7671–7676

12. Narimoto, T., Sakurai, K., Okamoto, A., Chatani, E., Hoshino, M., Hasegawa, K., Naiki, H. and Goto, Y. (2004) Conformational stability of amyloid fibrils of β_2-microglobulin probed by guanidine-hydrochloride-induced unfolding. FEBS Lett. **576**, 313–319

13. Goldschmidt, L., Teng, P.K., Riek, R. and Eisenberg, D. (2010) Identifying the amylome, proteins capable of forming amyloid-like fibrils. Proc. Natl. Acad. Sci. U.S.A. **107**, 3487–3492

14. Knowles, T.P.J., Waudby, C.A., Devlin, G.L., Cohen, S.I.A., Aguzzi, A., Vendruscolo, M., Terentjev, E.M., Welland, M.E. and Dobson, C.M. (2009) An analytical solution to the kinetics of breakable filament assembly. Science **326**, 1533–1537

15. Cohen, S.I.A., Vendruscolo, M., Welland, M.E., Dobson, C.M., Terentjev, E.M. and Knowles, T.P.J. (2011) Nucleated polymerization with secondary pathways. I. time evolution of the principal moments. J. Chem. Phys. **135**, 065105

16. Dill, K.A. (1990) Dominant forces in protein folding. Biochemistry **29**, 7133–7155

17. Chandler, D. (2005) Interfaces and the driving force of hydrophobic assembly. Nature **437**, 640–647

18. Sasahara, K., Naiki, H. and Goto, Y. (2005) Kinetically controlled thermal response of β_2-microglobulin amyloid fibrils. J. Mol. Biol. **352**, 700–711

19. Kardos, J., Yamamoto, K., Hasegawa, K., Naiki, H. and Goto, Y. (2004) Direct measurement of the thermodynamic parameters of amyloid formation by isothermal titration calorimetry. J. Biol. Chem. **279**, 55308–55314

20. Morel, B., Varela, L. and Conejero-Lara, F. (2010) The thermodynamic stability of amyloid fibrils studied by differential scanning calorimetry. J. Phys. Chem. B **114**, 4010–4019

21. Jeppesen, M.D., Hein, K., Nissen, P., Westh, P. and Otzen, D.E. (2010) A thermodynamic analysis of fibrillar polymorphism. Biophys. Chem. **149**, 40–46

22. Debye, P. and Hückel, E. (1923) The theory of electrolytes. I. Lowering of freezing point and related phenomena. Phys. Zeitschr. **24**, 185–206

23. Israelachvili, J. (1992) Intermolecular And Surface Forces, Academic Press, MA

24. Shammas, S.L., Knowles, T.P.J., Baldwin, A.J., Macphee, C.E., Welland, M.E., Dobson, C.M. and Devlin, G.L. (2011) Perturbation of the stability of amyloid fibrils through alteration of electrostatic interactions. Biophys. J. **100**, 2783–2791

25. Marshall, K.E., Hicks, M.R., Williams, T.L., Hoffmann, S.V., Rodger, A., Dafforn, T.R. and Serpell, L.C. (2010) Characterizing the assembly of the sup35 yeast prion fragment, GNNQQNY: structural changes accompany a fiber-to-crystal switch. Biophys. J. **98**, 330–338

26. Nelson, R., Sawaya, M.R., Balbirnie, M., Madsen, A.O., Riekel, C., Grothe, R. and Eisenberg, D. (2005) Structure of the cross-β spine of amyloid-like fibrils. Nature **435**, 773–778

27. Tartaglia, G.G., Pechmann, S., Dobson, C.M. and Vendruscolo, M. (2007) Life on the edge: a link between gene expression levels and aggregation rates of human proteins. Trends Biochem. Sci. **32**, 204–206

28. Chiti, F., Stefani, M., Taddei, N., Ramponi, G. and Dobson, C.M. (2003) Rationalization of the effects of mutations on peptide and protein aggregation rates. Nature **424**, 805–808

29. Fernandez-Escamilla, A.-M., Rousseau, F., Schymkowitz, J. and Serrano, L. (2004) Prediction of sequence-dependent and mutational effects on the aggregation of peptides and proteins. Nat. Biotechnol. **22**, 1302–1306

30. DuBay, K.F., Pawar, A.P., Chiti, F., Zurdo, J., Dobson, C.M. and Vendruscolo, M. (2004) Prediction of the absolute aggregation rates of amyloidogenic polypeptide chains. J. Mol. Biol. **341**, 1317–1326

31. Buell, A.K., Blundell, J.R., Dobson, C.M., Welland, M.E., Terentjev, E.M. and Knowles, T.P.J. (2010) Frequency factors in a landscape model of filamentous protein aggregation. Phys. Rev. Lett. **104**, 228101

32. Buell, A.K., Dhulesia, A., White, D.A., Knowles, T.P.J., Dobson, C.M. and Welland, M.E. (2012) Detailed analysis of the energy barriers for amyloid fibril growth. Angew. Chem. Int. Ed. Engl. **51**, 5247–5251

33. Shorter, J. and Lindquist, S. (2004) HSP104 catalyzes formation and elimination of self-replicating Sup35 prion conformers. Science **304**, 1793–1797

34. Cohen, S.I.A., Linse, S., Luheshi, L.M., Hellstrand, E., White, D.A., Rajah, L., Otzen, D.E., Vendruscolo, M., Dobson, C.M. and Knowles, T.P.J. (2013) Proliferation of amyloid-β42 aggregates occurs through a secondary nucleation mechanism. Proc. Natl. Acad. Sci. U.S.A. **110**, 9758–9763

35. Lomakin, A., Chung, D.S., Benedek, G.B., Kirschner, D.A. and Teplow, D.B. (1996) On the nucleation and growth of amyloid β-protein fibrils: detection of nuclei and quantitation of rate constants. Proc. Natl. Acad. Sci. U.S.A. **93**, 1125–1129

36. LeVine, H. (1993) Thioflavine T interaction with synthetic Alzheimer's disease β-amyloid peptides: detection of amyloid aggregation in solution. Protein Sci. **2**, 404–410

37. Berne, B.J. and Pecora, R. (2000) Dynamic Light Scattering: With Applications to Chemistry, Biology, and Physics, Dover Publication, NY

38. Hudson, S.A., Ecroyd, H., Kee, T.W. and Carver, J.A. (2009) The thioflavin T fluorescence assay for amyloid fibril detection can be biased by the presence of exogenous compounds. FEBS J. **276**, 5960–5972

39. Wang, Y.-Q., Buell, A.K., Wang, X.-Y., Welland, M.E., Dobson, C.M., Knowles, T.P.J. and Perrett, S. (2011) Relationship between prion propensity and the rates of individual molecular steps of fibril assembly. J. Biol. Chem. **286**, 12101–12107

40. Pedersen, J.S., Dikov, D., Flink, J.L., Hjuler, H.A., Christiansen, G. and Otzen, D.E. (2006) The changing face of glucagon fibrillation: structural polymorphism and conformational imprinting. J. Mol. Biol. **355**, 501–523

41. Giehm, L., Svergun, D.I., Otzen, D.E. and Vestergaard, B. (2011) Low-resolution structure of a vesicle disrupting α-synuclein oligomer that accumulates during fibrillation. Proc. Natl. Acad. Sci. U.S.A. **108**, 3246–3251

42. Knowles, T.P.J., Shu, W., Devlin, G.L., Meehan, S., Auer, S., Dobson, C.M. and Welland, M.E. (2007) Kinetics and thermodynamics of amyloid formation from direct measurements of fluctuations in fibril mass. Proc. Natl. Acad. Sci. U.S.A. **104**, 10016–10021

43. Xue, W.-F. and Radford, S.E. (2013) An imaging and systems modeling approach to fibril breakage enables prediction of amyloid behavior. Biophys. J. **105**, 2811–2819

44. Knowles, T.P.J., White, D.A., Abate, A.R., Agresti, J.J., Cohen, S.I.A., Sperling, R.A., Genst, E.J. D., Dobson, C.M. and Weitz, D.A. (2011) Observation of spatial propagation of amyloid assembly from single nuclei. Proc. Natl. Acad. Sci. U.S.A. **108**, 14746–14751

45. Ban, T., Hamada, D., Hasegawa, K., Naiki, H. and Goto, Y. (2003) Direct observation of amyloid fibril growth monitored by thioflavin T fluorescence. J. Biol. Chem. **278**, 16462–16465

46. Goldsbury, C., Kistler, J., Aebi, U., Arvinte, T. and Cooper, G.J. (1999) Watching amyloid fibrils grow by time-lapse atomic force microscopy. J. Mol. Biol. **285**, 33–39

47. Cremades, N., Cohen, S.I.A., Deas, E., Abramov, A.Y., Chen, A.Y., Orte, A., Sandal, M., Clarke, R.W., Dunne, P., Aprile, F.A. et al. (2012) Direct observation of the interconversion of normal and toxic forms of α-synuclein. Cell **149**, 1048–1059

48. Pinotsi, D., Buell, A.K., Galvagnion, C., Dobson, C.M., Schierle, G.S.K. and Kaminski, C.F. (2014) Direct observation of heterogeneous amyloid fibril growth kinetics via two-color super-resolution microscopy. Nano Lett. **14**, 339–345

49. Hasegawa, K., Ono, K., Yamada, M. and Naiki, H. (2002) Kinetic modeling and determination of reaction constants of Alzheimer's β-amyloid fibril extension and dissociation using surface plasmon resonance. Biochemistry **41**, 13489–13498

50. Hovgaard, M.B., Dong, M., Otzen, D.E. and Besenbacher, F. (2007) Quartz crystal microbalance studies of multilayer glucagon fibrillation at the solid–liquid interface. Biophys. J. **93**, 2162–2169

51. Buell, A.K., White, D.A., Meier, C., Welland, M.E., Knowles, T.P.J. and Dobson, C.M. (2010) Surface attachment of protein fibrils via covalent modification strategies. J. Phys. Chem. B **114**, 10925–10938

52. Buell, A.K., Hung, P., Salvatella, X., Welland, M.E., Dobson, C.M. and Knowles, T.P.J. (2013) Electrostatic effects in filamentous protein aggregation. Biophys. J. **104**, 1116–1126

53. Orte, A., Birkett, N.R., Clarke, R.W., Devlin, G.L., Dobson, C.M. and Klenerman, D. (2008) Direct characterization of amyloidogenic oligomers by single-molecule fluorescence. Proc. Natl. Acad. Sci. U.S.A. **105**, 14424–14429

54. Kellermayer, M.S.Z., Karsai, A., Benke, M., Soos, K. and Penke, B. (2008) Stepwise dynamics of epitaxially growing single amyloid fibrils. Proc. Natl. Acad. Sci. U.S.A. **105**, 141–144

55. Xue, W.-F., Homans, S.W. and Radford, S.E. (2008) Systematic analysis of nucleation-dependent polymerization reveals new insights into the mechanism of amyloid self-assembly. Proc. Natl. Acad. Sci. U.S.A. **105**, 8926–8931

56. Fändrich, M. (2007) Absolute correlation between lag time and growth rate in the spontaneous formation of several amyloid-like aggregates and fibrils. J. Mol. Biol. **365**, 1266–1270

57. Kashchiev, D. and Auer, S. (2010) Nucleation of amyloid fibrils. J. Chem. Phys. **132**, 215101

58. Garcia, G.A., Cohen, S.I.A., Dobson, C.M. and Knowles, T.P.J. (2014) Nucleation-conversion-polymerisation reactions of biological macromolecules with pre-nucleation clusters. Phys. Rev. E **89**, 032712

59. Campioni, S., Carret, G., Jordens, S., Nicoud, L., Mezzenga, R. and Riek, R. (2014) The presence of an air-water interface affects formation and elongation of α-synuclein fibrils. J. Am. Chem. Soc. **136**, 2866–2875

60. Zhu, M., Li, J. and Fink, A.L. (2003) The association of alpha-synuclein with membranes affects bilayer structure, stability, and fibril formation. J. Biol. Chem. **278**, 40186–40197

61. Lorenzen, N., Nielsen, S.B., Buell, A.K., Kaspersen, J.D., Arosio, P., Vad, B.S., Paslawski, W., Christiansen, G., Valnickova-Hansen, Z., Andreasen, M. et al. (2014) The role of stable α-synuclein oligomers in the molecular events underlying amyloid formation. J. Am. Chem. Soc. **136**, 3859–3868

62. Collins, S.R., Douglass, A., Vale, R.D. and Weissman, J.S. (2004) Mechanism of prion propagation: amyloid growth occurs by monomer addition. PLoS Biol. **2**, e321

63. Lorenzen, N., Cohen, S.I.A., Nielsen, S.B., Herling, T.W., Christiansen, G., Dobson, C.M., Knowles, T.P.J. and Otzen, D. (2012) Role of elongation and secondary pathways in S6 amyloid fibril growth. Biophys. J. **102**, 2167–2175

64. Kusumoto, Y., Lomakin, A., Teplow, D.B. and Benedek, G.B. (1998) Temperature dependence of amyloid β-protein fibrillization. Proc. Natl. Acad. Sci. U.S.A. **95**, 12277–12282

65. Qiang, W., Kelley, K. and Tycko, R. (2013) Polymorph-specific kinetics and thermodynamics of β-amyloid fibril growth. J. Am. Chem. Soc. **135**, 6860–6871

66. Ferkinghoff-Borg, J., Fonslet, J., Andersen, C.B., Krishna, S., Pigolotti, S., Yagi, H., Goto, Y., Otzen, D. and Jensen, M.H. (2010) Stop-and-go kinetics in amyloid fibrillation. Phys. Rev. E **82**, 010901

67. Tanaka, M., Chien, P., Naber, N., Cooke, R. and Weissman, J.S. (2004) Conformational variations in an infectious protein determine prion strain differences. Nature **428**, 323–328

68. DePace, A.H. and Weissman, J.S. (2002) Origins and kinetic consequences of diversity in Sup35 yeast prion fibers. Nat. Struct. Mol. Biol. **9**, 389–396

69. Ohhashi, Y., Kihara, M., Naiki, H. and Goto, Y. (2005) Ultrasonication-induced amyloid fibril formation of $β_2$-microglobulin. J. Biol. Chem. **280**, 32843–32848

70. Smith, J.F., Knowles, T.P.J., Dobson, C.M., Macphee, C.E. and Welland, M.E. (2006) Characterization of the nanoscale properties of individual amyloid fibrils. Proc. Natl. Acad. Sci. U.S.A. **103**, 15806–15811

71. Paparcone, R. and Buehler, M.J. (2011) Failure of Aβ(1–40) amyloid fibrils under tensile loading. Biomaterials **32**, 3367–3374

72. Ruschak, A.M. and Miranker, A.D. (2007) Fiber-dependent amyloid formation as catalysis of an existing reaction pathway. Proc. Natl. Acad. Sci. U.S.A. **104**, 12341–12346

73. Cohen, S.I.A., Rajah, L., Yoon, C.H., Buell, A.K., White, D.A., Sperling, R.A., Vendruscolo, M., Terentjev, E.M., Dobson, C.M., Weitz, D.A. and Knowles, T.P.J. (2014) Spatial propagation of protein polymerization. Phys. Rev. Lett. **112**, 098101

74. Zurdo, J., Guijarro, J.I., Jimenez, J.L., Saibil, H.R. and Dobson, C.M. (2001) Dependence on solution conditions of aggregation and amyloid formation by an SH3 domain. J. Mol. Biol. **311**, 325–340

75. Hill, S.E., Miti, T., Richmond, T. and Muschol, M. (2011) Spatial extent of charge repulsion regulates assembly pathways for lysozyme amyloid fibrils. PLoS ONE **6**, e18171

76. Marek, P.J., Patsalo, V., Green, D.F. and Raleigh, D.P. (2012) Ionic strength effects on amyloid formation by amylin are a complicated interplay among Debye screening, ion selectivity, and Hofmeister effects. Biochemistry **51**, 8478–8490

77. Bennion, B.J. and Daggett, V. (2003) The molecular basis for the chemical denaturation of proteins by urea. Proc. Natl. Acad. Sci. U.S.A. **100**, 5142–5147

78. Arakawa, T. and Timasheff, S.N. (1985) The stabilization of proteins by osmolytes. Biophys. J. **47**, 411–414

79. Zimmerman, S.B. and Trach, S.O. (1991) Estimation of macromolecule concentrations and excluded volume effects for the cytoplasm of *Escherichia coli*. J. Mol. Biol. **222**, 599–620

80. Minton, A.P. (1983) The effect of volume occupancy upon the thermodynamic activity of proteins: some biochemical consequences. Mol. Cell. Biochem. **55**, 119–140

81. van den Berg, B., Ellis, R.J. and Dobson, C.M. (1999) Effects of macromolecular crowding on protein folding and aggregation. EMBO J. **18**, 6927–6933

82. Seeliger, J., Werkmüller, A. and Winter, R. (2013) Macromolecular crowding as a suppressor of human IAPP fibril formation and cytotoxicity. PLoS ONE **8**, e69652

83. Munishkina, L.A., Cooper, E.M., Uversky, V.N. and Fink, A.L. (2004) The effect of macromolecular crowding on protein aggregation and amyloid fibril formation. J. Mol. Recognit. **17**, 456–464

84. Zhou, Z., Fan, J.-B., Zhu, H.-L., Shewmaker, F., Yan, X., Chen, X., Chen, J., Xiao, G.-F., Guo, L. and Liang, Y. (2009) Crowded cell-like environment accelerates the nucleation step of amyloidogenic protein misfolding. J. Biol. Chem. **284**, 30148–30158

85. White, D.A., Buell, A.K., Knowles, T.P.J., Welland, M.E. and Dobson, C.M. (2010) Protein aggregation in crowded environments. J. Am. Chem. Soc. **132**, 5170–5175

86. Shinohara, H., Inaguma, Y., Goto, S., Inagaki, T. and Kato, K. (1993) αB crystallin and HSP28 are enhanced in the cerebral cortex of patients with Alzheimer's disease. J. Neurol. Sci. **119**, 203–208

87. Fink, A.L. (1999) Chaperone-mediated protein folding. Physiol. Rev. **79**, 425–449

88. Xu, L.-Q., Wu, S., Buell, A.K., Cohen, S.I.A., Chen, L.-J., Hu, W.-H., Cusack, S.A., Itzhaki, L.S., Zhang, H., Knowles, T.P.J. et al. (2013) Influence of specific HSP70 domains on fibril formation of the yeast prion protein Ure2. Philos. Trans. R. Soc. Lond., B, Biol. Sci. **368**, 20110410

89. Narayan, P., Orte, A., Clarke, R.W., Bolognesi, B., Hook, S., Ganzinger, K.A., Meehan, S., Wilson, M.R., Dobson, C.M. and Klenerman, D. (2012) The extracellular chaperone clusterin sequesters oligomeric forms of the amyloid-β(1–40) peptide. Nat. Struct. Mol. Biol. **19**, 79–83

90. Shammas, S.L., Waudby, C.A., Wang, S., Buell, A.K., Knowles, T.P.J., Ecroyd, H., Welland, M.E., Carver, J.A., Dobson, C.M. and Meehan, S. (2011) Binding of the molecular chaperone αB-crystallin to Aβ amyloid fibrils inhibits fibril elongation. Biophys. J. **101**, 1681–1689

91. Knight, S.D., Presto, J., Linse, S. and Johansson, J. (2013) The BRICHOS domain, amyloid fibril formation, and their relationship. Biochemistry **52**, 7523–7531

92. Guilliams, T., El-Turk, F., Buell, A.K., O'Day, E.M., Aprile, F.A., Esbjrner, E.K., Vendruscolo, M., Cremades, N., Pardon, E., Wyns, L. et al. (2013) Nanobodies raised against monomeric α-synuclein distinguish between fibrils at different maturation stages. J. Mol. Biol. **425**, 2397–2411

93. Puchtler, H., Sweat, F. and Levine, M. (1962) On the binding of Congo Red by amyloid. J. Histochem. Cytochem. **10**, 355–364

94. Zhuang, Z.P., Kung, M.P., Hou, C., Skovronsky, D.M., Gur, T.L., Plössl, K., Trojanowski, J.Q., Lee, V.M. and Kung, H.F. (2001) Radioiodinated styrylbenzenes and thioflavins as probes for amyloid aggregates. J. Med. Chem. **44**, 1905–1914

95. Buell, A.K., Esbjöner, E.K., Riss, P.J., White, D.A., Aigbirhio, F.I., Toth, G., Welland, M.E., Dobson, C.M. and Knowles, T.P.J. (2011) Probing small molecule binding to amyloid fibrils. Phys. Chem. Chem. Phys. **13**, 20044–20052

96. Tjernberg, L.O., Näslund, J., Lindqvist, F., Johansson, J., Karlström, A.R., Thyberg, J., Terenius, L. and Nordstedt, C. (1996) Arrest of β-amyloid fibril formation by a pentapeptide ligand. J. Biol. Chem. **271**, 8545–8548

97. Ikenoue, T., Lee, Y.-H., Kardos, J., Saiki, M., Yagi, H., Kawata, Y. and Goto, Y. (2014) Cold denaturation of alpha-synuclein amyloid fibrils. Angew. Chem. Int. Ed. **126**, 1–7

© The Authors Journal compilation © 2014 Biochemical Society
Essays Biochem. (2014) 56, 41–52: doi: 10.1042/BSE0560041

3

Predicting aggregation-prone sequences in proteins

Greet De Baets*†, **Joost Schymkowitz***†[1] and **Frederic Rousseau***†[1]

**Switch Laboratory, VIB, University of Leuven, Herestraat 49 Box 802, 3000 Leuven, Belgium*
†Switch Laboratory, Department of Cellular and Molecular Medicine, University of Leuven, B-3000 Leuven, Belgium

Abstract

Owing to its association with a diverse range of human diseases, the determinants of protein aggregation are studied intensively. It is generally accepted that the effective aggregation tendency of a protein depends on many factors such as folding efficiency towards the native state, thermodynamic stability of that conformation, intrinsic aggregation propensity of the polypeptide sequence and its ability to be recognized by the protein quality control system. The intrinsic aggregation propensity of a polypeptide sequence is related to the presence of short APRs (aggregation-prone regions) that self-associate to form intermolecular β-structured assemblies. These are typically short sequence segments (5–15 amino acids) that display high hydrophobicity, low net charge and a high tendency to form β-structures. As the presence of such APRs is a prerequisite for aggregation, a plethora of methods have been developed to identify APRs in amino acid sequences. In the present chapter, the methodological basis of these approaches is discussed, as well as some practical applications.

Keywords:

β-aggregation, aggregation-prone region (APR), charge, hydrophobicity, sequence-based, β-sheet, structure-based, thermodynamic stability.

[1]*Correspondence may be addressed to either of these authors (email joost.schymkowitz@switch.vib-kuleuven.be or frederic.rousseau@switch.vib-kuleuven.be).*

Introduction

Misfolding of a polypeptide, either by deleterious mutations or stress conditions in the cell, can cause protein aggregation. For many years the manner in which monomer proteins stack into these aggregates has been investigated, i.e. which interactions initiate the intermolecular association resulting in an aggregate. Several models have been proposed, such as β-aggregation, native aggregation and 3D domain swapping. The latter posits that two or more protein chains exchange identical domains to form a strongly bound oligomer. β-Aggregation refers to the formation of β-structure by exposure of short APRs (aggregation-prone regions). No single model is likely to account for the properties of all aggregates formed from different (poly)peptides and under different conditions, but several lines of evidence suggest that β-aggregation is the most prevalent.

First of all, a study performed by Chiti et al. [1] illustrated that the aggregation rate of the α/β protein acylphosphatase is determined by two regions in the sequence. These regions have a high hydrophobicity and a high tendency to form β-sheet structures, pointing to aggregation driven by short APRs. Moreover, these regions are distinct from the folding nucleus, hinting at a competition between protein folding and aggregation. Next, the importance of these APRs to initiate aggregation was confirmed by several independent grafting studies where aggregation of an otherwise non-aggregating protein was induced through grafting of an APR from another protein. An example is the grafting of the mouse β2M (β$_2$-microglobulin) with the APR present in human β2M. In contrast with the wild-type mouse β2M, the chimaera which contains an APR readily aggregates [2]. Moreover, it has been shown that the vast majority of proteins known to be associated with aggregation diseases contains an APR that determines the intrinsic aggregation propensity of a polypeptide [3].

These APRs are usually composed of 5–15 successively placed hydrophobic amino acids with a high β-sheet propensity and a low net charge. Although most proteins possess one or several APRs, they are mostly protected from aggregation by being buried inside the hydrophobic core [4]. This points to another important determinant of effective aggregation, namely protein stability. It is only upon destabilization of a protein through, e.g. a mutation, that the APRs might be exposed and trigger aggregation (Figure 1). Examples are destabilizing mutations in SOD1 (superoxide dismutase 1), p53 and α-galactosidase resulting in protein aggregation.

Depending on the degree of β-sheet organization, protein aggregation can refer to the formation of different macroscopic forms. The two extremes are amyloid fibrils and

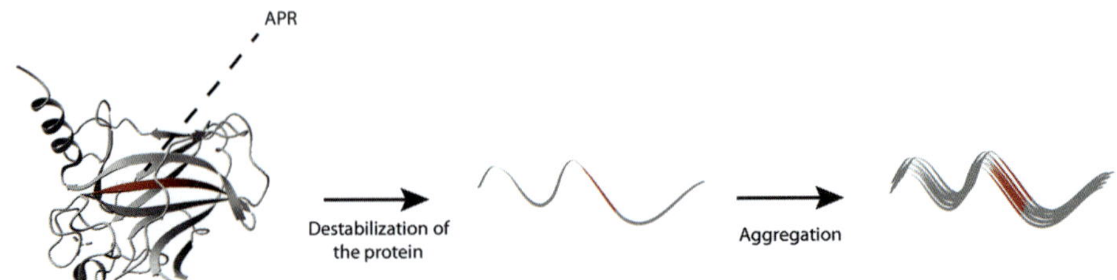

Figure 1. Schematic representation of protein aggregation through short stretches
In the folded state, the APR is buried in the globular native structure. Only upon destabilization the protein exposes an aggregation-prone region (APR). These APRs may align into an intermolecular β-sheet, nucleating the formation of a protein aggregate.

amorphous β aggregates, with a whole range of morphologies in between [5] (Figure 2). Amyloid fibrils are highly ordered and repetitive structures. In contrast, amorphous aggregates consist mostly of disordered polypeptide chains and show no macroscopic regularity using electron microscopy. Whether a protein will form an amorphous aggregate or an amyloid fibril depends on the amino acid sequence of the APR. In the case of amorphous aggregates, the only requirement is a short stretch with an overall high β-sheet propensity and neutral in charge [6]. In contrast, the less flexible amyloid fibrils are more position-specific with a very strict core and flanks that are more tolerant towards polar and charged residues [3].

Prediction of aggregation

As the presence of an APR is a requirement for the ubiquitous β-aggregation mechanism, several methods have been developed to determine the intrinsic aggregation propensity of a protein by detecting the APRs in its sequence (Figure 3, steps 1–3). The most common approaches evaluate either (i) intrinsic amino acid properties (sequence based) or (ii) the compatibility of the protein structural features with known amyloid fibril structures (structure based). As the structure-based methods are based on the structural information of amyloid fibrils, they are more specific for this type of aggregate. Machine-learning methods combining several predictors, e.g. AmylPred [7], form another approach. As these methods do not add additional physico-chemical or structural information, they are not discussed in this overview. For the alternative aggregation mechanisms such as 3D domain swapping and native protein aggregation, no methods have yet been developed.

General aggregation predictors

The main physico-chemical factors that promote aggregation of unfolded polypeptide chains have been characterized a decade ago: hydrophobicity, net charge, and propensity to form β-sheet and α-helical structure are correlated with aggregation propensity [8]. This original formula was extended with experimental variables such as protein concentration, solvent pH and ionic strength to predict the absolute aggregation rates of unstructured peptides and natively unfolded proteins [9]. On the basis of these initial findings, several methods have been developed that generate aggregation propensity profiles, enabling the identification of regions with high-intrinsic propensity for aggregation.

The 'Zyggregator' method initially started purely from these principles, but later versions also included more sophisticated measures, such as the spatial relationship between aggregation-prone residues and gatekeepers, i.e. residues opposing aggregation. An upgraded version of this method is available which includes protein flexibility and solvent accessibility. As such, it tries to compensate for the fact that under native conditions these APRs are buried inside stable structural elements, unable to form the specific intermolecular interactions required for aggregation [10]. 'TANGO', a statistical thermodynamics algorithm, is another algorithm used to identify the nucleation sites for aggregation by considering not only the factors described above, but also the competition between β-aggregate formation and other structural states such as α-helix, β-turn, β-strand and random coil [6]. Another method is 'SALSA' (Simple ALgorithm for Sliding Averages), which assumes a strong correlation between β-strand propensity and fibril formation. It calculates a mean β-strand propensity for each residue to identify the fibrillogenic hotspot [11]. On the other hand, 'AGGRESCAN' identifies aggregation

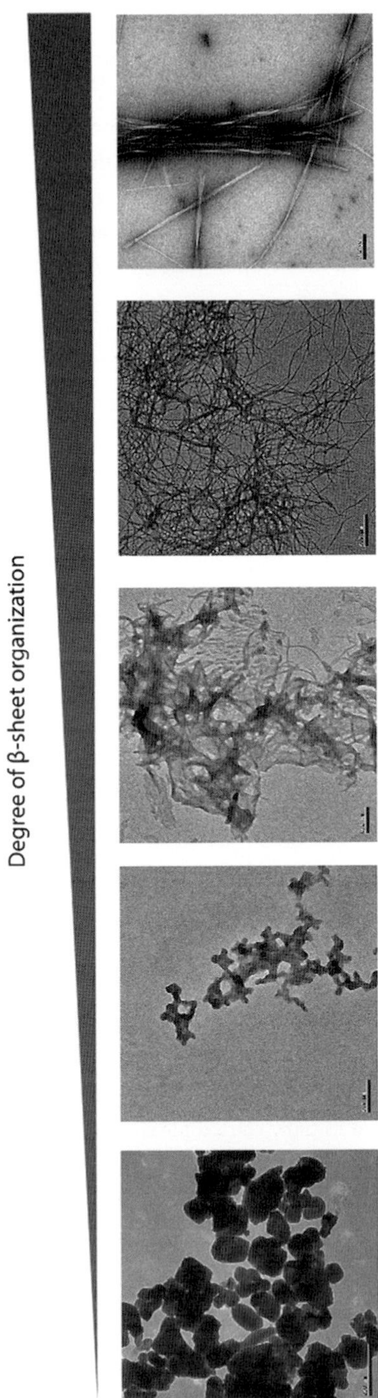

Figure 2. Transmission electron microscopy images of aggregating peptides
Selection of peptides displaying a wide range of morphologies: from a completely amorphous (bottom) to a highly ordered structure (top). From top to bottom, the scale bars are 0.2, 0.5, 0.2, 0.5 and 0.2 μm respectively.

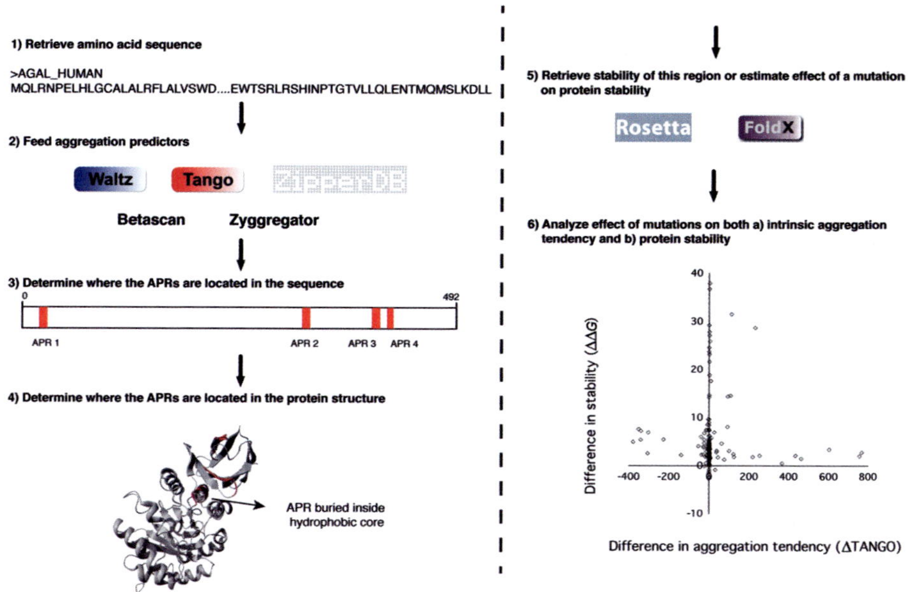

Figure 3. Workflow to determine whether a protein is prone to aggregation

hot spots relying on an aggregation propensity scale for each of the amino acids [12]. This scale is based on the relative solubility of point mutants of amyloid β-peptide in *Escherichia coli* [13]. Another method is 'FoldAmyloid' that predicts the amyloid fibril-forming regions based on the mean packing density. Segments with a strong packing density are considered amyloidogenic [14].

Amyloid-specific predictors

High-resolution structural studies of fibrils from a number of different peptides have revealed that APRs associate in an intermolecular way through formation of a cross-β spine [15]. In this model, the APR has a tendency to pack into a β-sheet and the fibril grows as more segments of identical molecules stack into the β-sheet. Transmission electron microscopy revealed that amyloids are straight unbranched fibrils with a diameter of 7–12 nm, made up by two to six protofilaments. Inside these protofilaments, intermolecular β-sheets perpendicular to the fibril axis are present, confirming the cross-β sheet motif. This motif is observed by X-ray reflections at 4.7 and 10 Å (1 Å = 0.1 nm), corresponding to the spacing between β-strands and the distance between adjacent β-sheets respectively [16]. Using microcrystal X-ray diffraction, Eisenberg and co-workers showed that amyloid protofibrils are stabilized by a steric zipper, indicating that the side chains of two identical β-sheets facing each other, intermesh in a zipper-like, tightly packed and highly complementary interface [15].

This wealth of structural information has been exploited by (i) employing homology modelling methods on the basis of this structural data or (ii) combining PSSM (position-specific scoring matrices) with such homology-modelling-based scores. However, as these predictors are based on structural information of amyloid fibrils, they are, in contrast with sequence-based predictors, more specific for the amyloid fibril.

'3D-profile method' [17] and 'PRE-AMYL' [18] are such structure-based methods that use the amyloid fibril structure as a template to define amino acid sequences compatible with the 3D cross-β-spine structure. By determining the probability that a protein segment fits in this conformation, they identify APRs.

'PASTA' (Prediction of Amyloid STructure Aggregation) is another method based on the assumption that β-strands constituting the amyloid fibril have a preference for an in-register parallel or anti-parallel arrangement with minimal energy. Creating a dataset with these strictly defined secondary structures allowed the calculation of a pairing energy for each possible pair of residues, which is then used to score all possible stretches [19]. The 'PIMA' (Peptide Interaction Matrix Analyzer) method is based on the same principle and threads each possible peptide stretch on to an in-register parallel or anti-parallel β-sheet structure [20]. 'BETASCAN' is another algorithm based on β-strands pairing in the amyloid core [21].

Our own 'WALTZ' combines the sequence-based and structure-based method by using sequence-based PSSM based on a dataset including both positive and negative peptides for fibril formation, a set of physicochemical properties, and structure-based PSSM [22].

Workflow of APR detection

Once the APRs are identified, it is crucial to investigate where the APRs reside in the protein structure (Figure 3, step 4). In most cases, these contribute to the thermodynamic stability of a protein and are buried inside the protein core. Therefore to estimate the effect of an amino acid change on the effective aggregation tendency, it is necessary to analyse the effect on (i) intrinsic aggregation tendency by using the aggregation predictors and (ii) protein stability by using force fields [23,24]. In Figure 3 (step 6), the effect of all known mutations in α-galactosidase on protein stability and aggregation tendency was analysed using SNPeffect [25] and their effect on both determinants was visualized using a MASS (Mutant Aggregation and Stability Spectrum) plot (Figure 3, step 6), i.e. a scatter plot of the effect on protein stability ($\Delta\Delta G$) versus the difference in aggregation tendency (ΔTANGO). This plot shows that the majority of the mutations does not alter the intrinsic aggregation propensity of a protein, but decrease the thermodynamic stability (positive $\Delta\Delta G$) of a protein. Since protein stability is a co-operative effect dependent on many residues, whereas aggregation only depends on few residues, we can conclude that mutations are much more likely to trigger aggregation by affecting stability than by increasing intrinsic aggregation.

Limitations of current prediction methods

All algorithms discussed so far have been inspired by and tested against experimental data obtained *in vitro*, where the protein aggregates are in a buffered solution in the absence of other proteins. In contrast, the cell is a complex environment, so the question arises whether the predictors are also valid in this context. A study by Chiti and co-workers illustrated that in most cases there is an agreement between the predictions and *in vivo* experiments [26], justifying the use of these predictors.

In contrast, a recent study [27] using scrambled versions of the aggregating stretch of Huntington protein, illustrates that the algorithms do vary in their ability to correctly identify the aggregating ones. They propose several reasons for the under- and over-prediction. A possible reason for overprediction is the high peptide concentrations used in the experimental system to train the algorithms. Moreover, there is also a poor understanding of how a peptide contributes to the aggregation kinetics. Protein aggregation depends on both primary and secondary nucleation processes. In the primary pathway, aggregate formation results from interaction between soluble monomers. If this nucleation step is inefficient, aggregation will not occur.

Additionally, for most approaches, the APRs identified computationally still need to become exposed by (partial) unfolding before they can actually nucleate protein aggregation. Therefore 3D relationships that exist in the folded state are highly relevant to determine whether a particular region is likely to become exposed in the first place. However, most methods do not take into account structural constraints and the modulatory context of the remaining protein. Therefore there is a need for extension of these APR-detection methods with reliable methods to estimate protein stability.

Application of APR predictors

Define APR present in a protein

The above-described methods are very useful to estimate whether a protein of interest is prone to aggregation and to define which region is responsible for this aggregation propensity. Identification of these APRs makes it possible to design mutations that avoid aggregation. As there are several methods available, based on different assumptions, it seems wise to test them all. In the following section two proteins known to aggregate are analysed.

Aβ (amyloid β-peptide): Aβ40 versus Aβ42

Deposition in the brain of Aβ, which is generated from the APP (amyloid precursor protein), is one of the main hallmarks of Alzheimer's disease. Proteolytic cleavage of APP can result in peptides of different lengths and longer variants seem to have an increased aggregation propensity. In this example, we investigate how well different predictors predict (i) the aggregation propensity of the Aβ peptide and (ii) the increased aggregation tendency with C-terminal elongation. Two sequence-based methods (TANGO and Zyggregator) and two structure-based methods (WALTZ and 3D profile) were used. In Figure 4, you may notice that all predictors estimate that the Aβ peptide has some aggregation tendency. However, WALTZ fails to predict any aggregation propensity in the C-terminal part of the peptide and is not capable of detecting an increased aggregation tendency following C-terminal elongation. As this elongation

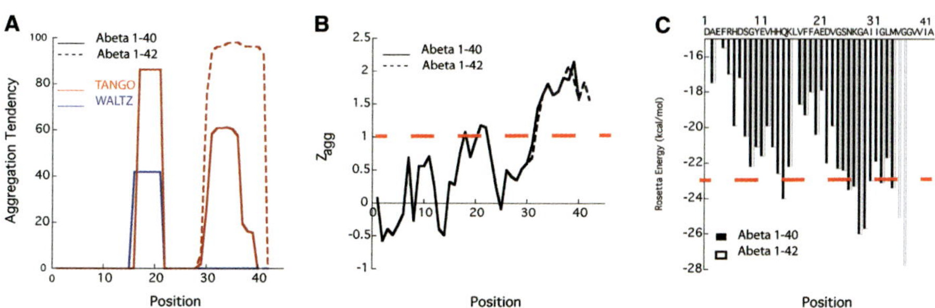

Figure 4. Predicted aggregation tendency of Aβ(40) and Aβ(42)
(**A**) TANGO and WALTZ, (**B**) Zyggregator and (**C**) 3D profile output for Aβ(40) and Aβ(42). A red line indicates the threshold for Zyggregator and 3D profile.

induces amorphous aggregation, this could explain why WALTZ, which is more specific for amyloid fibrils, did not predict this observation.

Tumour suppressor p53

p53 (also known as tumour suppressor p53) is a key regulator of the cell cycle and gets mutated in approximately 30% of all cancers. It was shown previously that the DNA-binding domain of p53 is conformationally unstable and studies in our laboratory confirmed that destabilizing mutations in this domain can result in the formation of cellular aggregates [28]. TANGO, Zyggregator and a 3D profile predict an APR around position 250 (APR1, sequence ILTIITL). Zyggregator and 3D profile also suggest another APR around position 120 (APR2, sequence SVTCTYS) (Figure 5). When analysing where these APRs reside in the protein structure, it is clear that APR1 is buried inside the hydrophobic core and needs to become exposed to trigger aggregation. WALTZ does not predict any of these APRs, which is again due to the amorphous nature of p53 aggregates [28]. In general, we can conclude that WALTZ is specific

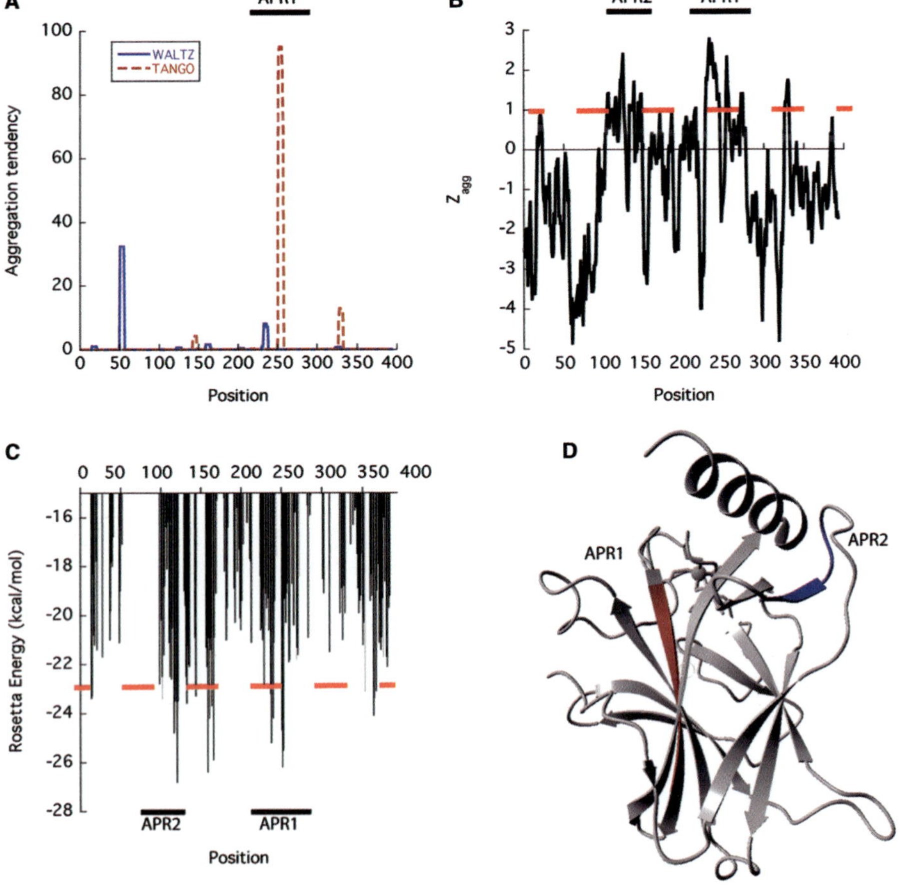

Figure 5. Predicted aggregation tendency of p53
(**A**) TANGO and WALTZ, (**B**) Zyggregator and (**C**) 3D profile output for p53. A red line indicates the threshold for Zyggregator and 3D profile. (**D**) The predicted APRs are indicated in the structure of p53 (PDB code 2AC0).

for amyloid fibrils, whereas the others predict APRs that can result in structures ranging from amorphous aggregates to amyloid fibrils.

Proteome-wide analysis of aggregation to detect evolutionary imprints

Using the power of the aggregation prediction algorithms described in the section above, the aggregation load of several proteomes has been analysed in detail with different methods. In all of these studies, a clear evolutionary pressure to counteract aggregation was apparent.

The first study illustrated that the vast majority of proteins in any proteome contains at least one and generally several APRs [29] that can nucleate aggregation by assembling into intermolecular β-structures. A first way to avoid misfolding and aggregation is proper folding into the compact structure [30]. However, in the case of IDPs (intrinsically disordered polypeptides), the whole backbone is exposed to the solvent, so folding cannot play its protective role. Therefore several specific sequence adaptations are present to maintain their solubility and prevent aggregation; these proteins have a high net charge and low hydrophobicity [31], a lower number of APRs [32], and higher proline content [33].

Another way to prevent aggregation is interrupting the contiguous stretches of hydrophobic residues by placement of charged side chains acting as gatekeepers [34]. Rousseau et al. [29] revealed a strong enrichment of charged residues (arginine, lysine, glutamic acid and aspartic acid) and proline at the flanks of these APRs. Their study showed that 90% of all APRs are capped with at least one gatekeeper residue (arginine, lysine, glutamic acid and aspartic acid, or proline), with a preference for positively charged residues at regions with the highest aggregation propensity. These gatekeepers counteract aggregation by (i) charge repulsion (arginine, lysine, glutamic acid and aspartic acid); (ii) being large and flexible (arginine and lysine); or (iii) being incompatible with the β-structure (proline and glycine). It is important to note that gatekeepers do not avoid aggregation, but reduce the aggregation rate sufficiently to tip the balance towards native protein folding.

The importance of strategic placement of charges to avoid aggregation was already illustrated by the observation that supercharged proteins are remarkably resistant to aggregation and refold efficiently [35]. Recent studies also discovered that gatekeepers facilitate the recognition of APRs by molecular chaperones, such as Hsp70 [36]. This Hsp70 system can slow down the aggregation process by allowing polypeptide chains to fold or by directing them to degradation. The observation that mutations disrupting gatekeeper patterns are more frequently disease-associated than neutral also points to their functional role [37].

Moreover, the extent to which selective pressure minimizes aggregation tendency is determined by the biological context. Using the aforementioned methods, several interesting observations were made. First, proteins forming oligomeric complexes have a lower aggregation propensity than those operating in free form [38]. As they constantly interact with other polypeptides, they are at increased risk of aggregation and therefore the aggregation tendency should be minimized. Comparably, the sequence similarity of APRs between different subunits is minimized in multi-domain proteins, also illustrating the sequence specificity of aggregation [39].

Secondly, essential proteins were found to have a lower aggregation propensity, emphasizing evolutionary pressure to minimize aggregation propensity [40].

Thirdly, Monsellier et al. [41] demonstrated that long proteins, with lower folding rates [42], have less pronounced aggregation peaks. The aggregation propensity seems to be inversely correlated with organism complexity [43], and evolutionary protection mechanisms are more pronounced in thermophilic compared with mesophilic proteins [44]. It was also shown that aggregation propensity inversely correlates with gene expression [45] and with protein turnover rate [46].

Conclusions

As aggregation is a detrimental process for the cell, considerable time has been invested to investigate which parameters affect the effective aggregation propensity of a protein and to consequently use this knowledge to identify proteins prone to aggregate. Although several aggregation mechanisms have been identified, β-aggregation seems to be the most prevalent mechanism. It is based on the formation of β-structure by exposure of short APRs. Nowadays, several methods are available to predict the presence of these APRs in a protein and it is advised to combine these to obtain a reliable result. Moreover, beside the presence of APRs, protein stability is another important determinant, which is often not taken into account. Development of next-generation aggregation predictors should therefore include a reliable estimation of thermodynamic stability [10].

Summary

- Besides 3D domain swapping and native aggregation, β-aggregation is the most prevalent.
- β-Aggregation is driven by exposure of APRs forming an intermolecular β-structure.
- APRs typically contain 5–15 successively placed hydrophobic amino acids with a high β-sheet propensity and a low net charge.
- Thermodynamic stability is another important parameter affecting the effective aggregation propensity.
- Several methods, either structure- or sequence-based, predict the presence of APRs.
- Presence of an APR is not the only prerequisite for aggregation, therefore measures of protein stability should be taken into account.

References

1. Chiti, F., Taddei, N., Baroni, F., Capanni, C., Stefani, M., Ramponi, G. and Dobson, C.M. (2002) Kinetic partitioning of protein folding and aggregation. Nat. Struct. Biol. **9**, 137–143
2. Ivanova, M.I., Sawaya, M.R., Gingery, M., Attinger, A. and Eisenberg, D. (2004) An amyloid-forming segment of β2-microglobulin suggests a molecular model for the fibril. Proc. Natl. Acad. Sci. U.S.A. **101**, 10584–10589
3. Lopez de la Paz, M. and Serrano, L. (2004) Sequence determinants of amyloid fibril formation. Proc. Natl. Acad. Sci. U.S.A. **101**, 87–92
4. Dobson, C.M. (2003) Protein folding and misfolding. Nature **426**, 884–890
5. Rousseau, F., Schymkowitz, J. and Serrano, L. (2006) Protein aggregation and amyloidosis: confusion of the kinds? Curr. Opin. Struct. Biol. **16**, 118–126
6. Fernandez-Escamilla, A.M., Rousseau, F., Schymkowitz, J. and Serrano, L. (2004) Prediction of sequence-dependent and mutational effects on the aggregation of peptides and proteins. Nat. Biotechnol. **22**, 1302–1306

7. Frousios, K.K., Iconomidou, V.A., Karletidi, C.M. and Hamodrakas, S.J. (2009) Amyloidogenic determinants are usually not buried. BMC Struct. Biol. **9**, 44

8. Chiti, F., Stefani, M., Taddei, N., Ramponi, G. and Dobson, C.M. (2003) Rationalization of the effects of mutations on peptide and protein aggregation rates. Nature **424**, 805–808

9. DuBay, K.F., Pawar, A.P., Chiti, F., Zurdo, J., Dobson, C.M. and Vendruscolo, M. (2004) Prediction of the absolute aggregation rates of amyloidogenic polypeptide chains. J. Mol. Biol. **341**, 1317–1326

10. Tartaglia, G.G., Pawar, A.P., Campioni, S., Dobson, C.M., Chiti, F. and Vendruscolo, M. (2008) Prediction of aggregation-prone regions in structured proteins. J. Mol. Biol. **380**, 425–436

11. Zibaee, S., Makin, O.S., Goedert, M. and Serpell, L.C. (2007) A simple algorithm locates β-strands in the amyloid fibril core of α-synuclein, Aβ, and tau using the amino acid sequence alone. Protein Sci. **16**, 906–918

12. Conchillo-Sole, O., de Groot, N.S., Aviles, F.X., Vendrell, J., Daura, X. and Ventura, S. (2007) AGGRESCAN: a server for the prediction and evaluation of "hot spots" of aggregation in polypeptides. BMC Bioinformatics **8**, 65

13. Sanchez de Groot, N., Pallares, I., Aviles, F.X., Vendrell, J. and Ventura, S. (2005) Prediction of "hot spots" of aggregation in disease-linked polypeptides. BMC Struct. Biol. **5**, 18

14. Galzitskaya, O.V., Garbuzynskiy, S.O. and Lobanov, M.Y. (2006) Prediction of amyloidogenic and disordered regions in protein chains. PLoS Comput. Biol. **2**, e177

15. Sawaya, M.R., Sambashivan, S., Nelson, R., Ivanova, M.I., Sievers, S.A., Apostol, M.I., Thompson, M.J., Balbirnie, M., Wiltzius, J.J., McFarlane, H.T. et al. (2007) Atomic structures of amyloid cross-β spines reveal varied steric zippers. Nature **447**, 453–457

16. Serpell, L.C., Sunde, M., Benson, M.D., Tennent, G.A., Pepys, M.B. and Fraser, P.E. (2000) The protofilament substructure of amyloid fibrils. J. Mol. Biol. **300**, 1033–1039

17. Thompson, M.J., Sievers, S.A., Karanicolas, J., Ivanova, M.I., Baker, D. and Eisenberg, D. (2006) The 3D profile method for identifying fibril-forming segments of proteins. Proc. Natl. Acad. Sci. U.S.A. **103**, 4074–4078

18. Zhang, Z., Chen, H. and Lai, L. (2007) Identification of amyloid fibril-forming segments based on structure and residue-based statistical potential. Bioinformatics **23**, 2218–2225

19. Trovato, A., Seno, F. and Tosatto, S.C. (2007) The PASTA server for protein aggregation prediction. Protein Eng. Des. Sel. **20**, 521–523

20. Bui, J.M., Cavalli, A. and Gsponer, J. (2008) Identification of aggregation-prone elements by using interaction-energy matrices. Angew. Chem. Int. Ed. Engl. **47**, 7267–7269

21. Bryan, Jr, A.W., Menke, M., Cowen, L.J., Lindquist, S.L. and Berger, B. (2009) BETASCAN: probable beta-amyloids identified by pairwise probabilistic analysis. PLoS Comput. Biol. **5**, e1000333

22. Maurer-Stroh, S., Debulpaep, M., Kuemmerer, N., Lopez de la Paz, M., Martins, I.C., Reumers, J., Morris, K.L., Copland, A., Serpell, L., Serrano, L. et al. (2010) Exploring the sequence determinants of amyloid structure using position-specific scoring matrices. Nat. Methods **7**, 237–242

23. Schymkowitz, J., Borg, J., Stricher, F., Nys, R., Rousseau, F. and Serrano, L. (2005) The FoldX web server: an online force field. Nucleic Acids Res. **33**, W382–W388

24. Rohl, C.A., Strauss, C.E., Misura, K.M. and Baker, D. (2004) Protein structure prediction using Rosetta. Methods Enzymol. **383**, 66–93

25. De Baets, G., Van Durme, J., Reumers, J., Maurer-Stroh, S., Vanhee, P., Dopazo, J., Schymkowitz, J. and Rousseau, F. (2012) SNPeffect 4.0: on-line prediction of molecular and structural effects of protein-coding variants. Nucleic Acids Res. **40**, D935–D939

26. Belli, M., Ramazzotti, M. and Chiti, F. (2011) Prediction of amyloid aggregation *in vivo*. EMBO Rep. **12**, 657–663

27. Roland, B.P., Kodali, R., Mishra, R. and Wetzel, R. (2013) A serendipitous survey of prediction algorithms for amyloidogenicity. Biopolymers **100**, 780–789

28. Xu, J., Reumers, J., Couceiro, J.R., De Smet, F., Gallardo, R., Rudyak, S., Cornelis, A., Rozenski, J., Zwolinska, A., Marine, J.C. et al. (2011) Gain of function of mutant p53 by coaggregation with multiple tumor suppressors. Nat. Chem. Biol. **7**, 285–295

29. Rousseau, F., Serrano, L. and Schymkowitz, J.W. (2006) How evolutionary pressure against protein aggregation shaped chaperone specificity. J. Mol. Biol. **355**, 1037–1047

30. Watters, A.L., Deka, P., Corrent, C., Callender, D., Varani, G., Sosnick, T. and Baker, D. (2007) The highly cooperative folding of small naturally occurring proteins is likely the result of natural selection. Cell **128**, 613–624

31. Uversky, V.N. and Fink, A.L. (2004) Conformational constraints for amyloid fibrillation: the importance of being unfolded. Biochim. Biophys. Acta 1**698**, 131–153

32. Linding, R., Schymkowitz, J., Rousseau, F., Diella, F. and Serrano, L. (2004) A comparative study of the relationship between protein structure and β-aggregation in globular and intrinsically disordered proteins. J. Mol. Biol. **342**, 345–353

33. Tompa, P. (2002) Intrinsically unstructured proteins. Trends Biochem. Sci. **27**, 527–533

34. Otzen, D.E., Kristensen, O. and Oliveberg, M. (2000) Designed protein tetramer zipped together with a hydrophobic Alzheimer homology: a structural clue to amyloid assembly. Proc. Natl. Acad. Sci. U.S.A. **97**, 9907–9912

35. Lawrence, M.S., Phillips, K.J. and Liu, D.R. (2007) Supercharging proteins can impart unusual resilience. J. Am. Chem. Soc. **129**, 10110–10112

36. Van Durme, J., Maurer-Stroh, S., Gallardo, R., Wilkinson, H., Rousseau, F. and Schymkowitz, J. (2009) Accurate prediction of DnaK-peptide binding via homology modelling and experimental data. PLoS Comput. Biol. **5**, e1000475

37. Reumers, J., Schymkowitz, J. and Rousseau, F. (2009) Using structural bioinformatics to investigate the impact of non synonymous SNPs and disease mutations: scope and limitations. BMC Bioinformatics **10**, S9

38. Chen, Y. and Dokholyan, N.V. (2008) Natural selection against protein aggregation on self-interacting and essential proteins in yeast, fly, and worm. Mol. Biol. Evol. **25**, 1530–1533

39. Wright, C.F., Teichmann, S.A., Clarke, J. and Dobson, C.M. (2005) The importance of sequence diversity in the aggregation and evolution of proteins. Nature **438**, 878–881

40. Tartaglia, G.G. and Caflisch, A. (2007) Computational analysis of the S. cerevisiae proteome reveals the function and cellular localization of the least and most amyloidogenic proteins. Proteins **68**, 273–278

41. Monsellier, E., Ramazzotti, M., Taddei, N. and Chiti, F. (2008) Aggregation propensity of the human proteome. PLoS Comput. Biol. **4**, e1000199

42. Ivankov, D.N., Garbuzynskiy, S.O., Alm, E., Plaxco, K.W., Baker, D. and Finkelstein, A.V. (2003) Contact order revisited: influence of protein size on the folding rate. Protein Sci. **12**, 2057–2062

43. Tartaglia, G.G., Pellarin, R., Cavalli, A. and Caflisch, A. (2005) Organism complexity anti-correlates with proteomic β-aggregation propensity. Protein Sci. **14**, 2735–2740

44. Thangakani, A.M., Kumar, S., Velmurugan, D. and Gromiha, M.S. (2012) How do thermophilic proteins resist aggregation? Proteins **80**, 1003–1015

45. Tartaglia, G.G., Pechmann, S., Dobson, C.M. and Vendruscolo, M. (2007) Life on the edge: a link between gene expression levels and aggregation rates of human proteins. Trends Biochem. Sci. **32**, 204–206

46. De Baets, G., Reumers, J., Delgado Blanco, J., Dopazo, J., Schymkowitz, J. and Rousseau, F. (2011) An evolutionary trade-off between protein turnover rate and protein aggregation favors a higher aggregation propensity in fast degrading proteins. PLoS Comput. Biol. **7**, e1002090

© The Authors Journal compilation © 2014 Biochemical Society
Essays Biochem. (2014) 56, 53–68: doi: 10.1042/BSE0560053

4

Protein folding, misfolding and quality control: the role of molecular chaperones

Katharina Papsdorf and Klaus Richter[1]

Department Chemie, Lehrstuhl für Biotechnologie, Lichtenbergstrasse 4, 85748 Garching, Germany

Abstract

Cells have to cope with stressful conditions and adapt to changing environments. Heat stress, heavy metal ions or UV stress induce damage to cellular proteins and disturb the balanced status of the proteome. The adjusted balance between folded and folding proteins, called protein homoeostasis, is required for every aspect of cellular functionality. Protective proteins called chaperones are expressed under extreme conditions in order to prevent aggregation of cellular proteins and safeguard protein quality. These chaperones co-operate during *de novo* folding, refolding and disaggregation of damaged proteins and in many cases refold them to their functional state. Even under physiological conditions these machines support protein homoeostasis and maintain the balance between *de novo* folding and degradation. Mutations generating unstable proteins, which are observed in numerous human diseases such as Alzheimer's disease, Huntington's disease, amyotrophic lateral sclerosis and cystic fibrosis, also challenge the protein quality control system. A better knowledge of how the protein homoeostasis system is regulated will lead to an improved understanding of these diseases and provide potential targets for therapy.

Keywords:

chaperone, heat-shock protein, Hsc70 (heat-shock cognate 70), Hsp90 (heat-shock protein 90), protein aggregation, protein folding, proteostasis.

[1]*To whom correspondence should be addressed (email klaus.richter@tum.de).*

Introduction: the protein folding challenge

The native state of functional proteins is a delicate, flexible and, in many cases, metastable conformation. Spontaneous folding to this native state was demonstrated in the early 1960s, when denatured proteins were successfully refolded in the absence of other cellular components [1]. This immediately posed the question of how this structure, representing an energetic minimum, is obtained. As it is impossible for the amino acid chain to sample all potential conformations on a reasonable timescale and then choose the most stable one, folding pathways had to be postulated [2]. Over the last decades, many of these pathways have been analysed to define critical intermediate structures on the way to the folded protein [3]. It also became apparent that not all proteins spontaneously fold into their native structure *in vitro*. Many proteins are trapped in local energy minima during the folding process and cannot overcome energy hurdles to proceed on to the correct form. Therefore alternative routes are taken and misfolded states are formed (Figure 1). Due to the exposure of hydrophobic patches, these misfolded states are prone to uncontrolled assembly reactions and aggregation [4].

Folding within the crowded environment of the cell is even more complex than in the test tube. Total protein concentrations in the cell are above 200 mg/ml, more than 1000-fold higher than in standard folding experiments [5]. One important difference though originates from co-translational folding, whereby the N-terminal portion of a polypeptide folds or interacts with chaperones while the unfinished protein is still attached to the ribosome or has not yet been synthesized. It can be envisioned that during evolution, folding pathways were optimized to function in co-operation with the protein synthesis machinery. This implies that important folding steps are generally performed while the unfinished protein is still attached to the ribosome. Ribosome-attached folding helper proteins, such as the NAC (nascent chain-associated complex) and the RAC (ribosome-associated complex), participate in this reaction and minimize the amount of misfolded proteins emanating from the ribosome [6,7] (Figure 2). However, it is estimated that even with the participation of NAC, only a fraction of the produced protein chains successfully reach the folded state, implying that the cell has to cope routinely with the problem of misfolded proteins [7]. Moreover, it also does not solve the

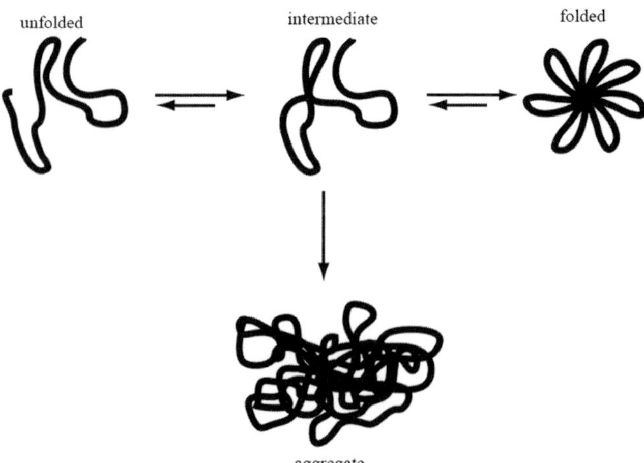

Figure 1. Model of protein aggregation as a result of protein instability

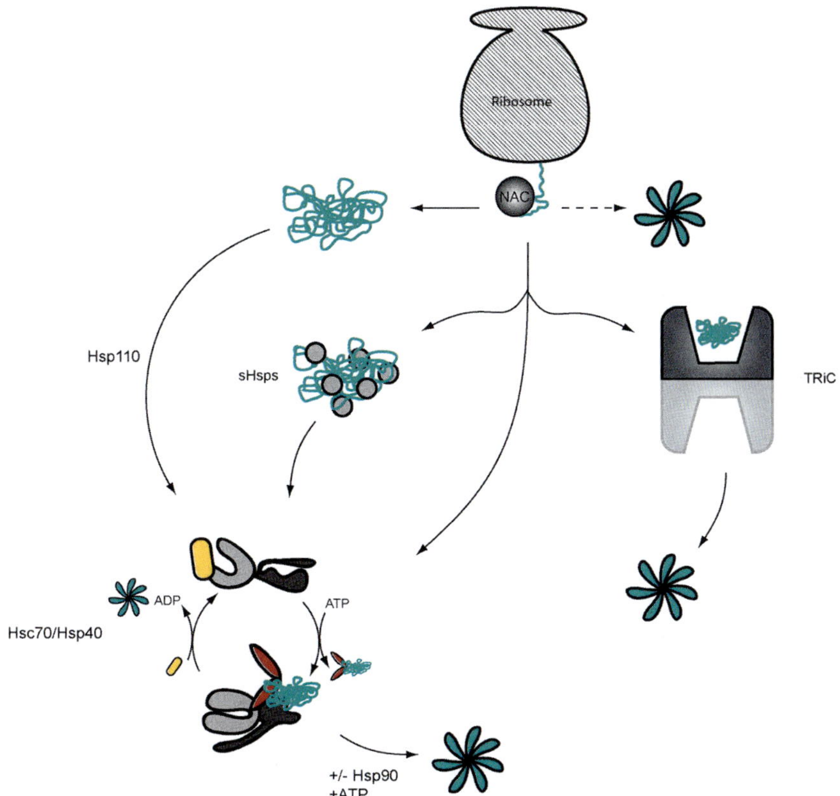

Figure 2. Cellular proteostasis system to control the production and folding of cytosolic proteins
Ribosome-associated chaperones of the NAC and the 'free' chaperones TRiC, Hsc70, Hsp90, Hsp110 and sHSPs, which control protein homoeostasis in the cytosol. Proteins (green) can follow several possible pathways, which lead from misfolded, aggregated or stabilized proteins to the native fold.

problems of cytosolic proteins that become unfolded during their function or during exposure to stressful conditions that then have to be repaired following this incident. To this end, sophisticated protein folding machines were developed.

Cellular proteostasis and quality control systems

It is necessary that cells continuously safeguard the functionality of their proteins and the general protein homoeostasis, termed proteostasis [8,9]. This is challenging even during normal growth periods, but in particular after exposure to harmful conditions, such as elevated temperatures [10] or contact with heavy metal ions [11,12], which compromise protein homoeostasis. Under these conditions, the cell induces the heat-shock response and expresses protective proteins, such as chaperones, to repair the damage. Similarly, tunicamycin and other compounds that interfere with glycosylation in the secretory pathway are very potent inducers of the UPR (unfolded protein response), which regulates the levels of chaperones in the secretory compartments [13,14].

Heat-shock proteins, or chaperones, were originally identified as being overexpressed in response to proteotoxic challenges, but are also found in the cytosol of unstressed cells. In all stress response pathways the primary signal may be the accumulation of damaged proteins, which results from overburdening the cell's quality control system. A misfolded protein has three different destinies: it can be refolded into the functional form, it can be degraded by the ubiquitin–proteasome system or it can be sequestered into inclusions. The expression of cytosolic heat-shock genes is regulated by the transcription factor Hsf1. Normally, chaperones like Hsp40 (heat-shock protein 40), Hsc70 (heat-shock cognate 70) and Hsp90 (heat-shock protein 90) bind to Hsf1 and prevent it from activating chaperone genes. When damaged proteins start to accumulate, they compete with Hsf1 for chaperone interaction. Hsf1 is released and induces production of further chaperones until homoeostasis has been re-established [9]. This feedback regulation based on complex formation between chaperones and Hsf1 is thought to be a basic circuit to control chaperone levels in the cell [15]. The coupling of the heat-shock response to the accumulation of unfolded proteins also best explains the observation that all species show a similar heat-shock response, if their body temperature briefly increases more than 10°C over their normal growth temperature. In the human genome, four Hsf-like proteins, named Hsf1–Hsf4, can be found. Besides heat stress, misbalanced proteostasis may also originate from other forms of stress. Some cells, which express very high amounts of proteins in a short time, such as antibody-generating B-cells, require high levels of ER (endoplasmic reticulum)-based Hsp70 (heat-shock protein 70) to support the production and secretion of correctly folded antibodies [16]. Also in fast growing cells, such as tumour cells, increased expression of the chaperone proteins Hsp70 and Hsp90 can be observed [17], indicating that quality control of protein synthesis and protein folding is a major challenge for quickly dividing cells.

The protein quality control system of the cell encompasses many other proteins, including the >500 proteins involved in the regulation of protein degradation. Furthermore, it is well established that aggregates or larger assemblies of misfolded proteins can be removed from the cell with the help of lysosomes. These organelles can degrade individual proteins, which are imported across the membrane, as well as larger structures, which are first surrounded by membranes and then fuse with lysosomes to induce degradation. The coating of aggregates with a membrane-containing structure is organized by the autophagic system, which is used by the cell to remove organelles and other large particles in a controlled manner [18].

Role of molecular chaperones in cellular quality control

Molecular chaperones are structurally diverse proteins that help other proteins obtain their native fold [19]. They assist during the folding process and prevent formation of unproductive intermediates. Their concentration is highest in the ER of protein-secreting cells, but their functional diversity is most extensive in the cytosol. The cytosolic chaperones of higher eukaryotes are grouped into classes based on their sizes and homologies and can be seen as individual machineries to perform protein-folding tasks [20]: Hsp60/CCT/TriC (heat-shock protein 60/chaperonin-containing T-complex protein/T-complex protein 1-containing ring complex), Hsp70/Hsp40, Hsp90, ClpX/Hsp100, Hsp110 and sHSPs (small heat-shock proteins) (Figure 2).

These proteins have been studied in detail in the last decades and models have been developed to understand the principles of their operation during folding of their protein substrates.

Hsp60/chaperonin system and caged protein folding

The best-studied molecular chaperone is the bacterial ring-like assembly GroEL/GroES, which belongs to the chaperonin family. The 14 subunits of GroEL and the lid-like GroES form a barrel-like structure that encapsulates the unfolded protein and supports its refolding in an isolated environment [21]. This isolation reduces contact with other metastable proteins and thus prevents aggregation. The extent of contact between unfolded proteins and GroEL, and the participation of certain loop structures of GroEL, is currently debated [22]. *In vitro*, GroEL/GroES refolds proteins after the addition of ATP [23]. During ATP hydrolysis, GroEL switches between exposure of hydrophobic and hydrophilic surfaces, thereby controlling the interaction with the client protein. GroEL folds approximately 35% of bacterial proteins [8,24]. In eukaryotes, GroEL is only found in mitochondria, whereas the cytosol contains a related but distinct protein, called CCT/TRiC, composed of eight homologous subunits and devoid of a lid-like cofactor [25,26] (Figure 3). TriC and GroEL differ in several ways, such as the absence of extensive hydrophobic regions in the inner chamber of TRiC [27] and closing of the folding chamber of TriC is not induced by client protein binding, but instead occurs upon ATP hydrolysis [28]. In general, TRiC is much more restricted in respect to its range of substrates and expression is barely increased upon heat shock. Substrates of TriC are primarily cytoskeletal proteins such as actin and tubulin [29,30]. The contribution to cellular quality control and proteostasis nevertheless becomes evident in nematodes, where a reduction in TRiC levels leads to the induction of the heat-shock response in muscle cells [31]. While this could be explained by TRiC's specific

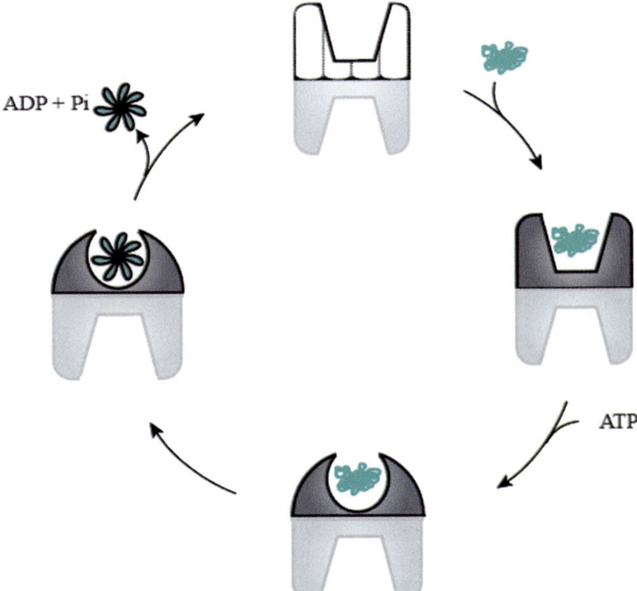

Figure 3. Model of CCT/TRiC function
TRiC (grey) binds and hydrolyses ATP after binding the unfolded protein. The cavity is closed in response to ATP hydrolysis and then releases the folded protein (green) into the cytosol.

role in muscle cells, where actin is essential and highly abundant, it could imply a more general involvement of TriC in protein quality control, which might also apply to other cell types.

Hsc70–Hsp40 and refolding to the native state

Constitutively expressed Hsc70 and the heat-shock-induced Hsp70 proteins are involved in most folding processes in eukaryotic cells. The human genome encodes 13 Hsp70s in the cytosolic compartment [32]. All Hsp70s contain an NBD (N-terminal ATP-binding domain), an SBD (substrate-binding domain) and a C-terminal lid region, which covers the substrate-binding groove of the SBD [33] (Figure 4). During ATP hydrolysis a linker region transmits the conformational changes from the NBD to the SBD [34,35]. The positioning of the lid domain is thus controlled by the hydrolysis reaction and switches between a closed and a wide-open position [36]. Substrate proteins bind to the ATP-bound form of the chaperone, but after hydrolysis the substrate lid closes to form a stable Hsp70–substrate complex [37]. Substrates are bound as extended polypeptide stretches containing at least one hydrophobic amino acid [38]. This complex is then slowly resolved by dissociation of ADP and substrate.

Nucleotide binding to Hsc70 is very tight, with dissociation constants in the nanomolar range [39]. Dissociation of the nucleotide is accelerated by NEFs (nucleotide exchange factors)

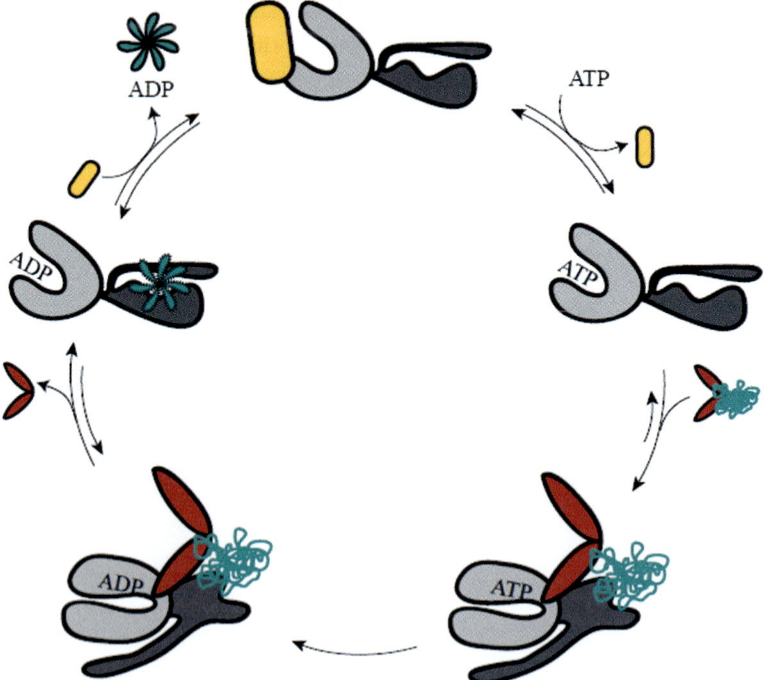

Figure 4. Model of the function of Hsc70 together with its cofactors
The client protein (green) is folded after initially binding to the open conformation of Hsc70 (grey). After ATP hydrolysis, which is triggered by the Hsp40/J-proteins (red), a folded client protein is released during the subsequent reopening of the chaperone. NEFs (yellow) facilitate the following ADP release and Hsc70 is able to re-enter the cycle. Reproduced with permission from [99]; Sun, L, Edelmann, F.T., Kaiser, C.J, Papsdorf, K., Gaiser, A.M. and Richter, K., (2012) The lid domain of *Caenorhabditis elegans* Hsc70 influences ATP turnover, cofactor binding and protein folding activity. PLoS ONE **7**, e33980

(see Figures 2 and 4). Several proteins have been shown to exert this function, including the BAG-domain-containing proteins, which interact with the NBD of Hsp70s and decrease the affinity for nucleotide [40]. Another class of Hsp70-regulating proteins are the J-domain-containing proteins, which include Hsp40s. The J-domain binds at the interface of the N-terminal domain and the SBD of Hsp70s (Figure 4) and accelerates nucleotide hydrolysis while slowing down the release of ADP [41,42]. Formation of the Hsp70–Hsp40 complex may be required during transfer of the protein substrate from Hsp40 to Hsp70. It is evident from *in vitro* folding assays that the presence of Hsp40 proteins is required for efficient refolding of denatured proteins by Hsc70.

Another class of cofactors are the TPR (tetratricopeptide) domain-containing proteins. In general, these cofactors, which associate with the C-terminus of Hsp70, control the targeting of Hsp70 to specific cellular processes that require its participation. TPR-domain-containing cofactors bind to the C-terminal tail of cytosolic Hsp70 proteins and influence the substrate specificity of the chaperone. Interesting in the context of protein quality control is the TPR-domain-containing protein CHIP, which couples an Hsc70-interacting TPR-domain with an E3-ligase domain [43] and influences to what extent proteins are refolded with the help of Hsc70 or degraded by the ubiquitin–proteasome system, thereby providing a connection between the chaperone-based protein folding system and protein degradation [44]. Thus Hsc70s are involved in many aspects of cellular quality control and are responsible for triage decisions leading to either refolding or degradation. Hsp70s also play a major part in folding reactions in the ER and other compartments by helping to transport proteins across membranes. Thus it is not very surprising to see strong induction of the heat-shock response after Hsc70 depletion [31]. Even the reduction in organelle-resident Hsp70s leads to induction of the cytosolic heat-shock response, implying that disruption of transport processes also affects the sensitive balance between protein folding and unfolding in the cytosol [31].

sHSPs and control of aggregation

Besides HSP40s, sHsps are the only ATP-independent chaperone class. sHSPs possess an extraordinary ability to bind unfolded peptide chains and suppress their aggregation [45]. The misfolded peptide chain remains bound to the sHSP and is released only after contact with the Hsp70/Hsp40 system [46]. In humans, some sHSPs are ubiquitously expressed, such as HSPB1 (heat-shock 27 kDa protein 1), whereas others are found in specific tissues, such as HSPB2 in heart and muscle tissues and HSPB4/alpha-crystallin in the eye lens [47]. Altogether, ten proteins of this class are encoded [48]. All sHSPs form oligomeric structures and share a common alpha-crystallin domain flanked by N- and C-terminal extensions. These extensions regulate oligomerization and are involved in client protein recognition. It is assumed that the oligomerization state of the sHSP controls its chaperone activity [49,50]. The chaperone activity of sHSPs is further regulated via temperature-dependent switches or phosphorylation [51].

Disaggregases for protein aggregates

In lower eukaryotes, plants, bacteria and mitochondria, Hsp100 proteins form another class of ATP-driven folding machines. Homologues of bacterial ClpB or yeast Hsp104 are not found in the cytosol of higher eukaryotes. Hsp100s are AAA-ATPases (ATPase associated with various cellular activities) with two nucleotide-binding sites. They form hexameric ring-like assemblies and many studies suggest that they perform unfolding reactions by pulling protein chains through the inner hole in their doughnut-like structure [52,53]. Mechanistic details of this reaction have not yet been elucidated, but this unfolding event may allow the subsequent refolding of the substrate protein to attain the current conformation [52,53]. It is well described that the Hsp70/Hsp40 system participates in the refolding of unfolded proteins in co-operation with Hsp100 proteins [54].

Apparently in higher eukaryotes, another chaperone is used for this purpose. Here Hsp110 performs the disaggregation function, in co-operation with Hsp70 and Hsp40. Interestingly, Hsp110 itself is a homologue of Hsc70, but apparently it has evolved to participate in the refolding of aggregates. Hsp110s, enlarged by certain loop structures in comparison with Hsp70s, perform holdase functions on client proteins and do not hydrolyse ATP [55–57]. They instead bind to Hsc70 and, similar to other NEFs, accelerate the release of nucleotide from the chaperone [58].

Hsp90 and stabilization of metastable clients

Among the chaperones, Hsp90 appears to have a special role as it is not thought to interact with unfolded or aggregating proteins, but is required to stabilize folded metastable proteins or intermediates (Figure 2). Hsp90 is a dimeric V-shaped molecular machine, which contains two ATP-binding sites at the respective N-termini; each monomer contains a 30 kDa middle domain and a C-terminal dimerization site [59]. Large conformational changes occur during ATP hydrolysis (Figure 5). These movements lead to the formation of defined Hsp90 conformations, which are required to initiate the ATP hydrolysis reaction [60]. One specific conformation is a ring-like structure, which is dimerized not only at the C-terminal sites, but also at the NBDs [59]. Substantial structural insight into these processes has been obtained from the crystal structures of the 'open' and 'closed' conformations of Hsp90, resolving movements during the ATPase reaction in atomic detail [59,61].

ATP binding and hydrolysis are required to stabilize the client proteins and prevent their degradation by the ubiquitin–proteasome system. Steroid hormone receptors are Hsp90 clients, as they depend on the chaperone to attain their hormone-binding state [62]. In the absence of the Hsp90 chaperone they are degraded very rapidly [63]. Hsp90 also forms complexes with protein kinases [64], transcription factors and E3 ligases, which are likewise targeted for degradation if Hsp90 is absent [65].

The role of Hsp90 in stabilizing important client proteins, which among many others include oncogenic protein kinases and transcription factors (a full list can be found at http://www.picard.ch) has led to the development of Hsp90 inhibitory molecules. Natural compound inhibitors include radicicol, geldanamycin and several variants of geldanamycin, such as macbecin and herbimycin [66,67]. These compounds bind to the N-terminal domain of Hsp90 with high affinity, preventing ATP from accessing its binding pocket [68,69]. The resulting inhibition disrupts the Hsp90/client protein complexes and leads to fast degradation of Hsp90 client proteins, and thus may be used to inhibit the growth of tumours which depends on mutated protein kinases or transcription factors [67].

Similar to Hsc70, Hsp90 has cofactors that control the hydrolysis reaction and the conformational states during the ATPase cycle (Figure 5). In addition to ATPase control, these proteins are also important for the correct folding and stability of defined Hsp90 client proteins. p23 and Sti1/Hop are supportive during the activation of steroid hormone receptors [70,71]. The kinase-specific Hsp90 cofactor Cdc37 is required for the formation of Hsp90/kinase complexes. Thus the further functionalization of the Hsp90 machine depends on these cofactors.

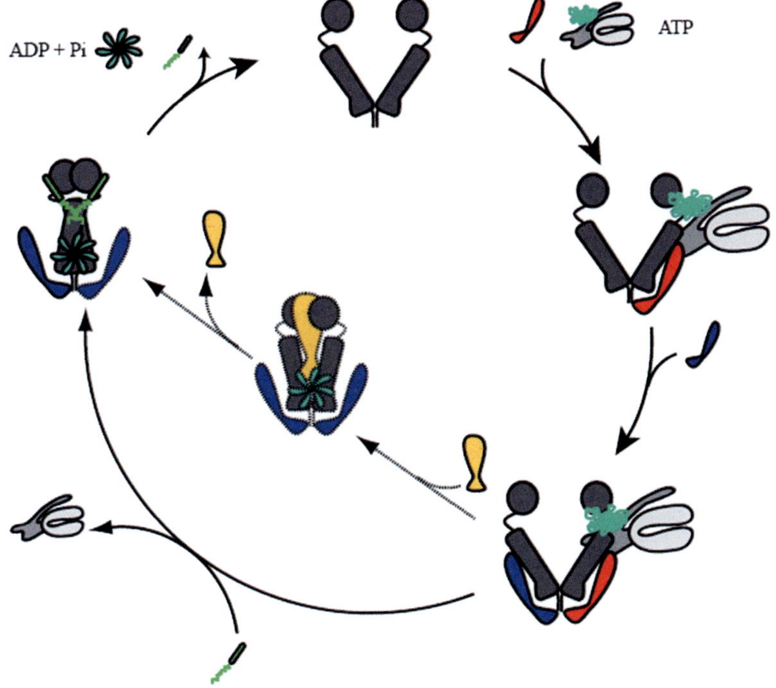

Figure 5. Model of the function of Hsp90 in co-operation with its cofactors
The client protein (green) is released after being folded during the cofactor-controlled ATPase cycle of Hsp90 (grey). Cofactor exchange is controlled by ATP hydrolysis. The cofactor Aha1 (yellow) is included, but may not be needed for all client proteins. Some client proteins are processed with the help of specialized cofactors, such as Cdc37 in the case of protein kinases. Sti1/Hop (red) connects the Hsp90 cycle to the Hsc70 system (light grey). PPIases (peptidylprolyl *cis–trans* isomerases) bind to Hsp90 in the following steps (blue). p23 (light green) is important during maturation of certain client proteins.

This is also exemplified by the protein Sti1/Hop, which serves as an adapter protein to connect the Hsp90 and Hsc70 machineries. It locks Hsp90 in an open conformation and facilitates client protein transition from the Hsp70/Hsp40 system to Hsp90. It is interesting to note that the number of TPR-domain-containing cofactors of Hsp90 and Hsc70 increases significantly between lower organisms and mammals, suggesting that during evolution a further development of Hsp90- and Hsc70-dependent functions occurred [72].

Protein aggregation diseases and neurodegeneration

Aggregation of proteins occurs *in vitro* and *in vivo*. Aggregation *in vivo* can occur spontaneously, if proteins do not fold correctly or are intrinsically unstable. In particular, mutations generating unstable proteins are responsible for many human protein aggregation pathologies, many of them neurodegenerative diseases [73]. For example, destabilizing SOD1 (superoxide dismutase 1) mutations are responsible for specific forms of amyotrophic lateral sclerosis [74], elongated polyglutamine stretches in huntingtin are responsible for Huntington's disease [75] and mutations in the Aβ peptide of the APP protein (amyloid precursor protein) [76] or the microtubule-associated tau protein are linked to Alzheimer's disease [77]. In many cases, aggregation-prone proteins are deposited as β-sheet-containing amyloids, but the origin of toxicity during the aggregation process is still unclear.

One class of proteins, which associate with and help to remodel aggregates are the molecular chaperones. These proteins, particularly the Hsp100 proteins ClpB in bacteria and Hsp104 in yeast, are able to extract peptide chains from aggregates and, together with Hsp70 and Hsp40, initiate the refolding of these proteins [78]. Hsp104 is found to be associated with assemblies of unfolded proteins [79] and appears to remodel these structures *in vivo*. Despite the potentially positive impact of these actions, toxicity of polyglutamine proteins in yeast is reduced and higher expression levels of these proteins are tolerated in the absence of Hsp104, implying that a direct beneficial effect has yet to be established [80,81]. As with Hsp104, the association of Hsc70 and Hsp40 with protein aggregates is well documented [82–84]. In higher eukaryotes, Hsp110 proteins, which are homologous to Hsp70s, appear to act as disaggregases [56]. Also, sHSPs are thought to influence the progression of aggregation and misfolding diseases such as Alzheimer's and Parkinson's [85]. It is likely that systems exist in all eukaryotes that are able to extract proteins from aggregates in order to refold them. Studies in eukaryotic model systems confirm that protein aggregation is enhanced if the chaperone systems are compromised [86]. This becomes evident in polyglutamine model systems, where faster aggregation can be observed if Hsc70 or Hsf1 are depleted [87]. Similarly, a stronger motility loss can be observed in SOD1 models after reduction or depletion of Hsf1 and certain Hsp40 homologues [88].

Chaperones, quality control and misfolding diseases

Besides neurodegenerative diseases, chaperones participate in general protein folding and quality control events in the cell and thus are involved in many other protein misfolding diseases. In particular, two examples highlight this contribution: the misfolding and degradation of the CFTR (cystic fibrosis transmembrane conductance regulator) receptor, leading to cystic fibrosis; and the recycling process of filamin, which is connected to the generation of myopathies. It is well established that mutations in the receptor and chloride channel CFTR can lead to cystic fibrosis. For example, the ΔF508 mutant of CFTR is expressed, but it fails to reach the plasma membrane in a correctly folded state and becomes degraded instead [89]. This process is closely related to the function of Hsp90, which together with its cofactor Aha1 controls the proper folding of the CFTR. Misfolded CFTR is degraded efficiently only in the presence of Aha1, and reductions in the level of Aha1 lead to less degradation and more functional CFTR in the plasma membrane [90]. Thus the reduction in quality control components in this particular case may prove beneficial for the health of the patients.

Another case where chaperones participate in cellular quality control is evident during the progression of myopathies. Hsp90, together with its cofactor UNC-45, participates in events that guarantee the functionality of the actin–myosin ultrastructure [91,92]. Hsp90 and UNC-45 help during the assembly of myosin filaments and in their absence, myosin tends to form intracellular aggregates, eventually leading to failure of the contractile function and loss of motility in nematodes, fruit flies, zebrafish and possibly also mammals [93,94]. Another chaperone-associated process ensures the recycling of filamin at muscle attachment sites. Here, the sHSP HSPB8, Hsc70 and its cofactors Bag3 and CHIP identify damaged filamin proteins, which are then degraded via autophagy and replaced. This process, termed CASA (chaperone-assisted selective autophagy), is controlled by the chaperones, which recognize the damaged protein and target it to the autophagosomes [95,96]. The 400 kDa filamin protein cannot undergo normal processing by the proteasome, thus the cellular quality control system has to take alternative routes to remove the protein and replace it with a new functional version. CFTR and filamin are only two of many examples in which chaperones and the cellular quality system are connected to the severity of diseases, making the cellular proteostasis system a promising target for drug development.

Conclusions

Based on the many studies investigating the role of molecular chaperones, it is evident that much of the work in the proteostasis system is performed by these ATP-driven machines. Thus it is important to fully understand their mechanism, as well as the specific changes they induce in their client proteins. This will ultimately help in the development of therapeutics that influence certain aspects of the proteostasis system in a controlled manner. This approach has progressed furthest with Hsp90 as natural compounds are available that can be used to influence the substrate turnover of specific Hsp90-dependent clients. Based on the original natural compounds, a large set of synthetic compounds has been developed, providing the prospect of bringing therapeutic compounds on to the market within the next few years. But also for Hsp70, compounds are being developed that influence its activities [97]. Likewise, screens have identified compounds that cause general activation of the heat-shock response by stimulating the transcription factor Hsf1 [98]. These approaches will allow the proteostasis system to be influenced in a more specific and defined manner and may one day allow treatment of misfolding diseases.

Summary

- Nature has provided the cell with a set of systems to control the quality of the cellular protein pool. These proteostasis systems include the folding helpers, the degradation system for soluble proteins based on ubiquitin attachment and proteasomal degradation and the different autophagic pathways.
- Chaperone proteins play a major role in these folding and degradation pathways.
- The most important eukaryotic chaperones are Hsp110, Hsp90, Hsc70–Hsp40, TriC and the sHSPs.
- Different chaperone classes hydrolyse ATP by vastly different mechanisms, but always couple conformational changes with the hydrolysis reaction.
- Some client proteins are entirely dependent on the chaperone machines during folding, whereas in other cases folding efficiency is only improved to a certain extent.
- Learning to influence this system will be a huge step forward in targeting the many diseases that originate from impaired quality control systems.

References

1. Anfinsen, C.B. and Haber, E. (1961) Studies on the reduction and re-formation of protein disulfide bonds. J. Biol. Chem. **236**, 1361–1363

2. Honig, B., Ray, A. and Levinthal, C. (1976) Conformational flexibility and protein folding: rigid structural fragments connected by flexible joints in subtilisin BPN. Proc. Natl. Acad. Sci. U.S.A. **73**, 1974–1978

3. Neudecker, P., Robustelli, P., Cavalli, A., Walsh, P., Lundström, P., Zarrine-Afsar, A., Sharpe, S., Vendruscolo, M. and Kay, L.E. (2012) Structure of an intermediate state in protein folding and aggregation. Science **336**, 362–366

4. Chiti, F. and Dobson, C.M. (2009) Amyloid formation by globular proteins under native conditions. Nat. Chem. Biol. **5**, 15–22

5. Gershenson, A. and Gierasch, L.M. (2011) Protein folding in the cell: challenges and progress. Curr. Opin. Struct. Biol. **21**, 32–41

6. Preissler, S. and Deuerling, E. (2012) Ribosome-associated chaperones as key players in proteostasis. Trends Biochem. Sci. **37**, 274–283

7. Frydman, J. (2001) Folding of newly translated proteins *in vivo*: the role of molecular chaperones. Annu. Rev. Biochem. **70**, 603–647

8. Kim, Y.E., Hipp, M.S., Hayer-Hartl, A.B.M. and Ulrich Hartl, F. (2013) Molecular chaperone functions in protein folding and proteostasis. Annu. Rev. Biochem. **82**, 323–355

9. Morimoto, R.I. (2011) The heat shock response: systems biology of proteotoxic stress in aging and disease. Cold Spring Harb. Symp. Quant. Biol. **76**, 91–99

10. Ashburner, M. and Bonner, J.J. (1979) The induction of gene activity in drosophilia by heat shock. Cell **17**, 241–254

11. Walsh, K.H. and Crabb, D.W. (1989) The heat-shock response in cultured cells exposed to ethanol and its metabolites. J. Lab. Clin. Med. **114**, 563–567

12. Yamada, H. and Koizumi, S. (1993) Induction of a 70-kDa protein in human lymphocytes exposed to inorganic heavy metals and toxic organic compounds. Toxicology **79**, 131–138

13. Brewer, J.W., Cleveland, J.L. and Hendershot, L.M. (1997) A pathway distinct from the mammalian unfolded protein response regulates expression of endoplasmic reticulum chaperones in non-stressed cells. EMBO J. **16**, 7207–7216

14. Haze, K., Yoshida, H., Yanagi, H., Yura, T. and Mori, K. (1999) Mammalian transcription factor ATF6 is synthesized as a transmembrane protein and activated by proteolysis in response to endoplasmic reticulum stress. Mol. Biol. Cell **10**, 3787–3799

15. Shi, Y., Mosser, D.D. and Morimoto, R.I. (1998) Molecular chaperones as HSF1-specific transcriptional repressors. Genes Dev. **12**, 654–666

16. Gass, J.N., Gifford, N.M. and Brewer, J.W. (2002) Activation of an unfolded protein response during differentiation of antibody-secreting B cells. J. Biol. Chem. **277**, 49047–49054

17. Protti, M.P., et al., Constitutive expression of the heat shock protein 72 kDa in human melanoma cells. Cancer Lett, 1994. 85(2), 211–216

18. Rubinsztein, D.C., Marino, G. and Kroemer, G. Autophagy and aging. Cell, 2011. 146(5), 682–695

19. Ellis, R.J., van der Vies, S.M. and Hemmingsen, S.M. (1989) The molecular chaperone concept. Biochem. Soc. Symp. **55**, 145–153

20. Walter, S. and Buchner, J. (2002) Molecular chaperones: cellular machines for protein folding. Angew. Chem. Int. Ed. Engl. **41**, 1098–1113

21. Todd, M.J., Viitanen, P.V. and Lorimer, G.H. (1994) Dynamics of the chaperonin ATPase cycle: implications for facilitated protein folding. Science **265**, 659–666

22. Clare, D.K., Vasishtan, D., Stagg, S., Quispe, J., Farr, G.W., Topf, M., Horwich, A.L. and Saibil, H.R. (2012) ATP-triggered conformational changes delineate substrate-binding and -folding mechanics of the GroEL chaperonin. Cell **149**, 113–123

23. Ellis, R.J. (2003) Protein folding: importance of the Anfinsen cage. Curr. Biol. **13**, R881–R883

24. Viitanen, P.V., Gatenby, A.A. and Lorimer, G.H. (1992) Purified chaperonin 60 (groEL) interacts with the nonnative states of a multitude of *Escherichia coli* proteins. Protein Sci. **1**, 363–369

25. Llorca, O., McCormack, E.A., Hynes, G., Grantham, J., Cordell, J., Carrascosa, J.L., Willison, K.R., Fernandez, J.J. and Valpuesta, J.M. (1999) Eukaryotic type II chaperonin CCT interacts with actin through specific subunits. Nature **402**, 693–696

26. Dunn, A.Y., Melville, M.W. and Frydman, J. (2001) Review: cellular substrates of the eukaryotic chaperonin TRiC/CCT. J. Struct. Biol. **135**, 176–184

27. Dekker, C., Roe, S.M., McCormack, E.A., Beuron, F., Pearl, L.H. and Willison, K.R. (2011) The crystal structure of yeast CCT reveals intrinsic asymmetry of eukaryotic cytosolic chaperonins. EMBO J. **30**, 3078–3090

28. Douglas, N.R., Reissmann, S., Zhang, J., Chen, B., Jakana, J., Kumar, R., Chiu, W. and Frydman, J. (2011) Dual action of ATP hydrolysis couples lid closure to substrate release into the group II chaperonin chamber. Cell **144**, 240–252

29. Dekker, C., Stirling, P.C., McCormack, E.A., Filmore, H., Paul, A., Brost, R.L., Costanzo, M., Boone, C., Leroux, M.R. and Willison, K.R. (2008) The interaction network of the chaperonin CCT. EMBO J. **27**, 1827–1839

30. Yam, A.Y., Xia, Y., Lin, H.T., Burlingame, A., Gerstein, M. and Frydman, J. (2008) Defining the TRiC/CCT interactome links chaperonin function to stabilization of newly made proteins with complex topologies. Nat. Struct. Mol. Biol. **15**, 1255–1262

31. Guisbert, E., Czyz, D.M., Richter, K., McMullen, P.D. and Morimoto, R.I. (2013) Identification of a tissue-selective heat shock response regulatory network. PLoS Genet. **9**, e1003466

32. Hageman, J., van Waarde, M.A., Zylicz, A., Walerych, D. and Kampinga, H.H. (2011) The diverse members of the mammalian HSP70 machine show distinct chaperone-like activities. Biochem. J. **435**, 127–142

33. Zhu, X., Zhao, X., Burkholder, W.F., Gragerov, A., Ogata, C.M., Gottesman, M.E. and Hendrickson, W.A. (1996) Structural analysis of substrate binding by the molecular chaperone DnaK. Science **272**, 1606–1614

34. Rist, W., Graf, C., Bukau, B. and Mayer, M.P. (2006) Amide hydrogen exchange reveals conformational changes in hsp70 chaperones important for allosteric regulation. J. Biol. Chem. **281**, 16493–16501

35. Swain, J.F., Dinler, G., Sivendran, R., Montgomery, D.L., Stotz, M. and Gierasch, L.M. (2007) Hsp70 chaperone ligands control domain association via an allosteric mechanism mediated by the interdomain linker. Mol. Cell **26**, 27–39

36. Zhuravleva, A., Clerico, E.M. and Gierasch, L.M. (2012) An interdomain energetic tugof-war creates the allosterically active state in Hsp70 molecular chaperones. Cell **151**, 1296–1307

37. Schlecht, R., Erbse, A.H., Bukau, B. and Mayer, M.P. (2011) Mechanics of Hsp70 chaperones enables differential interaction with client proteins. Nat. Struct. Mol. Biol. **18**, 345–351

38. Knarr, G., Gething, M.J., Modrow, S. and Buchner, J. (1995) BiP binding sequences in antibodies. J. Biol. Chem. **270**, 27589–27594

39. Arakawa, A., Handa, N., Shirouzu, M. and Yokoyama, S. (2011) Biochemical and structural studies on the high affinity of Hsp70 for ADP. Protein Sci. **20**, 1367–1379

40. Sondermann, H., Scheufler, C., Schneider, C., Hohfeld, J., Hartl, F.U. and Moarefi, I. (2001) Structure of a Bag/Hsc70 complex: convergent functional evolution of Hsp70 nucleotide exchange factors. Science **291**, 1553–1557

41. Russell, R., Wali Karzai, A., Mehl, A.F. and McMacken, R. (1999) DnaJ dramatically stimulates ATP hydrolysis by DnaK: insight into targeting of Hsp70 proteins to polypeptide substrates. Biochemistry **38**, 4165–4176

42. Gassler, C.S., Buchberger, A., Laufen, T., Mayer, M.P., Schröder, H., Valencia, A. and Bukau, B. (1998) Mutations in the DnaK chaperone affecting interaction with the DnaJ cochaperone. Proc. Natl. Acad. Sci. U.S.A. **95**, 15229–15234

43. Ballinger, C.A., Connell, P., Wu, Y., Hu, Z., Thompson, L.J., Yin, L.Y. and Patterson, C. (1999) Identification of CHIP, a novel tetratricopeptide repeatcontaining protein that interacts with heat shock proteins and negatively regulates chaperone functions. Mol. Cell. Biol. **19**, 4535–4545

44. Connell, P., Ballinger, C.A., Jiang, J., Wu, Y., Thompson, L.J., Höhfeld, J. and Patterson, C. (2001) The co-chaperone CHIP regulates protein triage decisions mediated by heat-shock proteins. Nat. Cell Biol. **3**, 93–96

45. Jakob, U., Gaestel, M., Engel, K. and Buchner, J. (1993) Small heat shock proteins are molecular chaperones. J. Biol. Chem. **268**, 1517–1520

46. Lee, G.J., Roseman, A.M., Saibil, H.R. and Vierling, E. (1997) A small heat shock protein stably binds heat-denatured model substrates and can maintain a substrate in a folding-competent state. EMBO J. **16**, 659–671

47. Garrido, C., Paul, C., Seigneuric, R. and Kampinga, H.H. (2012) The small heat shock proteins family: the long forgotten chaperones. Int. J. Biochem. Cell Biol. **44**, 1588–1592

48. Mymrikov, E.V., A.S. Seit-Nebi, and Gusev, N.B. (2011) Large potentials of small heat shock proteins. Physiol. Rev. **91**, 1123–1159

49. Haslbeck, M., Walke, S., Stromer, T., Ehrnsperger, M., White, H.E., Chen, S., Saibil, H.R. and Buchner, J. (1999) Hsp26: a temperature-regulated chaperone. EMBO J. **18**, 6744–6751

50. Franzmann, T.M., Wühr, M., Richter, K., Walter, S. and Buchner, J. (2005) The activation mechanism of Hsp26 does not require dissociation of the oligomer. J. Mol. Biol. **350**, 1083–1093

51. Lelj-Garolla, B. and Mauk, A.G. (2009) Self-association and chaperone activity of Hsp27 are thermally activated. J. Biol. Chem. **281**, 8169–8174

52. Weber-Ban, E.U., Reid, B.G., Miranker, A.D., Horwich, A.L. (1999) Global unfolding of a substrate protein by the Hsp100 chaperone ClpA. Nature **401**, 90–93

53. Schaupp, A., Marcinowski, M., Grimminger, V., Bösl, B. and Walter, S. (2007) Processing of proteins by the molecular chaperone Hsp104. J. Mol. Biol. **370**, 674–686

54. Haslbeck, M., Miess, A., Stromer, T., Walter, S. and Buchner, J. (2005) Disassembling protein aggregates in the yeast cytosol. The cooperation of Hsp26 with Ssa1 and Hsp104. J. Biol. Chem. **280**, 23861–23868

55. Oh, H.J., Chen, X. and Subjeck, J.R. (1997) Hsp110 protects heat-denatured proteins and confers cellular thermoresistance. J. Biol. Chem. **272**, 31636–31640

56. Rampelt, H., Kirstein-Miles, J., Nillegoda, N.B., Chi, K., Scholz, S.R., Morimoto, R.I. and Bukau, B. (2012) Metazoan Hsp70 machines use Hsp110 to power protein disaggregation. EMBO J. **31**, 4221–4235

57. Shaner, L., Sousa, R. and Morano, K.A. (2006) Characterization of Hsp70 binding and nucleotide exchange by the yeast Hsp110 chaperone Sse1. Biochemistry **45**, 15075–15084

58. Dragovic, Z., et al., Molecular chaperones of the Hsp110 family act as nucleotide exchange factors of Hsp70s. EMBO J, 2006. 25(11), 2519–2528

59. Ali, M.M., Broadley, S.A., Shomura, Y., Bracher, A. and Hartl, F.U. (2006) Crystal structure of an Hsp90-nucleotide-p23/Sba1 closed chaperone complex. Nature **440**, 1013–1017

60. Richter, K., Muschler, P., Hainzl, O. and Buchner, J. (2001) Coordinated ATP hydrolysis by the Hsp90 dimer. J. Biol. Chem. **276**, 33689–33696

61. Shiau, A.K., Harris, S.F., Southworth, D.R. and Agard, D.A. (2006) Structural Analysis of E. coli hsp90 reveals dramatic nucleotide-dependent conformational rearrangements. Cell **127**, 329–340

62. Smith, D.F. (1003) Dynamics of heat shock protein 90-progesterone receptor binding and the disactivation loop model for steroid receptor complexes. Mol. Endocrinol. **7**, 1418–1429

63. Segnitz, B. and Gehring, U. (1997) The function of steroid hormone receptors is inhibited by the hsp90-specific compound geldanamycin. J. Biol. Chem. **272**, 18694–18701

64. Whitelaw, M.L., Hutchison, K. and Perdew, G.H. (1991) A 50-kDa cytosolic protein complexed with the 90-kDa heat shock protein (hsp90) is the same protein complexed with pp60[v-src] hsp90 in cells transformed by the Rous sarcoma virus. J. Biol. Chem. **266**, 16436–16440

65. Taipale, M., Krykbaeva, I., Koeva, M., Kayatekin, C., Westover, K.D., Karras, G.I. and Lindquist, S. (2012) Quantitative analysis of HSP90-client interactions reveals principles of substrate recognition. Cell **150**, 987–1001

66. Sharma, S.V., Agatsuma, T. and Nakano, H. (1998) Targeting of the protein chaperone, HSP90, by the transformation suppressing agent, radicicol. Oncogene **16**, 2639–2645

67. Whitesell, L., Mimnaugh, E.G., De Costa, B., Myers, C.E. and Neckers, L.M. (1994) Inhibition of heat shock protein HSP90-pp60v-src heteroprotein complex formation by benzoquinone ansamycins: essential role for stress proteins in oncogenic transformation. Proc. Natl. Acad. Sci. U.S.A. **91**, 8324–8328

68. Stebbins, C.E., Russo, A.A., Schneider, C., Rosen, N., Hartl, F.U. and Pavletich, N.P. (1007) Crystal structure of an Hsp90-geldanamycin complex: targeting of a protein chaperone by an antitumor agent. Cell **89**, 239–250

69. Roe, S.M., Prodromou, C., O'Brien, R., Ladbury, J.E., Piper, P.W. and Pearl, L.H. (1999) Structural basis for inhibition of the Hsp90 molecular chaperone by the antitumor antibiotics radicicol and geldanamycin. J. Med. Chem. **42**, 260–266

70. Johnson, J.L., Beito, T.G., Krco, C.J. and Toft, D.O. (1994) Characterization of a novel 23-kilodalton protein of unactive progesterone receptor complexes. Mol. Cell. Biol. **14**, 1956–1963

71. Smith, D.F., Sullivan, W.P., Marion, T.N., Zaitsu, K., Madden, B., McCormick, D.J. and Toft, D.O. (1993) Identification of a 60-kilodalton stress-related protein, p60, which interacts with hsp90 and hsp70. Mol. Cell. Biol. **13**, 869–876

72. Haslbeck, V., Eckl, J.M., Kaiser, C.J., Papsdorf, K., Hessling, M. and Richter, K. (2013) Chaperone-interacting TPR proteins in *Caenorhabditis elegans*. J. Mol. Biol. **425**, 2922–2939

73. Voisine, C., Pedersen, J.S. and Morimoto, R.I. (2010) Chaperone networks: tipping the balance in protein folding diseases. Neurobiol. Dis. **40**, 12–20

74. Deng, H.X., Hentati, A., Tainer, J.A., Iqbal, Z., Cayabyab, A., Hung, W.Y., Getzoff, E.D., Hu, P., Herzfeldt, B., Roos, R.P. et al. (1993) Amyotrophic lateral sclerosis and structural defects in Cu,Zn superoxide dismutase. Science **261**, 1047–1051

75. Rubinsztein, D.C., Barton, D.E., Davison, B.C. and Ferguson-Smith, M.A. (1993) Analysis of the huntingtin gene reveals a trinucleotidelength polymorphism in the region of the gene that contains two CCG-rich stretches and a correlation between decreased age of onset of Huntington's disease and CAG repeat number. Hum. Mol. Genet. **2**, 1713–1715

76. Kang, J., Lemaire, H.G., Unterbeck, A., Salbaum, J.M., Masters, C.L., Grzeschik, K.H., Multhaup, G., Beyreuther, K. and Müller-Hill, B. (1987) The precursor of Alzheimer's disease amyloid A4 protein resembles a cell-surface receptor. Nature **325**, 733–736

77. Kosik, K.S., Joachim, C.L. and Selkoe, D.J. (1986) Microtubule-associated protein tau (tau) is a major antigenic component of paired helical filaments in Alzheimer disease. Proc. Natl. Acad. Sci. U.S.A. **83**, 4044–4048

78. Jana, N.R., Tanaka, M., Wang, G.-h. and Nukina, N. (2000) Polyglutamine length-dependent interaction of Hsp40 and Hsp70 family chaperones with truncated N-terminal huntingtin: their role in suppression of aggregation and cellular toxicity. Hum. Mol. Genet. **9**, 2009–2018

79. Kaganovich, D., Kopito, R. and Frydman, J. (2008) Misfolded proteins partition between two distinct quality control compartments. Nature **454**, 1088–1095

80. Giorgini, F., Guidetti, P., Nguyen, Q., Bennett, S.C. and Muchowski, P.J. (2005) A genomic screen in yeast implicates kynurenine 3- monooxygenase as a therapeutic target for Huntington disease. Nat. Genet. **37**, 526–531

81. Kaiser, C.J., Grötzinger, S.W., Eckl, J.M., Papsdorf, K., Jordan, S. and Richter, K. (2013) A network of genes connects polyglutamine toxicity to ploidy control in yeast. Nat. Commun. 4, 1571

82. Matsumoto, G., Kim, S. and Morimoto, R.I. (2006) Huntingtin and mutant SOD1 form aggregate structures with distinct molecular properties in human cells. J. Biol. Chem. **281**, 4477–4485

83. Escusa-Toret, S., Vonk, W.I. and Frydman, J. (2013) Spatial sequestration of misfolded proteins by a dynamic chaperone pathway enhances cellular fitness during stress. Nat. Cell Biol. **15**, 1231–1243

84. Park, S.H., Kukushkin, Y., Gupta, R., Chen, T., Konagai, A., Hipp, M.S., Hayer-Hartl, M. and Hartl, F.U. (2013) PolyQ proteins interfere with nuclear degradation of cytosolic proteins by sequestering the Sis1p chaperone. Cell **154**, 134–145

85. Sun, Y. and MacRae, T.H. (2005) The small heat shock proteins and their role in human disease. FEBS J. **272**, 2613–2627

86. Gidalevitz, T., Ben-Zvi, A., Ho, K.H., Brignull, H.R. and Morimoto, R.I. (2006) Progressive disruption of cellular protein folding in models of polyglutamine diseases. Science **311**, 1471–1474

87. Nollen, E.A., Garcia, S.M., van Haaften, G., Kim, S., Chavez, A., Morimoto, R.I. and Plasterk, R.H. (2004) Genome-wide RNA interference screen identifies previously undescribed regulators of polyglutamine aggregation. Proc. Natl. Acad. Sci. U.S.A. **101**, 6403–6408

88. Wang, J., Farr, G.W., Hall, D.H., Li, F., Furtak, K., Dreier, L. and Horwich, A.L (2009). An ALS-linked mutant SOD1 produces a locomotor defect associated with aggregation and synaptic dysfunction when expressed in neurons of *Caenorhabditis elegans*. PLoS Genet. **5**, e1000350

89. Youker, R.T., Walsh, P., Beilharz, T., Lithgow, T. and Brodsky, J.L. (2004) Distinct roles for the Hsp40 and Hsp90 molecular chaperones during cystic fibrosis transmembrane conductance regulator degradation in yeast. Mol. Biol. Cell **15**, 4787–4797

90. Wang, X., Venable, J., LaPointe, P., Hutt, D.M., Koulov, A.V., Coppinger, J., Gurkan, C., Kellner, W., Matteson, J., Plutner, H. et al. (2006) Hsp90 cochaperone Aha1 downregulation rescues misfolding of CFTR in cystic fibrosis. Cell **127**, 803–815

91. Venolia, L., Ao, W., Kim, S., Kim, C. and Pilgrim, D. (1999) unc-45 gene of *Caenorhabditis elegans* encodes a musclespecific tetratricopeptide repeat-containing protein. Cell Motil. Cytoskeleton **42**, 163–177

92. Barral, J.M., Hutagalung, A.H., Brinker, A., Hartl, F.U. and Epstein, H.F. (2002) Role of the myosin assembly protein UNC-45 as a molecular chaperone for myosin. Science **295**, 669–671

93. Etard, C., Behra, M., Fischer, N., Hutcheson, D., Geisler, R. and Strähle, U. (2007) The UCS factor Steif/Unc-45b interacts with the heat shock protein Hsp90a during myofibrillogenesis. Dev. Biol. **308**, 133–143

94. Gaiser, A.M., Kaiser, C.J.O., Haslbeck, V. and Richter, K. (2011) Downregulation of the Hsp90 system causes defects in muscle cells of *Caenorhabditis elegans*. PLoS ONE **6**, e25485

95. Arndt, V., Dick, N., Tawo, R., Dreiseidler, M., Wenzel, D., Hesse, M., Fürst, D.O., Saftig, P., Saint, R., Fleischmann, B.K. et al. (2010) Chaperone-assisted selective autophagy is essential for muscle maintenance. Curr. Biol. **20**, 143–148

96. Ulbricht, A., Arndt, V. and Hohfeld, J. (2013) Chaperone-assisted proteostasis is essential for mechanotransduction in mammalian cells. Commun. Integr. Biol. **6**, e24925

97. Chafekar, S.M., Wisén, S., Thompson, A.D., Echeverria, A., Walter, G.M., Evans, C.G., Makley, L.N., Gestwicki, J.E. and Duennwald, M.L. (2012) Pharmacological tuning of heat shock protein 70 modulates polyglutamine toxicity and aggregation. ACS Chem. Biol. **7**, 1556–1564

98. Calamini, B., Silva, M.C., Madoux, F., Hutt, D.M., Khanna, S., Chalfant, M.A., Saldanha, S.A., Hodder, P., Tait, B.D., Garza, D. et al. (2012) Small-molecule proteostasis regulators for protein conformational diseases. Nat. Chem. Biol. **8**, 185–196

99. Sun, L., Edelmann, F.T., Kaiser, C.J., Papsdorf, K., Gaiser, A.M. and Richter, K. (2012) The lid domain of *Caenorhabditis elegans* Hsc70 influences ATP turnover, cofactor binding and protein folding activity. PLoS ONE **7**, e33980

© The Authors Journal compilation © 2014 Biochemical Society
Essays Biochem. (2014) 56, 69–83: doi: 10.1042/BSE0560069

5

Insights into amyloid disease from fly models

Ko-Fan Chen and Damian C. Crowther[1]

University of Cambridge, Department of Genetics, Downing Street, Cambridge CB2 3EH, U.K.

Abstract

The formation of amyloid aggregates is a feature of most, if not all, polypeptide chains. *In vivo* modelling of this process has been undertaken in the fruitfly *Drosophila melanogaster* with remarkable success. Models of both neurological and systemic amyloid diseases have been generated and have informed our understanding of disease pathogenesis in two main ways. First, the toxic amyloid species have been at least partially characterized, for example in the case of the Aβ (amyloid β-peptide) associated with Alzheimer's disease. Secondly, the genetic underpinning of model disease-linked phenotypes has been characterized for a number of neurodegenerative disorders. The current challenge is to integrate our understanding of disease-linked processes in the fly with our growing knowledge of human disease, for the benefit of patients.

Keywords:

Drosophila *disease model, motor neuron, neurodegeneration, systemic amyloidosis, tauopathy, toxic oligomer.*

Introduction

The fruitfly *Drosophila melanogaster* has proven to be a powerful model organism for the study of amyloid proteinopathies. There are two main reasons for this success, first, there is a great deal of genetic and cell biological orthology between the fly and the human, and secondly, there are many powerful genetic tools that can be employed. The most prolific has been the

[1]To whom correspondence should be addressed (email dcc26@cam.ac.uk).

work on amyloid diseases that are restricted primarily to the central nervous system. These are characterized by a relatively small load of amyloid protein, but with the principal toxicity being derived from soluble amyloid precursor species. The fly has also been used to model human systemic amyloidoses where the pathology is related both to the bulk of protein deposition, as well as a contribution from a 'toxic oligomer' fraction.

Regardless of the particular amyloid disease being studied, the modelling work in flies has tended to group into a number of themes. These include the initial creation of a model where a particular protein, when aggregating, causes any of a wide range of fly phenotypes. Such experimental observations may be behavioural, related to longevity or alternatively linked to the microscopic or biochemical constituents of fly tissues. Once an initial model is created, follow-up studies are then able to answer more mechanistic questions, in particular what genes and proteins are involved in the pathogenesis. This often involves genetic screening for modifiers of the phenotypes and, of course, *Drosophila* is particularly well suited to such applications. Although occasionally such studies reveal insights that are of importance for fly biology, an example may be the role of aging in insect physiology [1,2], it is more often the case that investigators look to translate their findings to a human clinical context. In this case, the results in the fly usually require further experimental validation in mammalian cell culture and vertebrate model systems, often in the mouse, before interfacing with the clinic.

In the present chapter, we will describe tissue-specific amyloid disease models, focusing on nervous system disease and specifically on AD (Alzheimer's disease). We will also mention how flies have been used to model a localized non-neurological disorder of the pancreatic islets [IAPP (islet amyloid polypeptide) amyloidosis] that is linked to Type II diabetes. Finally, we will provide an introduction to the modelling of systemic amyloidoses in the fly.

Fly models of neurodegenerative diseases

The common neurodegenerative disorders are each characterized by particular amyloid-like protein aggregates that are either intracellular, such as tau tangles and α-synuclein containing Lewy bodies, or extracellular, such as β-amyloid plaques. These observations have stimulated interest in the molecular pathogenesis of such proteinopathies and whether there may be some processes that are common to all. Although the most powerful risk factor for most neurodegenerative disorders is advanced age, all else being equal, the balance of clinical risk is genetic. Despite intensive research, our understanding of both aging and the genetics of dementia is limited. Fly model systems have been used for the study of the genetics and pathological mechanisms of most of the amyloid neurodegenerative diseases, including models of AD, familial tauopathies, as well as prion, Parkinson's, Huntington's and motor neuron diseases [3–17] (Table 1).

Fly models of Aβ (amyloid β-peptide) toxicity in AD

There is a wealth of evidence that familial AD, which is inherited as an autosomal dominant condition and accounts for up to 5% of cases, is caused by the production of an aggregation-prone spectrum of Aβ peptides. In health, the endoproteolytic processing of the APP (amyloid precursor protein) (Figure 1) is achieved by a two-cleavage process, the second being performed by γ-secretase that releases predominantly a 40 amino acid peptide (Aβ_{40}). In disease, either the total amount of Aβ is increased or the sequence of the peptide is changed to make it more aggregation

Table 1. Summary of fly models for amyloid diseases

FUS, fused-in-sarcoma; PrP^{Sc}, disease-specific conformation of prion protein; TDP, transactive response DNA-binding protein.

Human disease modelled	Characteristic amyloid(-like) deposit	Experimental approach	Reference(s)
AD	β-Amyloid plaque and tau tangles	Human APP expression with β-secretase supplementation, Aβ peptide secretion, and combination of Aβ secretion and human tau expression	[3–8]
Tauopathies	Tau tangles	Wild-type and disease-linked variant tau expression, and pseudo-phosphorylated tau expression	[9,10]
Prion disease	PrP^{Sc} plaques	Wild-type and disease-linked variant PrP expression, and demonstration of oral infectivity	[11,12]
Parkinson's disease	Lewy bodies and Lewy neurite inclusions	Wild-type and disease-linked variant α-synuclein expression	[13]
Huntington's disease	Intranuclear inclusions	polyQ expression	[14,15]
Motor neuron disease	TDP-44 inclusions and FUS inclusions	TDP-43 and FUS expression	[16,17]

prone; most commonly the proportion of the 42 amino acid isoform (Aβ$_{42}$) is increased. There are mutations in three genes that account for almost all cases of familial AD and these are APP and presenilin-1 and -2; the last two gene products comprise the catalytic subunit of γ-secretase. In recent years, some concern has accumulated that aberrant production of Aβ may not explain the more common sporadic forms of AD, indeed these fears have been increased by the absence of familial AD genes from the GWAS (genome-wide association study) list that now includes 21 risk genes. However, strong support for the role of Aβ in the generation of AD comes from the finding that a distinct mutation in APP, that hinders proteolysis and hence Aβ production, protects against sporadic AD and also against benign age-related memory impairment [18].

The Aβ peptide is thought to contribute primarily to extracellular pathology, with aggregation occurring either in the extracellular space or alternatively in the lumina of intracellular vesicles. Peptide aggregates grow and eventually form the classical β-amyloid plaques that are a diagnostic feature of AD. In the fly, we can recreate some of the features of AD by driving the expression of Aβ in the brain or retina using one of two main strategies. The first approach most closely replicates the pathology in the human and involves the recreation, to a varying

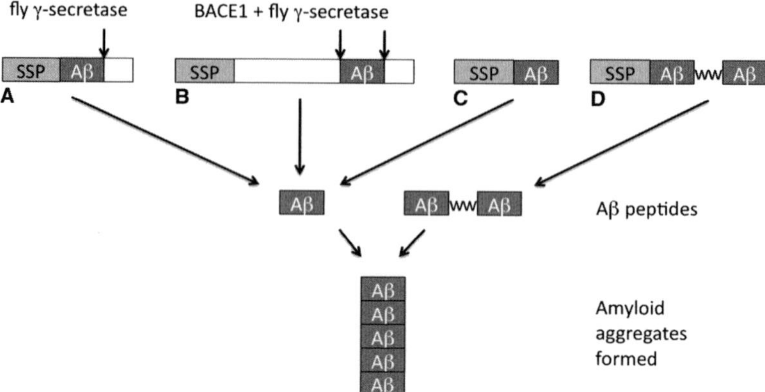

Figure 1. Transgenic constructs used to study the toxicity of Aβ
The first studies expressed truncated human APP (**A**) truncated at what would otherwise be the β-secretase cleavage site [3]. This model relies only on endogenous fly γ-secretase to release mature Aβ. Subsequently, models in which the human APP processing machinery is largely replicated involved making flies that are transgenic for both human APP and BACE1 (**B**) [5]. The aforementioned systems are useful for studying not only the toxicity of the generated Aβ, but also allow screening for secretase inhibitors. Alternatively, Aβ peptides of specific length and with desired sequences can be expressed downstream of an SSP (**C**) [4,6,7]. The Aβ peptides are typically coded for as monomers, but the generation of tandem Aβ peptides (**D**) may also be of interest [23]. The amyloid deposits in all model systems appear to be largely similar.

degree, of the full human APP processing pathway in the fly. To this end, human APP may be expressed along with human BACE1 (β-site amyloid precursor protein-cleaving enzyme 1) that is required to initiate proteolytic cleavage. Alternatively, BACE-1 can be dispensed with if truncated human APP is expressed instead of the full-length protein, yielding a functionally 'pre-cleaved' polypeptide. In both cases, the endogenous *Drosophila* γ-secretase activity generates sufficient Aβ to cause neurotoxic phenotypes. The second approach consists of expressing Aβ fused to an N-terminal SSP (secretion signal peptide). This simplified approach has the disadvantage that it may not generate Aβ in the correct subcellular compartment as do human neurone, but it provides the investigator with the ability to determine exactly which Aβ isoform is expressed in the fly's brain. To the degree that the two approaches have been compared, they seem to generate similar phenotypes in the fly (Figure 2) including Aβ deposition, neuronal and retinal degeneration and reduced longevity [4–7,19].

Fly models expressing Aβ have probed the mechanism of neurotoxicity in two main ways. The first has taken a biophysical approach and asked what features of the peptide are responsible for its aggregation behaviour and which aggregated species correlate most closely with toxic phenotypes [20]. In a systematic survey of single amino acid substitutions in the Aβ peptide, Luheshi and co-workers showed that, although the predicted propensity to form mature amyloid fibrils correlate well, there were certain Aβ variants, and the I31E/E22G Aβ$_{42}$ in particular, that showed surprisingly little toxicity considering their predicted and observed rates of amyloid fibril formation [21,22]. Such outliers were better accounted for, and the overall correlation with phenotype was better correlated, when the propensity to form prefibrillar, rather than fibrillar, species was considered [21].

The primary role of oligomeric species in mediating the toxicity of Aβ was further underlined by a study in which Aβ peptides were joined together into a single tandem Aβ using a

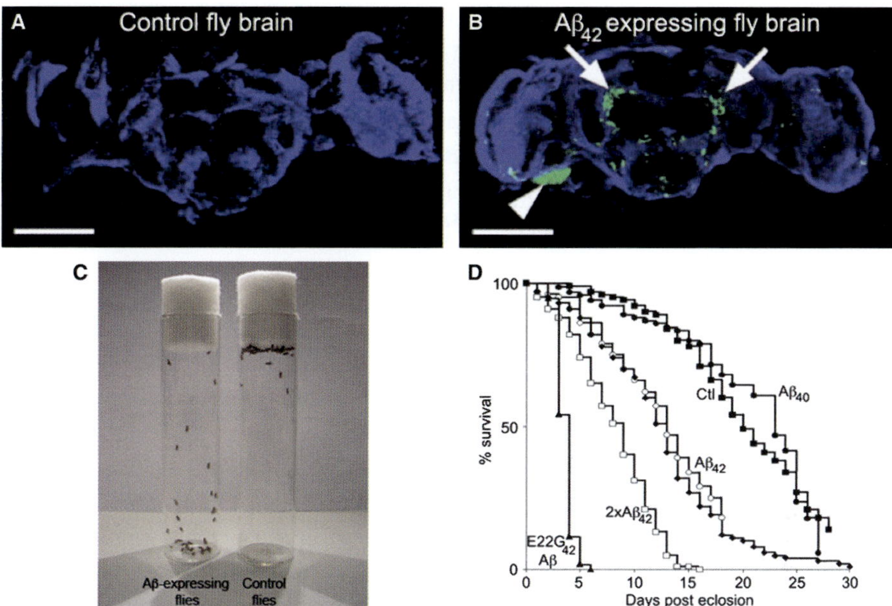

Figure 2. A selection of phenotypes from flies expressing Aβ peptides
Amyloid-binding dyes such as Thioflavin S, or here with luminescence-conjugated polythiophenes, exhibit little background staining in control flies (**A**, green staining absent) while clearly highlighting amyloid deposits (**B**, green staining and arrows). Fluorescence microscopy may be performed on brain sections; alternatively, confocal images of whole brain mounts are often more convenient. A number of behavioural phenotypes have been successfully used to monitor disease progression amongst which locomotor function is often assessed (**C**). Longevity analysis is often the gold-standard assay, measuring as it does the general functioning of the organism (**D**). In this Figure, we see that flies expressing single $A\beta_{42}$ transgenes ($A\beta_{42}$) die sooner than those carrying either $A\beta_{40}$ or control (Ctl) flies. Doubling the number of Aβ42 transgenes ($2 \times A\beta_{42}$) or expressing an aggregation-prone peptide variant (E22G $A\beta_{42}$) markedly reduces lifespan.

flexible glycine-rich linker peptide. The remarkable finding in that study was that, although both tandem $A\beta_{40}$ and tandem $A\beta_{42}$ both aggregated rapidly to form large amyloid-like deposits in the fly brain, only tandem $A\beta_{42}$ was toxic and this was linked to the copious amounts of oligomeric aggregates that were present. By contrast, tandem $A\beta_{40}$ was non-toxic and in fly brains, accordingly, $A\beta_{40}$ oligomers were essentially absent [23].

The second strategy for investigating the mechanism of Aβ neurotoxicity exploits the many tools that are available for undertaking genetic modifier screens in the fly. Two screens have been published that have used random insertion of enhancing transposon-like elements in to the fly genome, looking predominantly for dominant gain of gene function. Of the tens of genes implicated by these screens, a common thread is the importance of metal metabolism in mediating Aβ toxicity. Specifically, genes regulating copper [24] and iron [25] metabolism are highlighted while other functional themes include oxidative stress and transcriptional regulation. Typically, once a genetic screen has been completed, the fly can also be used to further investigate candidate genes. For example, the finding that copper-related genes were modifiers of Aβ toxicity was followed by studies in flies showing that oral copper chelation therapy [26] and the genetic knockdown of a high-affinity copper transporter [27] were both beneficial. Likewise, the chelation of iron, either by expressing the heavy and light chains of ferritin [25] or by feeding the flies with an iron-specific chelator also suppressed Aβ toxicity [28]. For both copper and iron, there is evidence that there may be two toxic modes of action for the metals: first, the metal may act to delay progression of oligomeric aggregates to less toxic larger Aβ amyloid species [27,28] and secondly, the metals may enhance the oxidative damage associated with amyloid deposition [25]. Whether these two mechanisms of amyloid toxicity are linked or independent of each other is not known.

Fly models of tau toxicity in AD

Of course, AD is not just an extracellular disease, but is characterized equally by cytoplasmic amyloid-like pathology involving hyperphosphorylated forms of the microtubule-binding protein tau. Although mutations in tau can themselves cause neurodegenerative diseases (such as fronto-temporal dementia with Parkinsonism [29]) the involvement in AD appears to be downstream of other predisposing factors, including Aβ accumulation. The fly has proven to be a powerful model organism for the study of tau toxicity, not least because of the clear rough eye phenotype that results when wild-type, but more so when mutant tau is expressed in the retina [9]. However, the expression of human tau alone does not lead to detectable amyloid-like neurofibrillary pathology. For this, GSK-3B (glycogen synthase kinase 3B) (*shaggy* in the fly) also needs to be up-regulated [30], supporting the role of kinase dysregulation in the development of mature tau pathology. Since these early studies, the popularity of the tau-expressing fly has grown rapidly, not least because the rough eye phenotype appears during development and so can be assessed upon eclosion (hatching) of the adult fly. In practical terms this means that the first round of genetic or pharmacological screening data can be acquired only 11 days following the initial mating of the parental flies, thus allowing the convenient screening of many (hundreds or even thousands) of conditions.

Consequently, systematic genetic modifier screening has become possible and these studies now comprise one of the two major applications of human tau-expressing flies. In the first screening studies, enhancing mobile genetic elements (EP elements) were used to randomly disrupt gene expression and the consequent changes in the rough eye were assessed [31]. In this way, Shulman and Feany [31] identified a number of kinases and phosphatases as modifiers, again supporting the pathogenic importance of tau phosphorylation. They also found components of apoptotic pathways and cytoskeletal components to be modifiers. In complementary studies, Blard et al. [32] and Fulga et al. [33] confirmed the importance of cytoskeletal components and additionally found chaperones to be highly represented modifiers.

These studies are beautiful examples of forward genetics, whereby a phenotype is created and then screening techniques are used to determine which genes are responsible. Recently, a related study design was used to illuminate the genetic data coming from GWASs in AD. By expressing RNAi constructs in the retina, alongside human Tau^{V337M}, the investigators found that nine out of 87 fly orthologues of human AD GWAS genes ($P < 10^{-4}$) resulted in synergistic toxicity [34]. Interestingly, this candidate RNAi screen highlighted *CD2AP*, a gene that had already been identified as carrying a risk for AD [35]. Furthermore, two genes, *FERMT2* and *CELF1* that were identified in the fly screen, were subsequently shown to possess genome-wide significance in the latest AD GWAS meta-analysis [36]. Lambert and colleagues also used clinical data alongside a fly model to show that the *Drosophila* orthologue of the AD GWAS gene, *BIN1*, is likely to be involved in mediating the tau toxicity [37]. The authors conclude that a subset of the proteins coded for by GWAS candidate genes are likely to modify AD risk through interactions with tau.

The second major application of tau-expressing flies has focused on understanding how phosphorylation disrupts the interaction between tau and microtubules and consequently favours neurotoxicity and the formation of amyloid-like inclusions that characterize AD. Initial work indicated that the mutation of 14 key serine and threonine phosphorylation sites to alanine markedly reduced tau toxicity in *Drosophila*. Conversely, the generation of a pseudo-phosphorylated tau variant (tau[E14]), with the same residues replaced with glutamate residues, significantly increased toxicity [38]. A more detailed dissection of the individual sites indicated that PAR1 (partitioning defective 1) kinase {the fly orthologue of the mammalian MARKs (microtubule affinity-regulating kinases) [39,40]}, by phosphorylating Ser^{262} and Ser^{356}, exerts a gate-keeping role and is required for the subsequent action of other kinases such as the fly orthologues of CDK5 and GSK-3 [41]. Phosphorylation at Ser^{262} reduces the affinity of human tau for microtubules and so it is conceivable that unbound tau is a preferred substrate for these kinases. In any case, these latter phosphorylation events constitute the diagnostically important epitopes of monoclonal antibodies such as AT8, AT100, AT180 and PHF1 and were each found to contribute rather uniformly to incremental tau toxicity using the fly as model system [42]. Interestingly, a study by Iijima-Ando et al. [43] has shown that depleting axons of their mitochondria in the fly brain results in increased PAR1 and consequent Ser^{262} phosphorylation. Previous reports have indicated that Aβ can reduce axonal mitochondria numbers and this points to the importance of PAR1 in linking Aβ with tau pathology [43]. Other workers have suggested that kinases including JNK [44,45] may be involved in Aβ toxicity, and in particular GSK-3B, in the form of its fly orthologue *shaggy*, may underpin tau hyperphosphorylation [10].

Fly models of combined Aβ and tau toxicity in AD

The link between Aβ and tau pathologies in AD has also been explored directly using fly models. Such studies have supported the role of Ser^{262} as a gatekeeper phosphorylation site; notably, flies carrying wild-type human tau exhibit synergistic toxicity when Aβ is co-expressed (Figure 3), an effect that is suppressed when the phosphorylation-resistant S262A substitution is introduced into tau [46]. The subsequent kinase cascade and tau hyperphosphorylation in the presence of Aβ also generates some of the clinically relevant phosphoepitopes on tau such as AT8 and AT180 [8].

Pancreatic islet amyloidosis

A characteristic feature of Type II diabetes is the accumulation of amyloid, composed of IAPP, in the pancreatic islets. IAPP is synthesized as prepro-hormone and serially cleaved to yield the mature peptide that is co-secreted with insulin. Whereas the physiological role of mature IAPP is to inhibit further insulin secretion, its oligomeric aggregates are also thought to contribute to islet β-cell loss in disease [47]. The IAPP from humans, other primates and cats is highly prone to form amyloid; by contrast rodent IAPP does not aggregate, the likely reason being a loss of sequence conservation at positions 20–29 [48]. With these findings in mind, Schultz et al. [49] created three lines of flies expressing either human pro-IAPP or else the mature isoforms of the human or mouse peptides. In this system the transgenic peptides were targeted for secretion from neurons of the central nervous system, using a signal peptide and

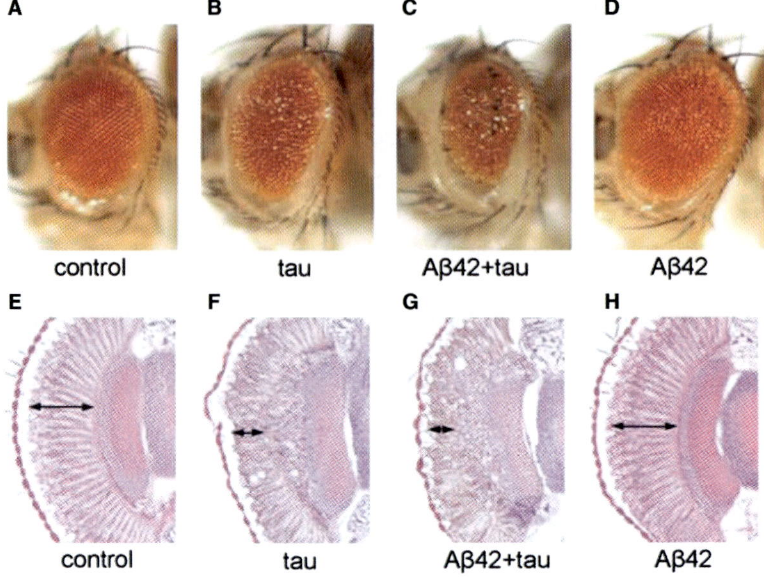

Figure 3. Expression of Aβ$_{42}$, tau or the both proteins together in the *Drosophila* retina

The external fly eye is composed of a regular array of photosensitive elements called ommatidia (**A**) that may be disrupted by Aβ$_{42}$ expression (**D**) and tau (**B**), but more so by both together (**C**). Similarly, there is a synthetic toxicity when the morphology of the retina is examined (**E–H**) [46].

the *elav^{c155}-gal4* driver. Remarkably, despite the deposition of amyloid in flies expressing both the pro-IAPP and the mature IAPP, only the former exhibited an associated reduction in longevity. As expected, the murine IAPP did not aggregate to form amyloid and was not significantly toxic to the flies. Although this study could not explain the peculiar toxicity of pro-IAPP in the fly, the disruption of pro-peptide cleavage in mammalian cell culture also results in amyloid deposition and cell death [50,51].

Drosophila models of systemic amyloidoses

In the systemic amyloidoses protein deposits are found in any or all of the viscera, connective tissue and blood vessels of the body except for the brain [52]. The polypeptides that constitute the amyloid deposits are varied and may accumulate both in the organ of synthesis and also at distant sites. With regard to *Drosophila* as a model organism, the specific organs involved may be different; however, the principle of local synthesis and distant accumulation and tissue toxicity may be maintained. In the clinic, systemic amyloidoses may be acquired as a consequence of a second disorder linked to the production of an amyloidogenic protein; examples include immunoglobulin light chain and serum amyloid A amyloidoses in chronic inflammatory disorders and haematological malignancies (amyloidoses tabulated in [53]). By contrast, hereditary amyloidosis results from sequence variation in a polypeptide that increases its propensity to misfold; examples include mutations in the genes for TTR (transthyretin) and lysozyme. More common than both of these forms are the sporadic forms of amyloidosis where the only risk factor is advanced age [54]; a good example of this is the common presence of TTR amyloid [55].

Classically, tissue dysfunction in systemic amyloidoses is considered to be a consequence of amyloid replacing functional tissue or else by changing the biophysical properties of organs such as the heart or blood vessels. In these respects, murine models have been informative because of their physiological proximity to humans. Fly modelling, on the other hand, has illuminated some of the defences that an organism has against amyloid, in the form of ER (endoplasmic reticulum) quality control systems. Moreover, the role of oligomeric aggregates in the neuropathic aspects of TTR amyloidosis has been particularly highlighted by fly results.

Lysozyme amyloidosis

Lysozyme is an important part of the human innate immune system, mediating as it does the hydrolysis of Gram-positive bacteria. In humans, it is abundant in secretions including saliva, tears and mucus; interestingly, in the fly, lysozyme functions predominantly as a digestive enzyme [56]. The first families in which lysozyme was linked to amyloidosis carried mutations coding for the I56T and D67H variants [57]; subsequent studies also linked the F57I variant to disease [58]. Taking advantage of the growing understanding of the structural biology of lysozyme, Kumita et al. [59] expressed two of these lysozyme variants in *Drosophila*. By expressing the destabilized lysozyme variants D67H and F57I, they found that the mutant proteins were expressed at much lower levels than wild-type, a finding that mirrored what had already been observed in yeast [60,61]. This is likely to be because stimulation of the UPR (unfolded protein response) results in ER-associated degradation and the removal of most of the unstable polypeptide. Despite this clearance of amyloidogenic peptides, the unstable lysozyme variants still caused a rough eye phenotype. One may conclude that the toxicity phenotypes are either a result of the UPR itself or else it may be the small fraction of mutant lysozyme that survives that is toxic. The latter seems likely, as clinical lysozyme amyloidosis is predominantly a visceral disease affecting tissues remote from its site of synthesis.

TTR amyloidosis

TTR is synthesized mainly in the liver and forms homotetramers that carry thyroxine in the circulation. The destabilization of TTR tetramers and the misfolding of the monomers are required for the formation of TTR amyloid. Such deposits are characteristic of both sporadic SSA (senile systemic amyloidosis) and FAP (familial amyloid polyneuropathy), both of which result in peripheral nerve damage and may be associated with cardiomyopathy. Although SSA is late onset and is linked to wild-type TTR, mutations in the gene underpin FAP and result in earlier onset, particularly in the Portuguese population [62]. To date, murine models of FAP replicate the visceral amyloid deposition, but have failed to show significant neuropathy [63–65], and consequently a *Drosophila* model has been developed [66]. By expressing the clinically important L55P and the artificially destabilized V14N/V16E variants, adult-onset neurodegeneration and TTR deposition were observed in the brains and retinas of flies. Notably, these TTR mutant organisms also exhibited neuropathological behaviours including abnormal wing posturing and flight defects, suggesting mutated TTR can travel from the cells of synthesis in the retina to distant sites via the circulation. Intriguingly, despite the larger quantity of TTR amyloid deposits detected in flies carrying two copies of the mutant transgene, as compared with those carrying a single copy, the heavier amyloid deposition was associated with less severe neurological phenotypes. Likewise, when tissue extracts were taken from the flies it was found that young flies with only one TTR transgene generated more

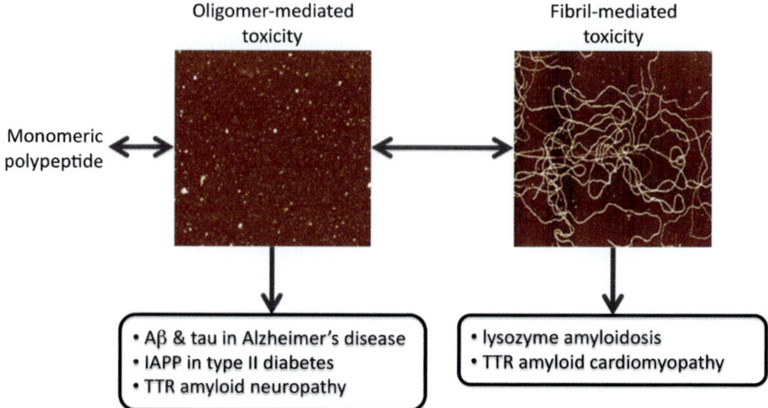

Figure 4. Fly models have allowed the investigation of the relative importance of oligomer- and fibril-mediated toxicity mechanisms
In this Figure, oligomers are shown causing predominantly tissue-specific and neuronal disorders while fibril deposition causes disease by replacing functional tissue or changing the biophysical characteristics of an organ. Re-used from [70]; William Blaine Stine, Jr, Karie N. Dahlgren, Grant K. Krafft, Mary Jo LaDu, (2002), In vitro characterization of conditions for amyloid-β peptide oligomerization and fibrillogenesis, Journal of Biological Chemistry, 278(13), 11612–22 Copyright © 2002, by the American Society for Biochemistry and Molecular Biology.

cytotoxic extracts when tested *in vitro* than those carrying two transgenes. The authors conclude that this surprising pattern of toxicity resulted from the incorporation of TTR into less toxic quasi-crystalline arrays of protein in the fat tissue of flies expressing high levels of the mutant proteins [67].

This protective sequestration of amyloidogenic protein in mature aggregates is mirrored by the subsequent finding that co-expression of serum amyloid P protein also reduced TTR toxicity, but this time by binding to and inactivating oligomeric aggregates without affecting overall amyloid formation [68]. The balance between fibrillar and oligomeric forms of TTR may hold the key to whether the consequences of accumulation are bulk amyloid deposition or else oligomer toxicity. The molecular environment in various tissues may hold the key and this is supported by a fly model showing that heparin can nucleate fibril formation, and consequently, alter the balance between TTR fibrils, which characterize cardiomyopathic infiltration, as compared with neuropathic cases where perhaps oligomeric toxicity is more important [69] (Figure 4).

Conclusions

The fly has proven to be a valuable model organism for the study of the full range of amyloid diseases because of the power of the genetic tools that are available and also because the speed and low costs allow many and varied experiments to be performed. Current approaches allow the dissection of pathological mechanisms using a mixture of unbiased genetic screens and targeted hypothesis-driven experiments. Neurological diseases have proven to be particularly well suited to study in the fly and the result has been a number of insights into the genetics and the role of protein aggregates in their pathogenesis. Fly models continue to play their role in the armoury of the biomedical scientist, complementing both mammalian *in vivo* models and cell-based systems.

Summary

- The expression of aggregation-prone polypeptides in *Drosophila* results in amyloid-disease-related phenotypes such as reduced longevity, developmental eye disruption and impaired locomotor behaviour.
- The systematic study of fly models can yield information about which aggregated states of polypeptides are most toxic, such as oligomers.
- Employing the genetic tools that are available to the fly biologist allow us to understand the genes underpinning disease-linked phenotypes.
- Integration of disease pathways in the fly with information in patients with the disease allows us to develop novel biomarkers and therapeutic interventions.

References

1. Jacobson, J., Lambert, A.J., Portero-Otín, M., Pamplona, R., Magwere, T., Miwa, S., Driege, Y., Brand, M.D. and Partridge, L. (2010) Biomarkers of aging in *Drosophila*. Aging Cell **9**, 466–477

2. Rogers, I., Kerr, F., Martinez, P., Hardy, J., Lovestone, S. and Partridge, L. (2012) Ageing increases vulnerability to Aβ42 toxicity in *Drosophila*. PLoS ONE **7**, e40569

3. Fossgreen, A., Brückner, B., Czech, C., Masters, C.L., Beyreuther, K. and Paro, R. (1998) Transgenic *Drosophila* expressing human amyloid precursor protein showg-secretase activity and blistered wing phenotype. Proc. Natl. Acad. Sci. U.S.A. **95**, 13703–13708

4. Finelli, A., Kelkar, A., Song, H.J., Yang, H. and Konsolaki, M. (2004) A model for studying Alzheimer's Aβ42-induced toxicity in *Drosophila melanogaster*. Mol. Cell. Neurosci. **26**, 365–375

5. Greeve, I., Kretzschmar, D., Tschape, J.A., Beyn, A., Brellinger, C., Schweizer, M., Nitsch, R.M. and Reifegerste, R. (2004) Age-dependent neurodegeneration and Alzheimer-amyloid plaque formation in transgenic *Drosophila*. J. Neurosci. **24**, 3899–3906

6. Iijima, K., Liu, H.P., Chiang, A.S., Hearn, S.A., Konsolaki, M. and Zhong, Y. (2004) Dissecting the pathological effects of human Aβ40 and Aβ42 in *Drosophila*: a potential model for Alzheimer's disease. Proc. Natl. Acad. Sci. U.S.A. **101**, 6623–6628

7. Crowther, D.C., Kinghorn, K.J., Miranda, E., Page, R., Curry, J.A., Duthie, F.A., Gubb, D.C. and Lomas, D.A. (2005) Intraneuronal Aβ, non-amyloid aggregates and neurodegeneration in a *Drosophila* model of Alzheimer's disease. Neuroscience **132**, 123–135

8. Folwell, J., Cowan, C.M., Ubhi, K.K., Shiabh, H., Newman, T.A., Shepherd, D. and Medher, A. (2009) Aβ exacerbates the neuronal dysfunction caused by human tau expression in a *Drosophila* model of Alzheimer's disease. Exp. Neurol. **223**, 401–409

9. Wittmann, C.W., Wszolek, M.F., Shulman, J.M., Salvaterra, P.M., Lewis, J., Hutton, M. and Feany, M.B. (2001) Tauopathy in *Drosophila*: neurodegeneration without neurofibrillary tangles. Science **293**, 711–714

10. Mudher, A., Shepherd, D., Newman, T.A., Mildren, P., Jukes, J.P., Squire, A., Mears, A., Drummond, J.A., Berg, S., MacKay, D. et al. (2004) GSK-3β inhibition reverses axonal transport defects and behavioural phenotypes in *Drosophila*. Mol. Psychiatry **9**, 522–530

11. Gavin, B.A., Dolph, M.J., Deleault, N.R., Geoghegan, J.C., Khurana, V., Feany, M.B., Dolph, P.J. and Supattapone, S. (2006) Accelerated accumulation of misfolded prion protein and spongiform degeneration in a *Drosophila* model of Gerstmann–Straussler–Scheinker syndrome. J. Neurosci. **26**, 12408–12414

12. Thackray, A.M., Muhammad, F., Zhang, C., Denyer, M., Spiropoulos, J., Crowther, D.C. and Bujdoso, R. (2012) Prion-induced toxicity in PrP transgenic *Drosophila*. Exp. Mol. Pathol. **92**, 194–201

13. Feany, M.B. and Bender, W.W. (2000) A *Drosophila* model of Parkinson's disease. Nature **404**, 394–398

14. Steffan, J.S., Bodai, L., Pallos, J., Poelman, M., McCampbell, A., Apostol, B.L., Kazantsev, A., Schmidt, E., Zhu, Y.Z., Greenwald, M. et al. (2001) Histone deacetylase inhibitors arrest polyglutamine-dependent neurodegeneration in *Drosophila*. Nature **413**, 739–743

15. Karpuj, M.V., Becher, M.W., Springer, J.E., Chabas, D., Youssef, S., Pedotti, R., Mitchell, D. and Steinman, L. (2002) Prolonged survival and decreased abnormal movements in transgenic model of Huntington disease, with administration of the transglutaminase inhibitor cystamine. Nat. Med. **8**, 143–149

16. Lagier-Tourenne, C., Polymenidou, M. and Cleveland, D.W. (2010) TDP-43 and FUS/TLS: emerging roles in RNA processing and neurodegeneration. Hum. Mol. Genet. **19**, R46–R64

17. Lanson, N.A.J., Maltare, A., King, H., Smith, R., Kim, J.H., Taylor, J.P., Lloyd, T.E. and Pandey, U.B. (2011) A *Drosophila* model of FUS-related neurodegeneration reveals genetic interaction between FUS and TDP-43. Hum. Mol. Genet. **20**, 2510–2523

18. Jonsson, T., Atwal, J.K., Steinberg, S., Snaedal, J., Jonsson, P.V., Bjornsson, S., Stefansson, H., Sulem, P., Gudbjartsson, D., Maloney, J. et al. (2012) A mutation in APP protects against Alzheimer's disease and age-related cognitive decline. Nature **488**, 96–99

19. Berg, I., Nilsson, K.P., Thor, S. and Hammarstrom, P. (2010) Efficient imaging of amyloid deposits in *Drosophila* models of human amyloidoses. Nat. Protoc. **5**, 935–944

20. Iijima, K., Chiang, H.C., Hearn, S.A., Hakker, I., Gatt, A., Shenton, C., Granger, L., Leung, A., Iijima-Ando, K. and Zhong, Y. (2008) Aβ42 mutants with different aggregation profiles induce distinct pathologies in *Drosophila*. PLoS ONE **3**, e1703

21. Luheshi, L.M., Tartaglia, G.G., Brorsson, A.C., Pawar, A.P., Watson, I.E., Chiti, F., Vendruscolo, M., Lomas, D.A., Dobson, C.M. and Crowther, D.C. (2007) Systematic *in vivo* analysis of the intrinsic determinants of amyloid β pathogenicity. PLoS Biol. **5**, e290

22. Brorsson, A.C., Bolognesi, B., Tartaglia, G.G., Shammas, S.L., Favrin, G., Watson, I., Lomas, D.A., Chiti, F., Vendruscolo, M., Dobson, C.M. et al. (201) Intrinsic determinants of neurotoxic aggregate formation by the amyloid β peptide. Biophys. J. **98**, 1677–1684

23. Speretta, E., Jahn, T.R., Tartaglia, G.G., Favrin, G., Barros, T.P., Imarisio, S., Lomas, D.A., Luheshi, L.M., Crowther, D.C. and Dobson, C.M. (2012) Expression in *Drosophila* of tandem amyloid beta peptides provides insights into links between aggregation and neurotoxicity. J. Biol. Chem. **287**, 20748–20754

24. Cao, W., Song, H.J., Gangi, T., Kelkar, A., Antani, I., Garza, D. and Konsolaki, M. (2008) Identification of novel genes that modify phenotypes induced by Alzheimer's β-amyloid overexpression in *Drosophila*. Genetics **178**, 1457–1471

25. Rival, T., Page, R.M., Chandraratna, D.S., Sendall, T.J., Ryder, E., Liu, B., Lewis, H., Rosahl, T., Hider, R., Camargo, L.M. et al. (2009) Fenton chemistry and oxidative stress mediate the toxicity of the β-amyloid peptide in a *Drosophila* model of Alzheimer's disease. Eur. J. Neurosci. **29**, 1335–1347

26. Singh, S.K., Sinha, P., Mishra, L. and Srikrishna, S. (2013) Neuroprotective role of a novel copper chelator against Aβ_{42} induced neurotoxicity. Int. J. Alzheimers Dis. **2013**, 567128

27. Lang, M., Fan, Q., Wang, L., Zheng, Y., Xiao, G., Wang, X., Wang, W., Zhong, Y. and Zhou, B. (2013) Inhibition of human high-affinity copper importer Ctr1 orthologous in the nervous system of *Drosophila* ameliorates Aβ42-induced Alzheimer's disease-like symptoms. Neurobiol. Aging **34**, 2604–2612

28. Liu, B., Moloney, A., Meehan, S., Morris, K., Thomas, S.E., Serpell, L.C., Hider, R., Marciniak, S.J., Lomas, D.A. and Crowther, D.C. (2011) Iron promotes the toxicity of amyloid β peptide by impeding its ordered aggregation. J. Biol. Chem. **286**, 4248–4256

29. Goedert, M. and Spillantini, M.G. (2000) Tau mutations in frontotemporal dementia FTDP-17 and their relevance for Alzheimer's disease. Biochim. Biophys. Acta **1502**, 110–121

30. Jackson, G.R., Wiedau-Pazos, M., Sang, T.K., Wagle, N., Brown, C.A., Massachi, S. and Geschwind, D.H. (2002) Human wild-type tau interacts with wingless pathway components and produces neurofibrillary pathology in *Drosophila*. Neuron **34**, 509–519

31. Shulman, J.M. and Feany, M.B. (2003) Genetic modifiers of tauopathy in *Drosophila*. Genetics **165**, 1233–1242

32. Blard, O., Feuillette, S., Bou, J., Chaumette, B., Frebourg, T., Campion, D. and Lecourtois, M. (2007) Cytoskeleton proteins are modulators of mutant tau-induced neurodegeneration in *Drosophila*. Hum. Mol. Genet. **16**, 555–566

33. Fulga, T.A., Elson-Schwab, I., Khurana, V., Steinhilb, M.L., Spires, T.L., Hyman, B.T. and Feany, M.B. (2007) Abnormal bundling and accumulation of F-actin mediates tau-induced neuronal degeneration *in vivo*. Nat. Cell Biol. **9**, 139–148

34. Shulman, J.M., Imboywa, S., Giagtzoglou, N., Powers, M.P., Hu, Y., Devenport, D., Chipendo, P., Chibnik, L.B., Diamond, A., Perrimon, N. et al. (2014) Functional screening in *Drosophila* identifies Alzheimer's disease susceptibility genes and implicates Tau-mediated mechanisms. Hum. Mol. Genet. **23**, 870–877

35. Hollingworth, P., Harold, D., Sims, R., Gerrish, A., Lambert, J.C., Carrasquillo, M.M., Abraham, R., Hamshere, M.L., Pahwa, J.S., Moskvina, V. et al. (2011) Common variants at ABCA7, MS4A6A/MS4A4E, EPHA1, CD33 and CD2AP are associated with Alzheimer's disease. Nat. Genet. **43**, 429–435

36. Lambert, J.C., Ibrahim-Verbaas, C.A., Harold, D., Naj, A.C., Sims, R., Bellenguez, C., Jun, G., DeStefano, A.L., Bis, J.C., Beecham, G.W. et al. (2013) Meta-analysis of 74,046 individuals identifies 11 new susceptibility loci for Alzheimer's disease. Nat Genet. **45**, 1452–1458

37. Chapuis, J., Hansmannel, F., Gistelinck, M., Mounier, A., Van Cauwenberghe, C., Kolen, K.V., Geller, F., Sottejeau, Y., Harold, D., Dourlen, P. et al. (2013) Increased expression of BIN1 mediates Alzheimer genetic risk by modulating tau pathology. Mol. Psychiatry **18**, 1225–1234

38. Steinhilb, M.L., Dias-Santagata, D., Mulkearns, E.E., Shulman, J.M., Biernat, J., Mandelkow, E.M. and Feany, M.B. (2007) S/P and T/P phosphorylation is critical for tau neurotoxicity in *Drosophila*. J. Neurosci. Res. **85**, 1271–1278

39. Drewes, G., Ebneth, A., Preuss, U., Mandelkow, E.M. and Mandelkow, E. (1997) MARK, a novel family of protein kinases that phosphorylate microtubule-associated proteins and trigger microtubule disruption. Cell **89**, 297–308

40. Trinczek, B., Brajenovic, M., Ebneth, A. and Drewes, G. (2003) MARK4 is a novel microtubule-associated proteins/microtubule affinity-regulating kinase that binds to the cellular microtubule network and to centrosomes. J. Biol. Chem. **279**, 5915–5923

41. Nishimura, I., Yang, Y., Lu, B. (2004) PAR-1 kinase plays an initiator role in a temporally ordered phosphorylation process that confers tau toxicity in *Drosophila*. Cell **116**, 671–682

42. Steinhilb, M.L., Dias-Santagata, D., Fulga, T.A., Felch, D.L. and Feany, M.B. (2007) Tau phosphorylation sites work in concert to promote neurotoxicity *in vivo*. Mol. Biol. Cell **18**, 5060–5068

43. Iijima-Ando, K., Sekiya, M., Maruko-Otake, A., Ohtake, Y., Suzuki, E., Lu, B. and Iijima, K.M. (2012) Loss of axonal mitochondria promotes tau-mediated neurodegeneration and Alzheimer's disease-related tau phosphorylation via PAR-1. PLoS Genet. **8**, e1002918

44. Tare, M., Modi, R.M., Nainaparampil, J.J., Puli, O.R., Bedi, S., Fernandez-Funez, P., Kango-Singh, M. and Singh, A. (2011) Activation of JNK signaling mediates amyloid-β-dependent cell death. PLoS ONE **6**, e24361

45. Hong, Y.K., Lee, S., Park, S.H., Lee, J.H., Han, S.Y., Kim, S.T., Jeon, S., Koo, B.S. and Cho, K.S. (2012) Inhibition of JNK/dFOXO pathway and caspases rescues neurological impairments in *Drosophila* Alzheimer's disease model. Biochem. Biophys. Res. Commun. **419**, 49–53

46. Iijima, K., Gatt, A. and Iijima-Ando, K. (2010) Tau Ser262 phosphorylation is critical for Aβ42-induced tau toxicity in a transgenic *Drosophila* model of Alzheimer's disease. Hum. Mol. Genet. **19**, 2947–2957

47. Gurlo, T., Ryazantsev, S., Huang, C.J., Yeh, M.W., Reber, H.A., Hines, O.J., O'Brien, T.D., Glabe, C.G. and Butler, P.C. (2010) Evidence for proteotoxicity in β cells in Type 2 diabetes: toxic islet amyloid polypeptide oligomers form intracellularly in the secretory pathway. Am. J. Pathol. **176**, 861–869

48. Betsholtz, C., Christmansson, L., Engstrom, U., Rorsman, F., Svensson, V., Johnson, K.H. and Westermark, P. (1989) Sequence divergence in a specific region of islet amyloid polypeptide (IAPP) explains differences in islet amyloid formation between species. FEBS Lett. **251**, 261–264

49. Schultz, S.W., Nilsson, K.P. and Westermark, G.T. (2011) *Drosophila melanogaster* as a model system for studies of islet amyloid polypeptide aggregation. PLoS ONE **6**, e20221

50. Paulsson, J.F. and Westermark, G.T. (2005) Aberrant processing of human proislet amyloid polypeptide results in increased amyloid formation. Diabetes **54**, 2117–2125

51. Marzban, L., Rhodes, C.J., Steiner, D.F., Haataja, L., Halban, P.A. and Verchere, C.B. (2006) Impaired NH_2-terminal processing of human proislet amyloid polypeptide by the prohormone convertase PC2 leads to amyloid formation and cell death. Diabetes **55**, 2192–2201

52. Pepys, M.B. (2006) Amyloidosis. Annu. Rev. Med. **57**, 223–241

53. Picken, M.M. (2010) Amyloidosis-where are we now and where are we heading? Arch. Pathol. Lab. Med. **134**, 545–551

54. Cornwell, G.G., Murdoch, W.L., Kyle, R.A., Westermark, P. and Pitkanen, P. (1983) Frequency and distribution of senile cardiovascular amyloid. A clinicopathologic correlation. Am. J. Med. **75**, 618–623

55. Dharmarajan, K. and Maurer, M.S. (2012) Transthyretin cardiac amyloidoses in older North Americans. J. Am. Geriatr. Soc. **60**, 765–774

56. Regel, R., Matioli, S.R. and Terra, W.R. (1998) Molecular adaptation of *Drosophila melanogaster* lysozymes to a digestive function. Insect Biochem. Mol. Biol. **28**, 309–319

57. Pepys, M.B., Hawkins, P.N., Booth, D.R., Vigushin, D.M., Tennent, G.A., Soutar, A.K., Totty, N., Nguyen, O., Blake, C.C., Terry, C.J. et al. (1993) Human lysozyme gene mutations cause hereditary systemic amyloidosis. Nature **362**, 553–557

58. Yazaki, M., Farrell, S.A. and Benson, M.D. (2003) A novel lysozyme mutation Phe57Ile associated with hereditary renal amyloidosis. Kidney Int. **63**, 1652–1657

59. Kumita, J.R., Helmfors, L., Williams, J., Luheshi, L.M., Menzer, L., Dumoulin, M., Lomas, D.A., Crowther, D.C., Dobson, C.M. and Brorsson, A.C. (2011) Disease-related amyloidogenic variants of human lysozyme trigger the unfolded protein response and disturb eye development in *Drosophila melanogaster*. FASEB J. **26**, 192–202

60. Kumita, J.R., Johnson, R.J., Alcocer, M.J., Dumoulin, M., Holmqvist, F., McCammon, M.G., Robinson, C.V., Archer, D.B. and Dobson, C.M. (2006) Impact of the native-state stability of human lysozyme variants on protein secretion by *Pichia pastoris*. FEBS J. **273**, 711–720

61. Whyteside, G., Alcocer, M.J., Kumita, J.R., Dobson, C.M., Lazarou, M., Pleass, R.J. and Archer, D.B. (2011) Native-state stability determines the extent of degradation relative to secretion of protein variants from *Pichia pastoris*. PLoS ONE **6**, e22692

62. Paggiaro, P.L., Dahle, R., Bakran, I., Frith, L., Hollingworth, K., Efthimiou, J. (1998) Multicentre randomised placebo-controlled trial of inhaled fluticasone proprionate in patients with chronic obstructive pulmonary disease. Lancet **351**, 773–780

63. Yi, S., Takahashi, K., Naito, M., Tashiro, F., Wakasugi, S., Maeda, S., Shimada, K., Yamamura, K. and Araki, S. (1991) Systemic amyloidosis in transgenic mice carrying the human mutant transthyretin (Met30) gene. Pathologic similarity to human familial amyloidotic polyneuropathy, type I. Am. J. Pathol. **138**, 403–412

64. Araki, S., Yi, S., Murakami, T., Watanabe, S., Ikegawa, S., Takahashi, K. and Yamarnura, K. (1994) Systemic amyloidosis in transgenic mice carrying the human mutant transthyretin (Met 30) gene. Pathological and immunohistochemical similarity to human familial amyloidotic polyneuropathy, type I. Mol. Neurobiol. **8**, 15–23

65. Sousa, M.M., Fernandes, R., Palha, J.A., Taboada, A., Vieira, P. and Saraiva, M.J. (2002) Evidence for early cytotoxic aggregates in transgenic mice for human transthyretin Leu55Pro. Am. J. Pathol. **161**, 1935–1948

66. Pokrzywa, M., Dacklin, I., Hultmark, D. and Lundgren, E. (2007) Misfolded transthyretin causes behavioral changes in a *Drosophila* model for transthyretin-associated amyloidosis. Eur. J. Neurosci. **26**, 913–924

67. Pokrzywa, M., Dacklin, I., Vestling, M., Hultmark, D., Lundgren, E. and Cantera, R. (2010) Uptake of aggregating transthyretin by fat body in a *Drosophila* model for TTR-associated amyloidosis. PLoS ONE **5**, e14343

68. Andersson, K., Pokrzywa, M., Dacklin, I. and Lundgren, E. (2013) Inhibition of TTR aggregation-induced cell death: a new role for serum amyloid P component. PLoS ONE **8**, e55766

69. Noborn, F., O'Callaghan, P., Hermansson, E., Zhang, X., Ancsin, J.B., Damas, A.M., Dacklin, I., Presto, J., Johansson, J., Saraiva, M.J. et al. (2011) Heparan sulfate/heparin promotes transthyretin fibrillization through selective binding to a basic motif in the protein. Proc. Natl. Acad. Sci. U.S.A. **108**, 5584–5589

70. Stine, Jr, W.B., Dahlgren, K.N., Krafft, G.A. and LaDu, M.J. (2003) *In vitro* characterization of conditions for amyloid-β peptide oligomerization and fibrillogenesis. J. Biol. Chem. **278**, 11612–11622

Essays Biochem. (2014) 56, 85–97: doi: 10.1042/BSE0560085

6

Yeast models for amyloid disease

Barry Panaretou* and Gary W. Jones[†1]

**Institute of Pharmaceutical Science, King's College London, Franklin-Wilkins Building, 150 Stamford Street, London SE1 9NH, U.K.*

†Department of Biology, National University of Ireland Maynooth, Maynooth, County Kildare, Ireland

Abstract

Saccharomyces cerevisiae (baker's yeast) is a well-established eukaryotic model organism, which has significantly contributed to our understanding of mechanisms that drive numerous core cellular processes in higher eukaryotes. Moreover, this has led to a greater understanding of the underlying pathobiology associated with disease in humans. This tractable model offers an abundance of analytical capabilities, including a vast array of global genetics and molecular resources that allow genome-wide screening to be carried out relatively simply and cheaply. A prime example of the versatility and potential for applying yeast technologies to explore a mammalian disease is in the development of yeast models for amyloid diseases such as Alzheimer's, Parkinson's and Huntington's. The present chapter provides a broad overview of high profile human neurodegenerative diseases that have been modelled in yeast. We focus on some of the most recent findings that have been developed through genetic and drug screening studies using yeast genomic resources. Although this relatively simple unicellular eukaryote seems far removed from relatively complex multicellular organisms such as mammals, the conserved mechanisms for how amyloid exhibits toxicity clearly underscore the value of carrying out such studies in yeast.

Keywords:

amyloid disease, amyloid toxicity, drug screening, genetic screening, Saccharomyces cerevisiae yeast model, α-synuclein.

[1]*To whom correspondence should be addressed (email gary.jones@nuim.ie).*

Introduction

Numerous human diseases are associated with the formation of amyloids, but until recently the downstream targets of amyloids have been poorly characterized. The bakers' yeast *Saccharomyces cerevisae* has been exploited as a platform to identify these targets. Even though most of the proteins that form disease-associated amyloids do not have counterparts native to yeast, ectopic expression of the corresponding genes in this model leads to toxicity. This has enabled genome-wide screening designed to identify enhancers and suppressors of this toxicity. The identity of these modulators of toxicity has subsequently permitted focus on specific aspects of cell biology that are disturbed by a specific amyloid. This has often been followed by identification of small molecules that both limit formation of an amyloid and abrogate its cytotoxic effects. Screening techniques applied to yeast have offered a dual advantage. First, they are inexpensive in comparison with similar strategies in other models. Secondly, they are executed rapidly given the relatively low generation time of this model coupled with a phenotype that is straightforward to measure, namely cell viability. The outcome is that within 10 years, this model has provided considerable insight regarding the underlying pathobiology associated with numerous disorders associated with amyloid, including PD (Parkinson's disease), AD (Alzheimer's disease) and HD (Huntington's disease).

Parkinson's disease

Aggregates of the pre-synaptic protein αsyn (α-synuclein) encoded by *SNCA*, have a well-established association with PD. These aggregates are a major component of Lewy bodies, ubiquitinated inclusions that are a hallmark of PD. Genetic pre-disposition to PD in humans has also been observed, which includes the A53T, A30P and E46K missense mutations of *SNCA*, as well as the duplication and triplication of *SNCA* itself (reviewed in [1]).

The dual utility of yeast as a model to characterize the underlying basis of SNCA-associated toxicity as well as a test bed for isolation of drugs that limit this toxicity, began with the finding that overexpression of both *SNCA* and the A53T mutant were toxic to yeast, with both forms localizing to the plasma membrane and then to intracellular inclusions (shown for wild-type αsyn in Figure 1). Moreover, αsyn expression in yeast leads to numerous effects on

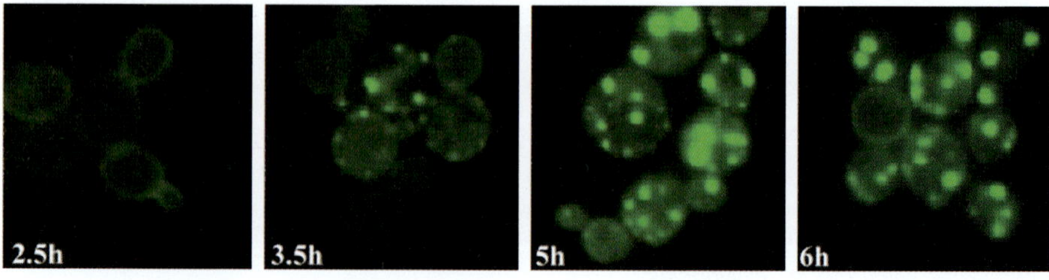

Figure 1. Aggregation of αsyn in yeast
Fluorescence microscopy visualizing αsyn–GFP (green fluorescent protein) at intervals (indicated in hours) after activating expression of two integrated copies of a cassette encoding the GFP fusion. Reproduced with permission from [46]: Gitler, A.D., Bevis, B.J., Shorter, J., Strathearn, K.E., Hamamichi, S., Su, L.J., Caldwell, K.A., Caldwell, G.A., Rochet, J.C. and McCaffery, J.M. et al. (2008) The Parkinson's disease protein α-synuclein disrupts cellular Rab homeostasis. Proc. Natl. Acad. Sci. U.S.A. **105**, 145–150. Copyright (2008) National Academy of Sciences, U.S.A.

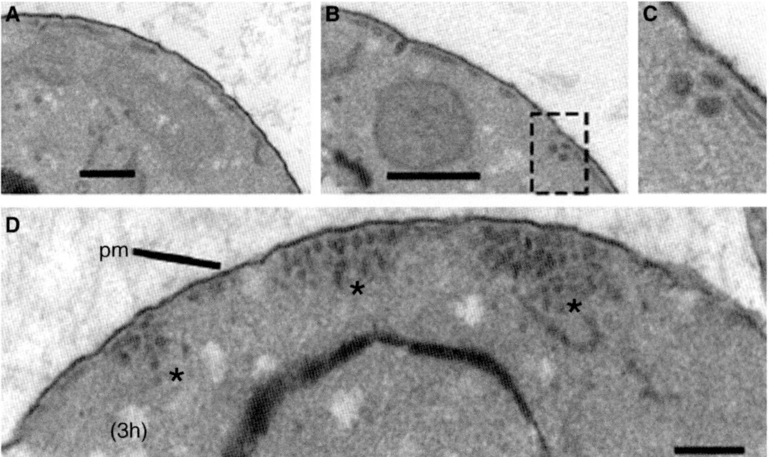

Figure 2. Expression of αsyn causes accumulation of transport vesicles

Electron microscopy of control strain (**A**), and (**B**) cells expressing one copy of αsyn–GFP (green fluorescent protein) at 3 hours after activating synthesis of the fusion. (**C**) A higher magnification of vesicles gathering at peripheral ER. (**D**) Excessive vesicle accumulation (asterisk) at the plasma membrane (pm) concomitant with expressing two integrated copies of a cassette encoding the αsyn–GFP fusion. Scale bars, 0.5 μm. Reproduced with permission from [46]: Gitler, A.D., Bevis, B.J., Shorter, J., Strathearn, K.E., Hamamichi, S., Su, L.J., Caldwell, K.A., Caldwell, G.A., Rochet, J.C. and McCaffery, J.M. et al. (2008) The Parkinson's disease protein α-synuclein disrupts cellular Rab homeostasis. Proc. Natl. Acad. Sci. U.S.A. **105**, 145–150. Copyright (2008) National Academy of Sciences, U.S.A.

cell physiology that have also been noted in neuronal models of PD, namely inhibition of protein degradation via the proteasome, abrogation of vesicle traffic (Figure 2), accumulation of lipid droplets, increase in the levels of ROS (reactive oxygen species) (reviewed in [2]), autophagy [3] and mitophagy [4]. This was followed by the two main types of genetic screening that are used to identify the underlying causes of toxicity associated with a given protein or drug, namely identification of (i) enhancers of αsyn toxicity by screening against the collection of strains representing deletes of all non-essential genes and (ii) enhancers and suppressors of αsyn toxicity, identified by overexpression of all genes. Screening the collection of non-essential gene deletes identified 86 mutants that displayed enhanced sensitivity to wild-type αsyn [5]. That, and another similar study [6], indicated that lipid metabolism and vesicle-mediated transport were the aspects of cell physiology that were most important in limiting the toxicity associated with expression of αsyn in yeast. Reinforcing the importance of vesicle-mediated transport was the finding that genes of this class were the largest and most potent suppressors to emerge from an overexpression screen, with the strongest suppressor of toxicity being the Ypt1 Rab GTPase-activating protein, which is essential for the ER (endoplasmic reticulum) to Golgi step of the secretory pathway. It was subsequently shown that overexpression of *RAB1* (the murine homologue of *YPT1*) limited the loss of dopaminergic neurons associated with αsyn toxicity in *Drosophila*, *Caenorhabditis elegans* and rat models of PD, further endorsing the use of the yeast model for the investigation of neurodegenerative disorders [7].

The stage was now set for exploiting the yeast model for rapid high-throughput screening of drugs that limit αsyn-associated toxicity, leading to identification of four tetrahydroquinolones [8], two flavonoids [9] and two cyclic peptides [10] that limited the toxicity of this amyloid.

The tetrahydroquinolones restored ER to Golgi traffic, and restored levels of ROS to wild-type levels. Moreover, these compounds also antagonized cell death in a rat PD model [8].

Unlike wild-type and A53T αsyn, A30P αsyn is only toxic when expressed at very high levels. Differences in toxicity may reflect the localization of the αsyns, because wild-type and A53T enter the secretory pathway, whereas A30P does not [11]. Not surprisingly, the stimulation of ER to Golgi transport limits wild-type and A53T αsyn toxicity, but has no effect on A30P toxicity. This infers the existence of a mechanism that clears cytosolic αsyn aggregates, and there is now an increasing body of evidence from yeast and other models that degradation in the vacuole via autophagy is primarily responsible for this, as opposed to disposal via the proteasome. For example, pharmacological inhibition of either process in yeast points to a greater contribution made by autophagy. Additionally, work using the yeast model indicates that autophagy is up-regulated by A30P αsyn [3], which is targeted to the vacuole for degradation [12].

A common feature of expression of all three αsyns in yeast is the subsequent elevation of ROS levels, a feature shared with all other models of PD. However, the extent of the role played by ROS in αsyn-associated cell death is not clear. In yeast expressing αsyn, there may be two 'waves' of toxicity. The first is the primary effects on pathways such as vesicle trafficking and autophagy. The second is the ROS that is generated as a consequence of the primary effects. This is plausible because limited expression of Ypt1 (which will limit ER to Golgi traffic) [13] and mutations that abrogate autophagy [14] both lead to accumulation of ROS in the absence of αsyn expression.

Alzheimer's disease

AD (Alzheimer's disease) is characterized by extracellular plaques composed of a 42-residue fragment, known as Aβ42, of APP (amyloid precursor protein). The Aβ42 peptide acts upstream of another hallmark of AD, namely the neurofibrillary tangles composed of the microtubule-binding protein tau. A yeast model of Aβ42-associated toxicity has been established by targeting the peptide to the secretory pathway, via N-terminal fusion to a signal peptide [15] (Figure 3). The cell wall limits secretion of the peptide, and as a result it is packaged into endocytic vesicles, thereby mimicking the localization of the peptide observed in neurons. Genome-wide screens in yeast led to identification of 23 suppressors and 17 enhancers of the impaired cell growth associated with Aβ42. Of these genes, 12 have human homologues, three of which play roles in clathrin-mediated endocytosis. One of these is *YAP1802*, the yeast homologue of *PICALM* (phosphatidylinositol-binding clathrin assembly protein) [15], which is one of the most statistically significant risk factors for AD identified from genome-wide association studies [16]. This indicated that one of the most toxic focal points of Aβ42 is the endocytic machinery, a notion that was validated with the finding that trafficking of a receptor from the yeast plasma membrane was significantly abrogated by Aβ42.

High-throughput drug screens have been applied to Aβ42 in yeast, but only against the peptide that is localized to the cytosol (i.e. lacking the signal sequence that allows transit through the secretory pathway). Such forms of the peptide are non-toxic, but they do form aggregates [17,18]. In order to achieve an observable readout for screening, these peptides are fused to a protein for which a convenient assay is available. In this case, the peptide is fused to an essential translation termination factor, the activity of which is determined *in vivo* by measuring the extent of protein synthesis termination at a premature stop codon. The assay is performed in a genetic background bearing a nonsense mutation in *ADE14*, a gene essential for

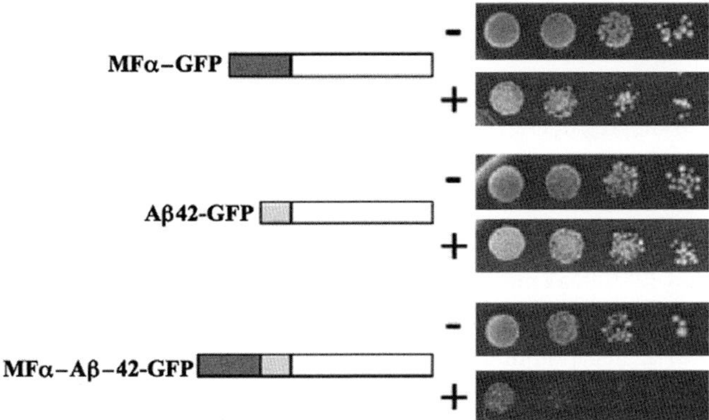

Figure 3. Establishing a toxicity model for Aβ42 peptide in yeast

Rectangular bars indicate fusion proteins: Aβ42 peptide (light grey), secretory signal of mating factor α (MFα) (dark grey) and GFP (green fluorescent protein) (white). Cultures spotted as serial dilutions from left to right on media that induce synthesis of the fusions (+) and controls where synthesis is not induced (–). Reproduced with permission from [15]: D'Angelo, F., Vignaud, H., Di Martino, J., Salin, B., Devin, A., Cullin, C. and Marchal, C. (2013) A yeast model for amyloid-β aggregation exemplifies the role of membrane trafficking and PICALM in cytotoxicity. Dis. Model Mech. **6**, 206–216.

biosynthesis of adenine. Fusion with Aβ42 peptide leads to translation termination factor aggregation, which in turn allows read-through of the premature stop codon, leading to cell growth in media that lack adenine [17]. Oligomerization of peptide debilitates function of the fusion. Consequently, a drug that inhibits oligomerization will re-establish function of the protein. Such a strategy was used to screen over 12000 compounds, two of which inhibited Aβ42 oligomer formation [19]. An additional advantage of this screen was that the Aβ42 fusion forms small soluble Aβ42 oligomers in yeast, which are now thought to be the toxic form of the peptide as opposed to larger fibrils and plaques [20]. Therefore the screen is biased towards identifying drugs that counter the toxic form of Aβ42.

ALS (amyotrophic lateral sclerosis) and frontotemporal dementias

Cytoplasmic inclusions of SOD1 (superoxide dismutase 1), the RNA-binding proteins TDP-43 (transactive response DNA binding protein-43) and FUS (fused-in-sarcoma), and OPTN (optineurin) have been independently associated with ALS (cited in [21]). FTLD (frontotemporal dementia lobar degeneration) is a generic term that describes a number of clinically similar disorders, with major subtypes linked to inclusions containing TDP-43 and FUS. The classification of these inclusions as amyloids is controversial at present. Binding of Thioflavin S is an indicator of amyloid, and this dye binds to inclusions in TDP-43 positive ALS, but does not bind to inclusions in TDP-43 positive FTLD (cited in [22]). Thioflavin S does not bind to SOD1 inclusions in ALS [23]. On the other hand, prion-like propagation (a characteristic typical of amyloid) is exhibited by mutant SOD1 aggregates in neuronal cells [24]. Nevertheless, the aggregation of these proteins can be modelled in yeast, where overepression of TDP-43, FUS (reviewed in [25]) and OPTN [21] is cytotoxic. Furthermore, elevated levels of TDP-43 led to its aggregation in the cytoplasm, preventing its localization to the nucleus, which reflects the localization of this protein in animal cell culture models [26]. The same is true for FUS [27].

RNA-binding proteins and proteins involved in metabolism of RNA were the largest class of enhancers and suppressors isolated from a genome-wide screen designed to identify modulators of TDP-43-associated toxicity. The strongest suppressor was absence of the RNA lariat de-branching enzyme, Dbr1. This prompted assessing the consequences of knocking down the human Dbr1 homologue in mammalian cell models, which led to abrogation of TDP-43-associated toxicity [28]. RNA metabolism genes were also identified in screens for modulators of FUS toxicity, but these did not overlap with modulators of TDP-43 toxicity, suggesting that disease caused by aggregation of these proteins is due to perturbation of different aspects of RNA biology [29]. Screens designed to identify modulators of toxicity associated with OPTN have not been reported yet.

The controversy relating to whether protein aggregates in ALS are amyloids extends to the yeast model. There are several reports indicating that FUS, TDP-43 and OPTN form non-amyloid aggregates in yeast [21,25], but there are also opposing reports [30]. Biophysical characteristics and binding to amyloid-specific dyes are the usual assays performed here. However, the finding that Btn2 in yeast is a modulator of both aggregation and toxicity associated with OPTN *in vivo*, suggests that OPTN aggregates may share features with amyloids, given that Btn2 also limits propagation of prions in yeast [21].

Huntington's disease

HD is a fatal neurodegenerative disorder that results from polyQ (polyglutamine) expansion in the htt (huntingtin) protein. Expansion of polyQ beyond 39 copies results in htt protein aggregation and disease onset. *Saccharomyces cerevisiae* does not contain an htt orthologue, so developing a model for HD relied on overexpression of fragments of the huntingtin gene in yeast. Initial experiments to establish a yeast model of HD were only capable of reproducing htt aggregation, but did not produce cellular toxicity [31]. Subsequently, it was discovered that sequence context within the htt plasmid constructs could influence toxicity as could the presence or absence of cellular aggregates of naturally occurring yeast proteins. The reasons behind such findings are beyond the scope of the present chapter, but a comprehensive review of modelling HD in yeast addresses these issues (see [32]).

A variety of genetic and chemical modifier screens using yeast HD models have been carried out and have identified genes that can enhance and reduce the toxicity of htt aggregation while also identifying potential small molecule inhibitors of toxicity (reviewed fully in [32]). In the present chapter, the focus will be on recent major findings that identified two cellular metabolic pathways that significantly influence htt toxicity. The most informative genetic screens in yeast have used a toxic HD model expressing polyQ of length 103 (Q103) and non-toxic Q25 as the negative control. A genetic screen for yeast gene deletions that suppressed the toxicity of Q103 identified genes involved in the kynurenine pathway of tryptophan degradation (Figure 4) as playing a role in htt toxicity [33]. Among 28 suppressors initially identified was *Δbna4*. The *BNA4* gene encodes KMO (kynurenine 3-monooxygenase) and is required for the production of toxic metabolites 3-HK (3-hydroxykynurenine) and QUIN (quinolinic acid) (Figure 4). Deletion of certain other genes encoding enzymes in the kynurenine pathway also suppressed Q103 toxicity in yeast (Figure 5). Levels of 3-HK and QUIN were increased in the

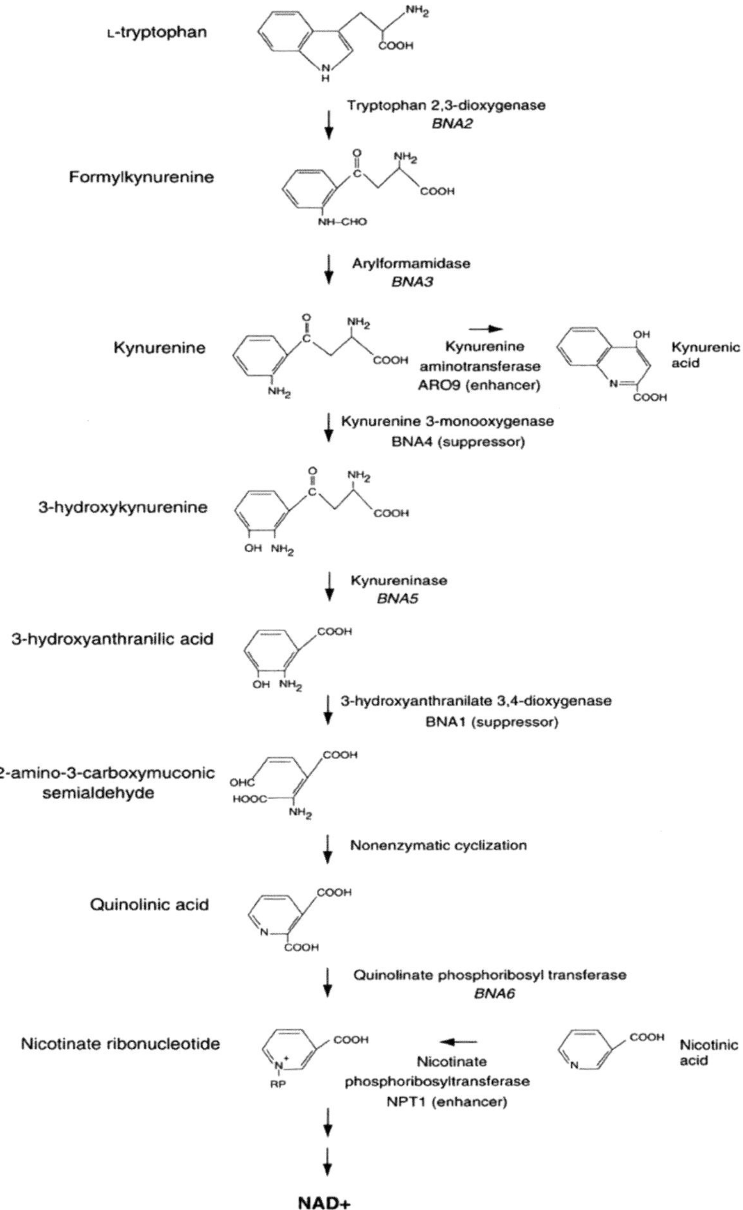

Figure 4. Genetic analysis of the kynurenine pathway in Q103-mediated toxicity
Schematic representation of the kynurenine pathway in yeast and mammals. The arrows represent enzymatic steps and the corresponding yeast gene encoding each enzyme is listed. Yeast deletions that enhance or suppress toxicity are indicated accordingly. Reprinted with permission from [33], Macmillan Publishers Ltd: [*Nature Genetics*] (**37**, 526–531), copyright (2005).

yeast model, which mirrors findings for mammalian models and HD patients [34]. However, in the *Δbna4* strain these metabolites were not present and corresponding increases in levels of ROS, believed to be a major factor in HD neurodegeneration, did not occur. Thus the Q103 HD model identified KMO as a new potential therapeutic target for HD, which importantly has been further validated in *Drosophila* and mouse models [35,36].

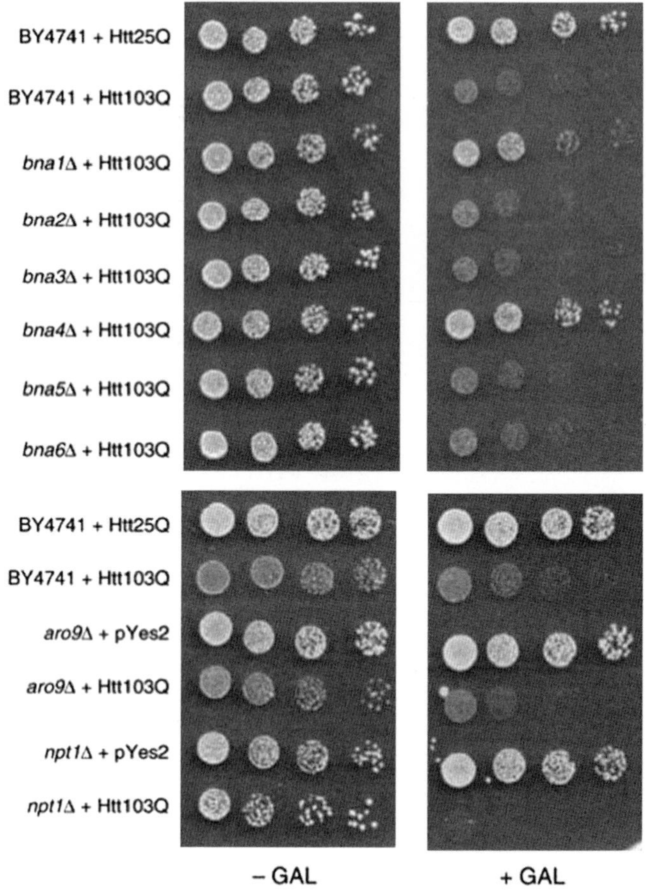

Figure 5. Influence of the kynurenine pathway gene deletions on Q103 toxicity as assessed using yeast spot growth assays

Of particular note is the suppression of Q103 toxicity by deletion of *BNA4* and *BNA1* genes and enhancement of Q103 toxicity by deletion of *ARO9* and *NPT1* genes. GAL, galactose. Reprinted with permission from [33], Macmillan Publishers Ltd: [*Nature Genetics*] (**37**, 526–531), copyright (2005).

Following the design of a high-throughput screening protocol (Figure 6A), Mason et al. [37] identified yeast genes that when overexpressed could abrogate toxicity of Q103 [37]. From this overexpression screen, a variety of yeast genes with human orthologues were identified as influencing Q103 toxicity when overexpressed. Of particular significance was the identification of overexpression of yeast genes encoding GPxs (glutathione peroxidases) as suppressing Q103 toxicity (Figure 6B). GPxs are conserved antioxidant enzymes that catalyse the reduction of hydrogen peroxide and reduce the accumulation of ROS in the cell. It appears that GPx suppression of Q103 toxicity is primarily due to counteracting the production of ROS. Importantly, these exciting results in the yeast system also held true for *Drosophila* and mammalian tissue culture HD models [37]. GPx mimetic drugs are available and are well tolerated in humans, which enhances further this metabolic pathway as a potential target for HD therapeutics.

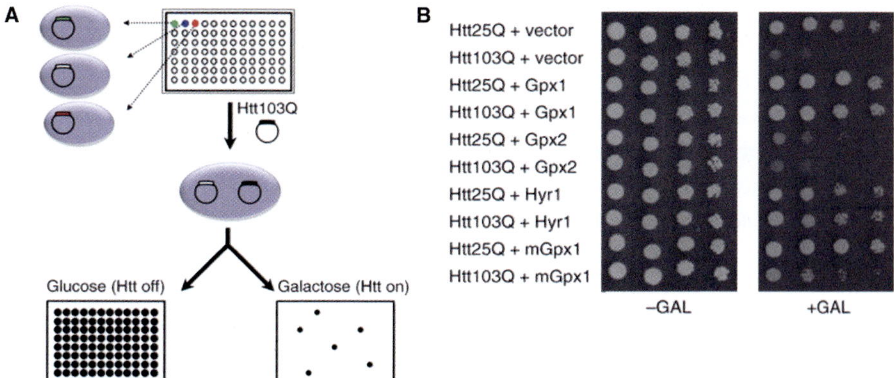

Figure 6. Suppression of Q103 toxicity in yeast by gene overexpression
(**A**) Schematic representation of the genome-wide systematic open reading frame (ORF) expression screen in yeast. Yeast ORFs were overexpressed in conjunction with Q103 by induction in the presence of galactose (GAL) (each ORF and Q103 under control of *GAL1* promoter). ORFs showing suppression of Q103 toxicity in a 96-well plate assay primary screen were analysed further. (**B**) Suppression of Q103 toxicity by overexpression of GPx. Gpx1 and Hyr1 (also called Gpx3), as well as a mitochondrial mGpx1, can efficiently suppress Q103 toxicity as assessed using yeast spot growth assays. Reprinted with permission from [37], Macmillan Publishers Ltd: [*Nature Genetics*] (**45**, 1249–1254), copyright (2013).

Prion disease

Aggregation of the PrP^C (normal cellular prion protein) into insoluble amyloid is the cause of a variety of mammalian neurodegenerative diseases termed TSEs (transmissible spongiform encephalopathies) or prion diseases [38]. Once PrP^C has converted into PrP^{Sc} (disease-specific conformation of prion protein), the protein is now infectious and able to convert soluble molecules of the same type into the insoluble prion form. PrP^C is connected to the plasma membrane through a GPI (glycosylphosphatidylinositol) anchor, which is added following glycosylation and processing in the ER. Although such post-translational modifications may suggest a major stumbling block in using *S. cerevisiae* to assess functional and structural aspects of PrP^C conversion into the prion form, studies have demonstrated that when PrP^C is expressed in yeast it can adopt PrP^{Sc}-like conformations [39,40]. These results suggest that yeast can be exploited as a model system for studying the formation and propagation of mammalian prions.

Although *S. cerevisiae* does not contain an orthologue of mammalian PrP^C, it has been shown to possess a number of proteins that have the capability to propagate as prions. Naturally occurring yeast prions form amyloid and are viewed as good models for studying prion propagation (reviewed in Chapter 14 by Reed Wickner). Owing to the modular nature of PFDs (prion-forming domains) in yeast prion proteins, researchers have taken the approach of replacing the PFD of the best-characterized yeast prion protein Sup35, with prion-forming regions of mammalian PrP^C. These chimaeric proteins have then been assayed for prion-forming ability in yeast [41,42]. Originally, it was reported that the PFD of mammalian prion protein could confer prion-forming ability on the Sup35 protein, and the chimaeric protein, although relatively mitotically unstable, possessed similar properties to the native Sup35 protein, both in terms of functionality and prion properties [41]. Recent findings suggest that interpretation of results using PrP-Sup35 chimaeras should be treated with some caution, as protein instability is a major complicating factor for such constructs. A reduction in the available amounts of functional soluble Sup35 protein will produce similar phenotypes related to those exhibited by Sup35 prion formation [42].

It is fair to say that the application of yeast genetics for investigations of mammalian prion diseases, through the analysis of PrP^C expression in *S. cerevisiae*, has not been as productive or informative as for other yeast-based neurodegenerative disease models.

Although not strictly modelling of a human amyloid disease, one area of major success that is particularly noteworthy has been the application of yeast prion genetics to mammalian prion diseases in terms of drug screening. Such screens are aimed at identifying novel compounds that cure yeast prions, which can then be analysed further in mammalian prion systems. The rationale behind such an approach being that both mammalian and yeast prions form amyloid so drugs may be found that inhibit conserved cellular processes in amyloid formation. Through such screens new yeast prion curing drugs such as 6-aminophenanthridine, guanabenz and imiquimod have been identified. Following screening in yeast, these drugs have also been shown to be active against mammalian prions [43–45].

Conclusions

The contribution of yeast genetics to our current understanding of the toxicity of amyloid to the cell cannot be underestimated. Genetic screens in yeast have identified key genetic modulators of amyloid toxicity and have been responsible for the identification of potential novel therapeutic classes of drugs that are active against amyloid toxicity. Importantly, key findings in yeast also translate through to metazoan models of neurodegenerative diseases.

A major challenge for the future is to integrate, as fully as possible, the major findings from the amyloid-toxicity genetic screens carried out in yeast. Currently, researchers have focused on characterizing only a few subsets of the genes/proteins that have been identified in such screens. Most of the genetic screens touched upon in the present chapter identified many genes involved in a variety of cellular pathways (some seemingly unrelated), which could influence amyloid toxicity. The most effective therapeutic approaches for amyloid diseases will be developed from the most complete understanding of how amyloid interacts *in vivo* with cellular components. Fortunately, the "awesome power of yeast genetics", as well as other established yeast technologies, provides the ideal experimental environment for studying the complex nature of amyloid systems biology.

Summary

- Yeast is an excellent model for initial screening for cellular factors that influence amyloid toxicity. These findings can then be carried forward and tested in other eukaryotic models.
- For a given amyloid, enhancers and suppressors identified in yeast genetics screens act in the same way across the eukaryotic lineage.
- At the level of cell physiology, there is no universal pathway that is disturbed by amyloid. Different amyloids poison the cell in different ways.
- Small molecule inhibitors of amyloid-associated toxicity identified in yeast also abrogate the toxicity observed in metazoan models.

References

1. Klein, C. and Westenberger, A. (2012) Genetics of Parkinson's disease. Cold Spring Harb. Perspect. Med. **2**, a008888
2. Tenreiro, S. and Outeiro, T.F. (2010) Simple is good: yeast models of neurodegeneration. FEMS Yeast Res. **10**, 970–979
3. Petroi, D., Popova, B., Taheri-Talesh, N., Irniger, S., Shahpasandzadeh, H., Zweckstetter, M., Outeiro, T.F. and Braus, G.H. (2012) Aggregate clearance of α-synuclein in *Saccharomyces cerevisiae* depends more on autophagosome and vacuole function than on the proteasome. J. Biol. Chem. **287**, 27567–27579
4. Sampaio-Marques, B., Felgueiras, C., Silva, A., Rodrigues, M., Tenreiro, S., Franssens, V., Reichert, A.S., Outeiro, T.F., Winderickx, J. and Ludovico, P. (2012) SNCA (α-synuclein)-induced toxicity in yeast cells is dependent on sirtuin 2 (Sir2)-mediated mitophagy. Autophagy **8**, 1494–1509
5. Willingham, S., Outeiro, T.F., DeVit, M.J., Lindquist, S.L. and Muchowski, P.J. (2003) Yeast genes that enhance the toxicity of a mutant huntingtin fragment or α-synuclein. Science **302**, 1769–1772
6. Zabrocki, P., Bastiaens, I., Delay, C., Bammens, T., Ghillebert, R., Pellens, K., De Virgilio, C., Van Leuven, F. and Winderickx, J. (2008) Phosphorylation, lipid raft interaction and traffic of α-synuclein in a yeast model for Parkinson. Biochim. Biophys. Acta **1783**, 1767–1780
7. Cooper, A.A., Gitler, A.D., Cashikar, A., Haynes, C.M., Hill, K.J., Bhullar, B., Liu, K., Xu, K., Strathearn, K.E., Liu, F. et al. (2006) α-Synuclein blocks ER-Golgi traffic and Rab1 rescues neuron loss in Parkinson's models. Science **313**, 324–328
8. Su, L.J., Auluck, P.K., Outeiro, T.F., Yeger-Lotem, E., Kritzer, J.A., Tardiff, D.F., Strathearn, K.E., Liu, F., Cao, S., Hamamichi, S. et al. (2010) Compounds from an unbiased chemical screen reverse both ER-to-Golgi trafficking defects and mitochondrial dysfunction in Parkinson's disease models. Dis. Model Mech. **3**, 194–208
9. Griffioen, G., Duhamel, H., Van Damme, N., Pellens, K., Zabrocki, P., Pannecouque, C., van Leuven, F., Winderickx, J. and Wera, S. (2006) A yeast-based model of α-synucleinopathy identifies compounds with therapeutic potential. Biochim. Biophys. Acta **1762**, 312–318
10. Kritzer, J.A., Hamamichi, S., McCaffery, J.M., Santagata, S., Naumann, T.A., Caldwell, K.A., Caldwell, G.A. and Lindquist, S. (2009) Rapid selection of cyclic peptides that reduce alpha-synuclein toxicity in yeast and animal models. Nat. Chem. Biol. **5**, 655–663
11. Dixon, C., Mathias, N., Zweig, R.M., Davis, D.A. and Gross, D.S. (2005) α-Synuclein targets the plasma membrane via the secretory pathway and induces toxicity in yeast. Genetics **170**, 47–59
12. Flower, T.R., Clark-Dixon, C., Metoyer, C., Yang, H., Shi, R., Zhang, Z. and Witt, S.N. (2007) YGR198w (YPP1) targets A30P α-synuclein to the vacuole for degradation. J. Cell Biol. **177**, 1091–1104
13. Ayer, A., Fellermeier, S., Fife, C., Li, S.S., Smits, G., Meyer, A.J., Dawes, I.W. and Perrone, G.G. (2012) A genome-wide screen in yeast identifies specific oxidative stress genes required for the maintenance of sub-cellular redox homeostasis. PLoS ONE **7**, e44278
14. Suzuki, S.W., Onodera, J. and Ohsumi, Y. (2011) Starvation induced cell death in autophagy-defective yeast mutants is caused by mitochondria dysfunction. PLoS ONE **6**, e17412
15. D'Angelo, F., Vignaud, H., Di Martino, J., Salin, B., Devin, A., Cullin, C. and Marchal, C. (2013) A yeast model for amyloid-β aggregation exemplifies the role of membrane trafficking and PICALM in cytotoxicity. Dis. Model Mech. **6**, 206–216
16. Treusch, S., Hamamichi, S., Goodman, J.L., Matlack, K.E., Chung, C.Y., Baru, V., Shulman, J.M., Parrado, A., Bevis, B.J., Valastyan, J.S. et al. (2011) Functional links between Aβ toxicity, endocytic trafficking, and Alzheimer's disease risk factors in yeast. Science **334**, 1241–1245
17. Bagriantsev, S. and Liebman, S. (2006) Modulation of Aβ$_{42}$ low-n oligomerization using a novel yeast reporter system. BMC Biol. **4**, 32

18. von der Haar, T., Josse, L., Wright, P., Zenthon, J. and Tuite, M.F. (2007) Development of a novel yeast cell-based system for studying the aggregation of Alzheimer's disease-associated Aβ peptides *in vivo*. Neurodegener Dis. **4**, 136–147

19. Park, S.K., Pegan, S.D., Mesecar, A.D., Jungbauer, L.M., LaDu, M.J. and Liebman, S.W. (2011) Development and validation of a yeast high-throughput screen for inhibitors of $A\beta_{42}$ oligomerization. Dis. Model Mech. **4**, 822–831

20. Walsh, D.M. and Selkoe, D.J. (2004) Oligomers on the brain: the emerging role of soluble protein aggregates in neurodegeneration. Protein Pept. Lett. **11**, 213–228

21. Kryndushkin, D., Ihrke, G., Piermartiri, T.C. and Shewmaker, F. (2012) A yeast model of optineurin proteinopathy reveals a unique aggregation pattern associated with cellular toxicity. Mol. Microbiol. **86**, 1531–1547

22. Bigio, E.H., Wu, J.Y., Deng, H.X., Bit-Ivan, E.N., Mao, Q., Ganti, R., Peterson, M., Siddique, N., Geula, C., Siddique, T. and Mesulam, M. (2013) Inclusions in frontotemporal lobar degeneration with TDP-43 proteinopathy (FTLD-TDP) and amyotrophic lateral sclerosis (ALS), but not FTLD with FUS proteinopathy (FTLD-FUS), have properties of amyloid. Acta Neuropathol. **125**, 463–465

23. Kerman, A., Liu, H.N., Croul, S., Bilbao, J., Rogaeva, E., Zinman, L., Robertson, J. and Chakrabartty, A. (2010) Amyotrophic lateral sclerosis is a non-amyloid disease in which extensive misfolding of SOD1 is unique to the familial form. Acta Neuropathol. **119**, 335–344

24. Munch, C., O'Brien, J. and Bertolotti, A. (2011) Prion-like propagation of mutant superoxide dismutase-1 misfolding in neuronal cells. Proc. Natl. Acad. Sci. U.S.A. **108**, 3548–3553

25. Kryndushkin, D. and Shewmaker, F. (2011) Modeling ALS and FTLD proteinopathies in yeast: an efficient approach for studying protein aggregation and toxicity. Prion **5**, 250–257

26. Johnson, B.S., McCaffery, J.M., Lindquist, S. and Gitler, A.D. (2008) A yeast TDP-43 proteinopathy model: Exploring the molecular determinants of TDP-43 aggregation and cellular toxicity. Proc. Natl. Acad. Sci. U.S.A. **105**, 6439–6444

27. Kryndushkin, D., Wickner, R.B. and Shewmaker, F. (2011) FUS/TLS forms cytoplasmic aggregates, inhibits cell growth and interacts with TDP-43 in a yeast model of amyotrophic lateral sclerosis. Protein Cell **2**, 223–236

28 Armakola, M., Higgins, M.J., Figley, M.D., Barmada, S.J., Scarborough, E.A., Diaz, Z., Fang, X., Shorter, J., Krogan, N.J., Finkbeiner, S. et al. (2012) Inhibition of RNA lariat debranching enzyme suppresses TDP-43 toxicity in ALS disease models. Nat. Genet. **44**, 1302–1309

29. Sun, Z., Diaz, Z., Fang, X., Hart, M.P., Chesi, A., Shorter, J. and Gitler, A.D. (2011) Molecular determinants and genetic modifiers of aggregation and toxicity for the ALS disease protein FUS/TLS. PLoS Biol. **9**, e1000614

30. Fushimi, K., Long, C., Jayaram, N., Chen, X., Li, L. and Wu, J.Y. (2011) Expression of human FUS/TLS in yeast leads to protein aggregation and cytotoxicity, recapitulating key features of FUS proteinopathy. Protein Cell **2**, 141–149

31. Krobitsch, S. and Lindquist, S. (2000) Aggregation of huntingtin in yeast varies with the length of the polyglutamine expansion and the expression of chaperone proteins. Proc. Natl. Acad. Sci. U.S.A. **97**, 1589–1594

32. Mason, R.P. and Giorgini, F. (2011) Modeling Huntington disease in yeast: perspectives and future directions. Prion **5**, 269–276

33. Giorgini, F., Guidetti, P., Nguyen, Q., Bennett, S.C. and Muchowski, P.J. (2005) A genomic screen in yeast implicates kynurenine 3-monooxygenase as a therapeutic target for Huntington disease. Nat. Genet. **37**, 526–531

34. Thevandavakkam, M.A., Schwarcz, R., Muchowski, P.J. and Giorgini, F. (2010) Targeting kynurenine 3-monooxygenase (KMO): implications for therapy in Huntington's disease. CNS Neurol. Disord. Drug Targets **9**, 791–800

35. Campesan, S., Green, E.W., Breda, C., Sathyasaikumar, K.V., Muchowski, P.J., Schwarcz, R., Kyriacou, C.P. and Giorgini, F. (2011) The kynurenine pathway modulates neurodegeneration in a *Drosophila* model of Huntington's disease. Curr. Biol. **21**, 961–966

36. Zwilling, D., Huang, S.Y., Sathyasaikumar, K.V., Notarangelo, F.M., Guidetti, P., Wu, H.Q., Lee, J., Truong, J., Andrews-Zwilling, Y., Hsieh, E.W. et al. (2011) Kynurenine 3-monooxygenase inhibition in blood ameliorates neurodegeneration. Cell **145**, 863–874

37. Mason, R.P., Casu, M., Butler, N., Breda, C., Campesan, S., Clapp, J., Green, E.W., Dhulkhed, D., Kyriacou, C.P. and Giorgini, F. (2013) Glutathione peroxidase activity is neuroprotective in models of Huntington's disease. Nat. Genet. **45**, 1249–1254

38. Aguzzi, A. and Calella, A.M. (2009) Prions: protein aggregation and infectious diseases. Physiol. Rev. **89**, 1105–1152

39. Ma, J. and Lindquist, S. (1999) *De novo* generation of a PrPSc-like conformation in living cells. Nat. Cell Biol. **1**, 358–361

40. Dong, J., Bloom, J.D., Goncharov, V., Chattopadhyay, M., Millhauser, G.L., Lynn, D.G., Scheibel, T. and Lindquist, S. (2007) Probing the role of PrP repeats in conformational conversion and amyloid assembly of chimeric yeast prions. J. Biol. Chem. **282**, 34204–34212

41. Tank, E.M., Harris, D.A., Desai, A.A. and True, H.L. (2007) Prion protein repeat expansion results in increased aggregation and reveals phenotypic variability. Mol. Cell. Biol. **27**, 5445–5455

42. Josse, L., Marchante, R., Zenthon, J., von der Haar, T. and Tuite, M.F. (2012) Probing the role of structural features of mouse PrP in yeast by expression as Sup35-PrP fusions. Prion **6**, 201–210

43. Bach, S., Talarek, N., Andrieu, T., Vierfond, J.M., Mettey, Y., Galons, H., Dormont, D., Meijer, L., Cullin, C. and Blondel, M. (2003) Isolation of drugs active against mammalian prions using a yeast-based screening assay. Nat. Biotechnol. **21**, 1075–1081

44. Tribouillard-Tanvier, D., Dos Reis, S., Gug, F., Voisset, C., Beringue, V., Sabate, R., Kikovska, E., Talarek, N., Bach, S., Huang, C. et al. (2008) Protein folding activity of ribosomal RNA is a selective target of two unrelated antiprion drugs. PLoS ONE **3**, e2174

45. Oumata, N., Nguyen, P.H., Beringue, V., Soubigou, F., Pang, Y., Desban, N., Massacrier, C., Morel, Y., Paturel, C., Contesse, M.A. et al. (2013) The Toll-like receptor agonist imiquimod is active against prions. PLoS ONE **8**, e72112

46. Gitler, A.D., Bevis, B.J., Shorter, J., Strathearn, K.E., Hamamichi, S., Su, L.J., Caldwell, K.A., Caldwell, G.A., Rochet, J.C., McCaffery, J.M. et al. (2008) The Parkinson's disease protein α-synuclein disrupts cellular Rab homeostasis. Proc. Natl. Acad. Sci. U.S.A. **105**, 145–150

© The Authors Journal compilation © 2014 Biochemical Society
Essays Biochem. (2014) 56, 99–110: doi: 10.1042/BSE0560099

7

Amyloid β-peptide and Alzheimer's disease

David Allsop[1] and Jennifer Mayes

Division of Biomedical and Life Sciences, Faculty of Health and Medicine, Lancaster University, Lancaster LA1 4YQ, U.K.

Abstract

One of the hallmarks of AD (Alzheimer's disease) is the formation of senile plaques in the brain, which contain fibrils composed of Aβ (amyloid β-peptide). According to the 'amyloid cascade' hypothesis, the aggregation of Aβ initiates a sequence of events leading to the formation of neurofibrillary tangles, neurodegeneration, and on to the main symptom of dementia. However, emphasis has now shifted away from fibrillar forms of Aβ and towards smaller and more soluble 'oligomers' as the main culprit in AD. The present chapter commences with a brief introduction to the disease and its current treatment, and then focuses on the formation of Aβ from the APP (amyloid precursor protein), the genetics of early-onset AD, which has provided strong support for the amyloid cascade hypothesis, and then on the development of new drugs aimed at reducing the load of cerebral Aβ, which is still the main hope for providing a more effective treatment for AD in the future.

Keywords:
amyloid cascade, genetics, oligomer, secretase, senile plaque, treatment.

Introduction to Alzheimer's disease

In 1907, Alois Alzheimer, a German neurologist, published an account of a 51-year-old female patient, Auguste Deter, who suffered from severe memory and language problems, disorientation, hallucinations and aggressive behaviour. When Alzheimer carried out a histological examination of this patient's brain following her death, he found extensive thinning of the

[1]To whom correspondence should be addressed (email d.allsop@lancaster.ac.uk).

cerebrocortical grey matter, along with the presence of numerous focal lesions between nerve cells, and dense bundles of fibrils inside nerve cells. This combination of presenile dementia (onset <65 years of age) with 'senile plaques' and 'neurofibrillary tangles' (see Figure 1) came to be known as AD (Alzheimer's disease), a term that was later broadened to include senile forms of dementia (onset >65 years) with similar neuropathological findings [1,2].

AD is progressive in nature, showing gradual but irreversible cognitive decline, leading to instrumental signs of aphasia (loss of speech and poor word recognition), apraxia (inability to make voluntary movements) and agnosia (lack of recognition of objects) [2]. The early stage is characterized by vague-to-moderate loss of cognitive function, which advances to severe memory deficit accompanied by loss of functional independence and an increase in behavioural problems. Mean survival time following initial diagnosis is around 8 years.

The major risk factor for AD is simply getting old. The majority of cases are sporadic in onset, but approximately 5% of them show clear autosomal dominant inheritance. By and large, fAD (familial AD) corresponds to early-onset disease, whereas sporadic AD is synonymous with late-onset disease. Other risk factors include reduced reserve capacity of the brain (small brain size and low educational achievement), head injury and vascular disease. Symptoms often present with higher severity and progress more rapidly in the presenile form of AD [2].

Critical to current diagnosis and treatment strategies is the fact that neurodegeneration is thought to commence 20–30 years prior to the onset of symptoms [2]. MCI (mild cognitive impairment) is a condition where an individual shows greater than expected memory impairment, but not severe enough for a diagnosis of dementia. Approximately 12% of individuals with MCI have been found to 'convert' into AD each year [3]. This fact, along with reports of the presence of early AD neuropathological changes in some individuals with MCI, has led to the strong belief that a subpopulation of MCI cases represents a preclinical phase of AD [4].

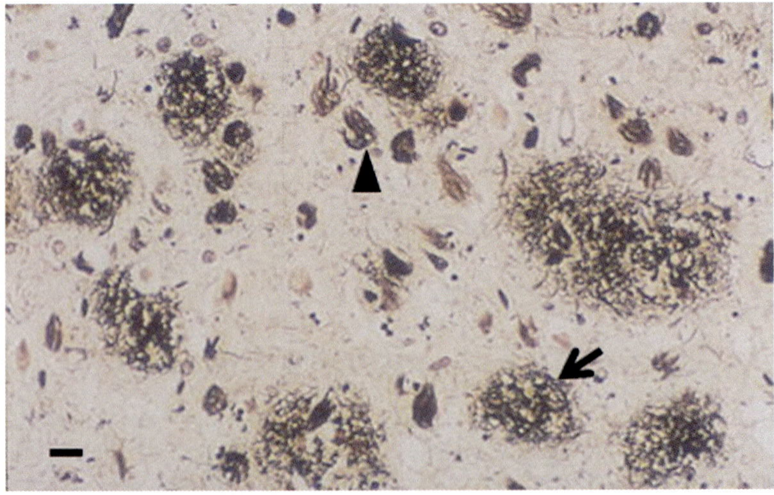

Figure 1. Histopathology of AD
Senile plaques (arrow) and neurofibrillary tangles (arrowhead) are detected by silver staining of a section of brain cortex (scale bar, 10 μM). Image courtesy of Professor D.M.A. Mann (University of Manchester, U.K.).

AD is the leading cause of dementia in the elderly and afflicts approximately 11% of people over the age of 65 years, rising to 32% of those over the age of 85 [5]. With an aging population, due to an ever increasing life expectancy, its prevalence is set to increase dramatically. In 2010 there were 36 million cases of AD worldwide, and this number is expected to approximately double every 20 years to 66 million in 2030 and 115 million in 2050 [6]. Currently available drugs for AD [the actetylcholinesterase inhibitors donepezil, rivastigmine and galantamine, and the NMDA (*N*-methyl-D-aspartate) receptor antagonist memantine] can only temporarily alleviate the symptoms of the disease [2,7]. Hence there is a great need for the development of more effective treatments. Even so, research into dementia has been grossly underfunded compared with other major public health concerns, such as cancer and heart disease [8].

Neuropathological changes

AD can be considered to be a localized form of brain amyloid disease (amyloidosis). It is one of several different 'protein misfolding disorders' that target the brain, with other examples being Parkinson's disease, prion disease (e.g. Creutzfeldt–Jacob disease), motor neuron disease (sometimes referred to as amyotrophic lateral sclerosis) and Huntington's disease. In each of these diseases, the progressive death of neurons occurs in different parts of the brain/central nervous system, with the consequent presentation of the relevant neurological symptoms.

In AD, the amyloid deposits are found mainly at the centre of senile plaques, where they accumulate in the form of radiating fibrils, surrounded by abnormal nerve cell processes and activated microglial cells. Their principal component is a 39–43 amino acid peptide, termed Aβ (amyloid β-peptide) [9]. Antibodies against Aβ can be used to detect these amyloid deposits *in vivo* (Figure 2A), and synthetic Aβ peptides will spontaneously aggregate into amyloid fibrils *in vitro* (Figure 2B). The neurofibrillary tangles on the other hand consist of filaments inside nerve cells that can occupy most of the cytoplasm and enter the nerve cell processes.

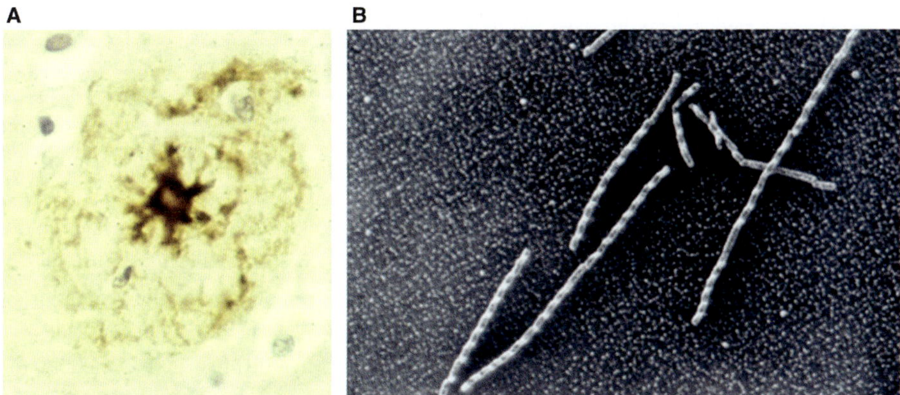

Figure 2. Role of Aβ in amyloid and senile plaque formation
This peptide can be detected at the centre of the senile plaque by immunostaining (**A**), and assembles *in vitro* into 10-nm-diameter amyloid fibrils, detected by electron microscopy with rotary metal shadowing (**B**). The image in (**B**) is courtesy of Dr David Howlett (King's College London, U.K.).

They are composed of a microtubule-associated protein called tau, which aggregates into PHFs (paired helical filaments), consisting of two 10 nm filaments wound around each other in the form of a double helix [1,10].

In addition to the hallmark plaques and tangles, the neuropathological features of AD include a substantial loss of brain weight, enlargement of the fluid-filled ventricles in the brain, an inflammatory response involving activation of glial cells, widespread and early oxidative damage, and extensive neuronal/synaptic degeneration, resulting in defects in a number of neurotransmitter systems including the brain's acteylcholine (cholinergic) system [2]. Amyloid fibrils composed of Aβ can also accumulate in the cerebral blood vessels, where they can lead to brain haemorrhage [1,2,9,11].

The amyloid precursor protein

Aβ is a 39–43 amino acid peptide that is found, even in healthy individuals, in the brain, blood, cerebrospinal fluid and in other tissues. In AD it becomes misfolded and self-associates to form extensive amyloid deposits. Aβ40 is the major Aβ species, and Aβ42 is a minor species that aggregates much more readily *in vitro* into amyloid fibrils and is heavily enriched in senile plaques ([1,12] and references within).

Aβ is generated from a larger precursor protein, usually referred to as the APP (amyloid precursor protein). This protein is a type 1 integral membrane glycoprotein (spanning the membrane once, and with an extracellular N-terminus). Alternative splicing of APP mRNA leads to multiple different length isoforms of APP being created. The largest isoform, APP770, has both a KPI (kunitz-type protease inhibitor) domain and an OX-2 antigen domain. There is some evidence to suggest that Aβ is formed preferentially from APP695, which lacks both of these domains, and is the predominant isoform present in human brain. The Aβ domain of APP lies partially embedded in the plasma membrane, with 12–14 residues residing inside the transmembrane domain and the remaining 28 residues residing outside of the membrane [2,13].

The physiological function of APP is still uncertain, but its potential roles have been suggested to include intracellular calcium regulation [14], regulation of cell growth [15], vesicle transport along axons [16] and metal ion homoeostasis [13]. Structurally, the large extracellular N-terminal region of APP contains a metal-binding domain, which is assumed by some researchers to be critical to its biological function. This domain has a strong affinity for copper ions ($K_d \approx 10$ nM) [13]. APP-knockout mice show raised levels of copper in the liver and brain, and, conversely, brain copper levels are diminished in APP transgenic mice, supporting a role for APP in metal (copper) homoeostasis [17,18].

APP is cleaved by proteolysis at three major sites in the molecule: cleavage at the α-secretase site (between residues 16–17 of the Aβ region) precludes the formation of Aβ, whereas sequential cleavage at the β- and γ-secretase sites is responsible for the generation of Aβ [1,2] (Figure 3).

Several zinc metalloproteinases belonging to the ADAM (a disintegrin and metalloproteinase) family have been identified as potential α-secretases, capable of cleaving APP at the α-site. However, even though a number of ADAMs have been implicated in this role, ADAM10 has emerged as the strongest candidate and is thought to be most physiologically relevant in the pathogenesis of AD [19]. The major β-secretase has been identified as an integral membrane aspartic protease called BACE1 (β-site APP-cleaving enzyme 1) [20]. An

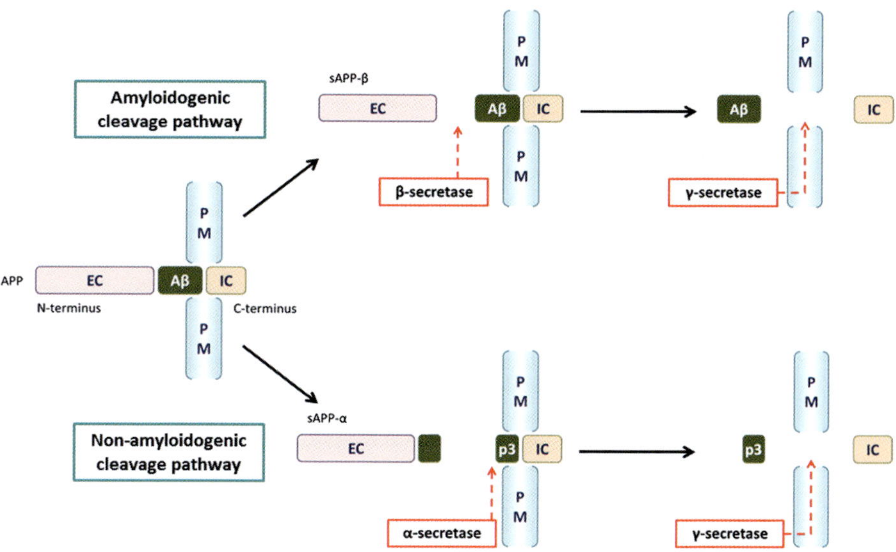

Figure 3. APP processing pathways
Proteolytic processing of APP is dependent on an initial cleavage by either α-secretase or β-secretase, followed by the action of γ-secretase. In the amyloidogenic pathway, APP is initially cleaved by β-secretase, and the Aβ fragment is formed, potentially leading to its aggregation. This is not the case for the non-amyloidogenic pathway, where APP is initially cleaved by α-secretase. EC, extracellular protein fragment; IC, intracellular protein fragment; PM, plasma membrane.

intramembrane protein complex has been identified as γ-secretase [21]. It is composed of four essential components: the proteins nicastrin, PEN-2 (presenilin enhancer 2), APH-1 (anterior pharynx defective 1) and presenilin (see below), which contributes the active site. This enzyme shows some heterogeneity in the exact site of APP cleavage, so that the Aβ peptide can be of varying lengths [1,2,21].

Following its formation, Aβ can be degraded by proteolysis or cleared from the brain into the peripheral blood circulation, through the BBB (blood–brain barrier). Neprilysin, IDE (insulin-degrading enzyme), ECE (endothelin-converting enzyme) and ACE (angiotensin-converting enzyme) have all been reported to be capable of degrading Aβ. The efflux of Aβ across the BBB is mediated by the LRP (low-density lipoprotein receptor-related protein). This is balanced by the action of RAGE (receptor for advanced glycation end products) which mediates its influx back into the brain [12,22].

It is likely that sporadic AD is due to an imbalance in the proteolytic events related to APP/Aβ or an inadequate clearance of Aβ from the brain.

Genetics of AD

The first genetic mutation identified for fAD was in the gene for APP, located on chromosome 21. Further studies have so far identified 25 pathogenic mutations of the APP gene, but together these mutations account for less than 1% of AD cases [23].

The disease-causing mutations in the gene for APP result in amino acid substitutions that are either clustered around the β- and γ-cleavage sites, or involve residues within Aβ that are

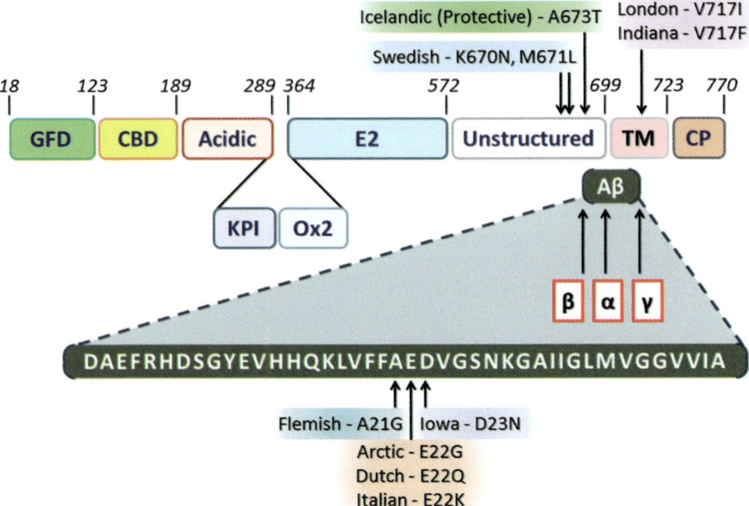

Figure 4. Some of the pathogenic amino acid substitutions resulting from mutations in the APP gene associated with fAD
Disease-causing mutations in the gene for APP result in amino acid substitutions clustered around each of the secretase cleavage sites. The domains of APP are shown, including positions where the KPI and OX-2 domains can be removed by alternative mRNA splicing events. The fragment that forms the Aβ peptide is shown (coloured olive green), with the cleavage sites for the secretases (α-secretase, β-secretase and γ-secretase) also indicated. The numbers represent the residue boundaries of each domain. Acidic, domain rich in acidic residues; CBD, copper-binding domain; CP, cytoplasmic tail; E2, glycosylated domain; GFD, growth factor domain; TM, transmembrane domain.

important for its self-association and aggregation (Figure 4). Consequently, they either increase the amount of Aβ released from APP, or promote Aβ aggregation. Multiple mutations around the γ-secretase cleavage site (T714I, V715M, V715A, I716V, V717I and V717L) specifically cause increased production of the more amyloidogenic Aβ42 compared with Aβ40. Those substitutions clustered around residues 21–23 of Aβ [A21G (Flemish), E22G (Arctic), E22Q (Dutch), E22K (Italian) and D23N (Iowa)] lead to either AD or to cerebral haemorrhage [1,11].

The idea that increased Aβ production causes AD is supported by *in vivo* gene dosage evidence from Down's syndrome patients. These individuals develop senile plaques and neurofibrillary tangles at an early age due to an extra copy of part or the whole of chromosome 21 (trisomy 21). Consequently, they have three copies of the gene for APP, resulting in overproduction of Aβ and accelerated plaque deposition, subsequently leading to tangle formation [1,24]. Moreover, some cases of fAD are also due to APP gene duplication [11].

The majority of fAD cases are explained by mutations in the highly homologous genes for presenilin 1 and presenilin 2 (*PSEN1* and *PSEN2*) located on chromosomes 14 and 1 respectively. These gene mutations cause altered APP processing and up-regulation of Aβ generation, especially of Aβ42 [2,11]. Recently, it has been determined that Alzheimer's original case, Auguste Deter, actually had a presenilin 1 (F176L) mutation [25].

All of this evidence from genetic studies implicates the involvement of APP processing events, especially those resulting in the generation of Aβ, as being central to the pathogenic pathways leading to AD [1,2,24]. This has been greatly reinforced recently by the finding of a rare variant (A673T) of APP that actually protects against AD and age-related cognitive impairment by inhibiting proteolytic cleavage at the β-secretase site and reducing Aβ production [26].

One of the most common risk factors for late-onset AD is the possession of the APOE (apolipoprotein E) ε4 allele located on chromosome 19. The allele exists in two other major forms, APOE ε2 and APOE ε3. Individuals who are heterozygous for APOE ε4 are three times more likely to develop AD, and individuals who are homozygous for APOE ε4 are eight times more likely to develop AD than individuals with no APOE ε4 allele. Possession of each APOE ε4 allele lowers AD onset by around 10 years, and results in increased senile plaque density [27].

ApoE is the major apolipoprotein expressed in the brain. It is a lipid and cholesterol transporter needed for the recycling of membrane lipids and for neuronal repair. ApoE4 is less efficient than the other variants at performing these functions, strengthening links between vascular disease, fat intake and AD. ApoE4 has also been suggested to increase risk of AD because it is less able to cope with Aβ-induced oxidative stress than the other isoforms [28]. As noted above, apoE4 has also been found to promote Aβ fibrillization and deposition into plaques [29]. However, apoE4 is also a risk factor for other neurodegenerative diseases, and so the effects of apoE4 in AD are likely to be both Aβ dependent and independent.

A rare missense mutation in the gene encoding TREM2 (triggering receptor expressed on myeloid cells 2) also confers a significant risk of late-onset AD [30]. This protein has an anti-inflammatory role in the brain, and so this reinforces the importance of pro-inflammatory processes, which have long been suspected of playing a significant role in AD pathogenesis, and could be a consequence of senile plaque formation.

Amyloid cascade hypothesis

The 'amyloid cascade' hypothesis proposes that an imbalance between the production and/or clearance of Aβ, leading to its accumulation and aggregation in the brain, is central to both sporadic and fAD [1,2,9,24]. Genetic evidence for this hypothesis has been paramount (see above), but there has also been an increased emphasis on problems related to the clearance of Aβ (due to reduced proteolytic degradation, reduced perivascular drainage or less microglial clearance) in sporadic AD [2]. This is supported by the finding that 'soluble Aβ' is present at a considerably higher level in the brains of victims of AD than in healthy control brains [12]. It should be noted here that Aβ could act as a direct neurotoxin and/or as a trigger that sets off other damaging processes, including tau pathology and neurofibrillary tangle formation.

The amyloid cascade hypothesis has proved to be resilient, although some revisions have been made [12]. In particular, emphasis has shifted away from amyloid fibrils as the predominant toxic form of Aβ and towards smaller and more soluble aggregates, which may include a variety of structures, referred to as soluble oligomers, ADDLs (amyloid β-derived diffusible ligands) or protofibrils [31] (Figure 5). This change in thinking has been prompted to some extent by the finding that the relationship between the numbers of senile plaques and the severity of dementia is poor, as well as by the finding that small soluble oligomers seem to be more toxic than fibrillar Aβ and, in addition, have potent effects on learning and memory in animals [31]. The precise nature of these neurotoxic, soluble oligomers remains unclear, however, due to the fact Aβ aggregates produced experimentally are often highly polymorphic and dynamic, with an inbuilt tendency to aggregate into higher-order structures. Also, detecting Aβ oligomers with any confidence in the human brain is highly problematic.

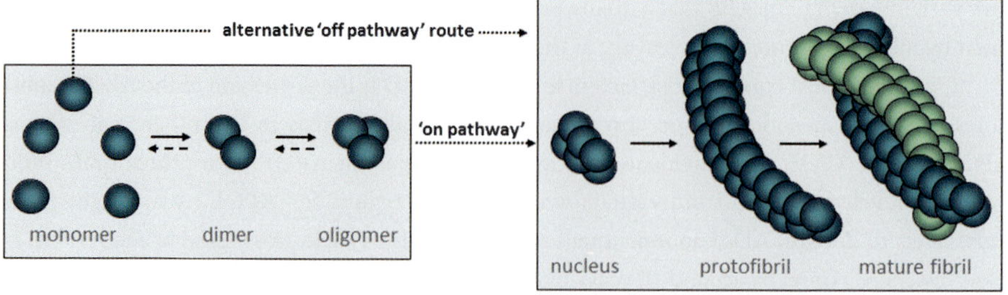

Figure 5. Schematic diagram showing the aggregation of monomeric Aβ into oligomers and amyloid fibrils

The oligomers can be either 'on pathway' or 'off pathway' with respect to amyloid fibril formation. In the former case, they are early intermediates on the pathway leading to fibre formation, whereas, in the latter case, the monomers assemble directly into the 'nucleus' required to initiate fibril formation, and the oligomers are formed on a separate pathway. In either case, the small oligomeric forms of Aβ are now thought to be more potent as brain toxins.

Development of new therapies for AD

Not surprisingly, the development of drugs which could alter the course of AD has been largely focused on reducing the load of cerebral Aβ [2,7] (Figure 6). These strategies, which include modulation of secretase action, immunotherapy and inhibition of Aβ aggregation, have so far yielded disappointing results in clinical trials [7]. However, in our opinion, this has been largely due to issues with trial design in combination with low efficacy, poor bioavailability or unwanted side effects, rather than any inherent problem with the amyloid hypothesis itself.

Inhibiting the action of BACE1 seems to be highly attractive, given the fact that BACE1-knockout mice do not produce any Aβ [32]. However, APP is not the only substrate for BACE1, and the development of BACE1 inhibitors has proved to be inherently problematic for medicinal chemists owing to its wide substrate-binding domain, along with the need to develop inhibitors that cross the BBB, although this has been overcome to some extent [7]. There is also the possibility that Aβ could have an important physiological function in the brain and so blocking its formation may not be desirable.

The γ-secretase enzyme has always been an unlikely drug target, because of its complexity, and the fact that it is involved in Notch processing, which plays an important role in cancer and cell differentiation. Notch-sparing γ-secretase 'modulators' (reviewed in [7,33]) are in clinical development, but they might not succeed because of the unavoidable accumulation of neurotoxic C-terminal fragments of APP, resulting from the continued action of the α- and β-secretases.

Direct immunization with Aβ or passive immunization with anti-Aβ antibodies has been found to prevent and/or reverse amyloid plaque deposition in brains of transgenic mice, but when applied to humans this approach has been plagued by adverse pro-inflammatory effects involving a detrimental T-cell-mediated brain response (reviewed in [7,34]). Another consideration with any approach, such as this, which targets senile plaques, is the fact that breaking down pre-existing amyloid deposits from patients with relatively advanced AD could result in the release of toxic forms of Aβ into the brain.

The critical event that initiates AD is likely to be the misfolding and aggregation of Aβ and so this would seem to be the most logical drug target. Aβ aggregation is a purely

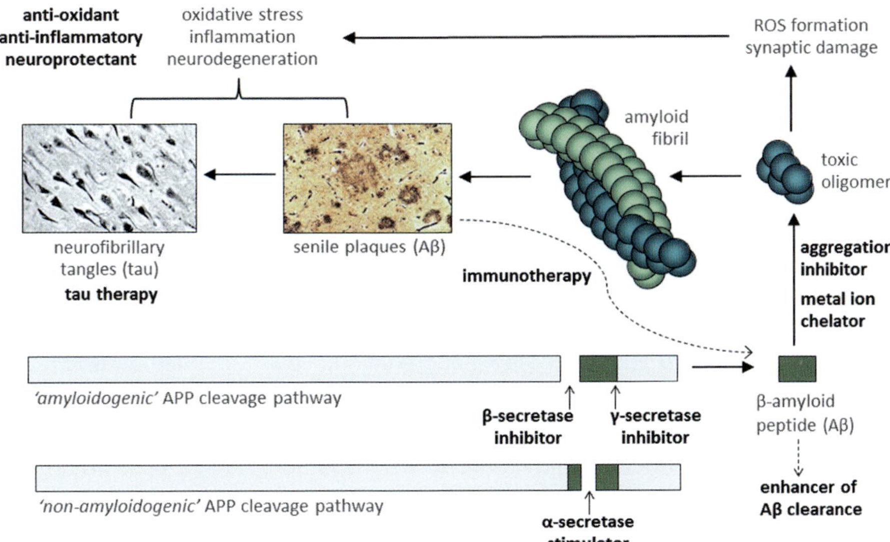

Figure 6. Possible new approaches to the therapy of Alzheimer's disease
These approaches include drugs targeted at the secretase cleavage enzymes, as well as inhibitors of Aβ aggregation and enhancers of Aβ clearance. The 'immunotherapy' approach involves passive or active immunization against Aβ, and results in inhibition of new plaque formation and/or the clearance of pre-existing plaques. More 'downstream' approaches involve tau modulators (inhibitors of tangle formation), anti-oxidants, anti-inflammatory drugs or neuroprotectants.

pathological phenomenon, and so this approach should not suffer from any serious side effects. However, developing potent, selective and bioavailable aggregation inhibitors represents a formidable challenge. Tramiprosate (Alzhemed) failed in clinical trials, but this drug was designed to interfere with the binding of proteoglycans to Aβ, and is not a proven inhibitor of toxic Aβ oligomer formation [7].

For all of these types of drug therapy to be most effective, they would have to be applied early on during the course of the disease, preferably at the MCI stage before too much irreversible damage has been done to the brain. This could be one of the major problems with the drug trials carried out to date, which have been on more advanced cases of AD. Molecular biomarkers (related to Aβ and tau) and brain imaging techniques already permit identification of those people with MCI who will go on to develop dementia with a reasonable degree of certainty [4], and it is likely that this population will soon become the main target for drug trials, leading to greater optimism for the future development of an effective preventative therapy for AD.

Summary

- AD, the most common cause of dementia, is a localized form of brain amyloidosis, involving the accumulation of Aβ fibrils within senile plaques.
- The only drugs currently available for AD are actetylcholinesterase inhibitors and memantine, which temporarily alleviate symptoms, but do not provide a cure.

- Aβ is generated from APP by BACE1 and γ-secretase (a mutienzyme complex composed of nicastrin, PEN-2, APH-1 and presenilin), whereas cleavage of APP by α-secretase (the strongest candidate for which is ADAM10) precludes the formation of Aβ.
- Aβ can be degraded by proteolysis or cleared from the brain into the blood, and there is mounting evidence that sporadic (late-onset) AD is caused by reduced clearance of Aβ from the brain.
- Rare genetic forms of early-onset AD are due to mutations in the genes for APP, presenilin 1 or presenilin 2, all of which increase the amount of Aβ released from APP, or promote Aβ aggregation.
- Alzheimer's original case (Auguste Deter) had a presenilin 1 (F176L) mutation.
- The most common genetic risk factors for sporadic AD are possession of the APOE ε4 allele, which increases senile plaque density, and a rare missense mutation in the gene encoding TREM2, which has an anti-inflammatory role in the brain.
- Emphasis has shifted away from amyloid fibrils as the predominant toxic form of Aβ and towards smaller 'oligomers'.
- The development of disease-modifying drugs for AD has been largely focused on modulation of secretase action, immunotherapy and inhibition of Aβ aggregation, in order to reduce the load of cerebral Aβ.
- So far, clinical trials of these drugs have produced disappointing results, but there is now a move towards testing new drugs at the early MCI stage, which provides some hope for a future preventative therapy.

Thanks to all former and current colleagues who have worked or collaborated with us on Aβ and Alzheimer's disease. Work in David Allsop's laboratory was recently supported by EU Framework 7, the Wellcome Trust, Alzheimer's Society UK, Alzheimer's Research UK, Eleanor Peel Trust, Joy Welch Foundation and The Sir John Fisher Foundation. Jennifer Mayes is particularly grateful for support for the last 4 years from The Sir John Fisher Foundation.

References

1. Selkoe, D.J. (2001) Alzheimer's disease: genes, proteins, and therapy. Physiol. Rev. **81**, 741–766
2. Blennow, K., de Leon, M.J. and Zetterberg, H. (2006) Alzheimer's disease. Lancet **368**, 387–403
3. Petersen, R.C. (2004) Mild cognitive impairment as a diagnostic entity. J. Int. Med. **256**, 183–194
4. Eckerström, C., Olsson, E., Bjerke, M., Malmgren, H., Edman, A., Wallin, A. and Nordlund, A. (2013) A combination of neuropsychological, neuroimaging, and cerebrospinal fluid markers predicts conversion from mild cognitive impairment to dementia. J. Alzheimers Dis. **36**, 421–431
5. Thies, W. and Bleiler, L. (2013) 2013 Alzheimer's disease facts and figures. Alzheimers Dement. **9**, 208–245

6. Alzheimer's Disease International: World Alzheimer Report 2009. Alzheimer's Disease International, London. Available at: http://www.alz.co.uk/research/files/WorldAlzheimerReport.pdf (Accessed 5 September 2013)

7. Anand, R., Gill, K.D. and Mahdi, A.A. (2014) Therapeutics of Alzheimer's disease: past, present and future. Neuropharmacology **76**, 27–50

8. Dementia 2010: the economic burden of dementia and associated research funding in the United Kingdom. Health Economics Research Centre, University of Oxford, Oxford. Available at: http://www.herc.ox.ac.uk/pubs/downloads/dementiafullreport (Accessed 5 September 2013)

9. Glenner, G.G. and Wong, C.W. (1984) Alzheimer's disease: initial report of the purification and characterization of a novel cerebrovascular amyloid protein. Biochem. Biophys. Res. Commun. **120**, 885–890

10. Kidd, M. (1963) Paired helical filaments in electron microscopy of Alzheimer's disease. Nature **197**, 192–193

11. Schellenberg, G.D. and Montine, T.J. (2012) The genetics and neuropathology of Alzheimer's disease. Acta Neuropath. **124**, 305–323

12. Hardy, J. and Selkoe, D.J. (2002) The amyloid hypothesis of Alzheimer's disease: progress and problems on the road to therapeutics. Science **297**, 353–356

13. Barnham, K.J., McKinstry, W.J., Multhaup, G., Galatis, D., Morton, C.J., Curtain, C.C., Williamson, N.A., White, A.R., Hinds, M.G., Norton, R.S. et al. (2003) Structure of the Alzheimer's disease amyloid precursor protein copper binding domain. A regulator of neuronal copper homeostasis. J. Biol. Chem. **278**, 17401–17407

14. Mattson, M.P., Cheng, B., Culwell, A.R., Esch, F.S., Lieberburg, I. and Rydel, R.E. (1993) Evidence for excitoprotective and intraneuronal calcium-regulating roles for secreted forms of the β-amyloid precursor protein. Neuron **10**, 243–254

15. Small, D.H., Nurcombe, V., Reed, G., Clarris, H., Moir, R., Beyreuther, K. and Masters, C.L. (1994) A heparin-binding domain in the amyloid protein precursor of Alzheimer's disease is involved in the regulation of neurite outgrowth. J. Neurosci. **14**, 2117–2127

16. Gunawardena, S. and Goldstein, L.S. (2001) Disruption of axonal transport and neuronal viability by amyloid precursor protein mutations in *Drosophila*. Neuron **32**, 389–401

17. Maynard, C.J., Cappai, R., Volitakis, I., Cherny, R.A., White, A.R., Beyreuther, K., Masters, C.L., Bush, A.I. and Li, Q.X. (2002) Overexpression of Alzheimer's disease amyloid-β opposes the age-dependent elevations of brain copper and iron. J. Biol. Chem. **277**, 44670–44676

18. White, A.R., Reyes, R., Mercer, J.F., Camakaris, J., Zheng, H., Bush, A.I., Multhaup, G., Beyreuther, K., Masters, C.L. and Cappai, R. (1999) Copper levels are increased in the cerebral cortex and liver of APP and APLP2 knockout mice. Brain Res. **842**, 439–444

19. Allinson, T.M., Parkin, E.T., Turner, A.J. and Hooper, N.M. (2003) ADAMs family members as amyloid precursor protein α-secretases. J. Neurosci. Res. **74**, 342–352

20. Vassar, R., Bennett, B.D., Babu-Khan, S., Kahn, S., Mendiaz, E.A., Denis, P., Teplow, D.B., Ross, S., Amarante, P., Loeloff, R. et al. (1999) β-Secretase cleavage of Alzheimer's amyloid precursor protein by the transmembrane aspartic protease BACE. Science **286**, 735–741

21. Smolarkiewicz, M., Skrzypczak, T. and Wojtaszek, P. (2013) The very many faces of presenilins and the γ-secretase complex. Protoplasma **250**, 997–1011

22. Tanzi, R.E., Moir, R.D. and Wagner, S.L. (2004) Clearance of Alzheimer's Aβ peptide: the many roads to perdition. Neuron **43**, 605–608

23. Lambert, J.C. and Amouyel, P. (2007) Genetic heterogeneity of Alzheimer's disease: complexity and advances. Psychoneuroendocrinology **32**, S62–S70

24. Hardy, J. and Allsop, D. (1991) Amyloid deposition as the central event in the aetiology of Alzheimer's disease. Trends Pharmacol. Sci. **12**, 383–388

25. Müller, U., Winter, P. and Graeber, M.B. (2013) A presenilin 1 mutation in the first case of Alzheimer's disease. Lancet Neurol. **12**, 129–130

26. Jonsson, T., Atwa, J.K. Steinberg, S., Snaedal, J., Jonsson, P.V., Bjornsson, S., Stefansson, H., Sulem, P., Gudbjartsson, D., Maloney, J. et al. (2012) A mutation in APP protects against Alzheimer's disease and age-related cognitive decline. Nature **488**, 96–99

27. Corder, E.H., Saunders, A.M., Strittmatter, W.J., Schmechel, D.E., Gaskell, P.C., Small, G.W., Roses, A.D., Haines, J.L. and Pericak-Vance, M.A. (1993) Gene dose of apolipoprotein E type 4 allele and the risk of Alzheimer's disease in late onset families. Science **261**, 921–923

28. Lauderback, C.M., Kanski, J., Hackett, J.M., Maeda, N., Kindy, M.S. and Butterfield, D.A. (2002) Apolipoprotein E modulates Alzheimer's Aβ(1–42)-induced oxidative damage to synaptosomes in an allele-specific manner. Brain Res. **924**, 90–97

29. Holtzman, D.M., Bales, K.R., Tenkova, T., Fagan, A.M., Parsadanian, M., Sartorius, L.J., Mackey, B., Olney, J., McKeel, D., Wozniak, D. and Paul, S.M. (2000) Apolipoprotein E isoform-dependent amyloid deposition and neuritic degeneration in a mouse model of Alzheimer's disease. Proc. Natl. Acad. Sci. U.S.A. **97**, 2892–2897

30. Jiang, T., Yu, J.T., Zhu, X.C. and Tan, L. (2013) TREM2 in Alzheimer's disease. Mol. Neurobiol. **48**, 180–185

31. Walsh, D.M. and Selkoe, D.J. (2007) Aβ oligomers: a decade of discovery. J. Neurochem. **101**, 1172–1184

32. Luo, Y., Bolon, B., Kahn, S., Bennett, B.D., Babu-Khan, S., Denis, P., Fan, W., Kha, H., Zhang, J., Gong, Y. et al. (2001) Mice deficient in BACE1, the Alzheimer's β-secretase, have normal phenotype and abolished β-amyloid generation. Nature Neurosci. **4**, 231–232

33. Golde, T.E., Koo, E.H., Felsenstein, K.M., Osborne, B.A. and Miele, L. (2013) γ-Secretase inhibitors and modulators. Biochim. Biophys. Acta **1828**, 2898–2907

34. Delrieu, J., Ousset, P.J., Caillaud, C. and Vellas, B. (2012) Clinical trials in Alzheimer's disease: immunotherapy approaches. J. Neurochem. **120**, S186–S193

© The Authors Journal compilation © 2014 Biochemical Society
Essays Biochem. (2014) 56, 111–123: doi: 10.1042/BSE0560111

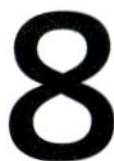

The physiology and pathology of microtubule-associated protein tau

Jian-Zhi Wang[1], Xinya Gao and Zhi-Hao Wang

Pathophysiology Department, Key Laboratory of Ministry of the People's Republic of China for Neurological Disorders, Tongji Medical College, Huazhong University of Science and Technology, Wuhan 430030, P.R. China

Abstract

Tau belongs to the family of microtubule-associated proteins predominantly expressed in neurons where they play an important role in promoting microtubule assembly and stabilizing microtubules. In addition, tau proteins interact with other cytoskeletal elements to allow spacing between microtubules. Recent studies have shown that tau is also actively involved in regulating cell viability and activity. Translated from a single gene located on chromosome 17q21, six isoforms of tau are produced by alternative splicing in adult human brain. Due to multiple post-translational modifications, heterogeneous tau species with a wide range of apparent molecular masses have been observed by denaturing polyacrylamide-gel electrophoresis. Since tau gene mutations and abnormal post-translational modifications have been detected in over 20 neurodegenerative disorders, namely the tauopathies, tau has gained widespread attention as a target protein in Alzheimer's disease and other neurodegenerative disorders. In the present chapter, research progress regarding physiology and pathology of tau is reviewed, particularly in terms of the role of post-translational modification.

Keywords:
Alzheimer's disease, hyperphosphorylation, neurodegeneration, tau, tauopathies.

[1]*To whom correspondence should be addressed (email wangjz@mails.tjmu.edu.cn).*

Introduction

Tau protein was discovered in the mid-1970s when searching for the factors involved in microtubule formation. Tau proteins are predominantly expressed in neurons of the brain and very low levels have also been detected in astrocytes and oligodendrocytes of the CNS (central nervous system). Normally, tau proteins are located in neuronal axons. As a major microtubule-associated protein, the primary function of tau is to modulate microtubule dynamics and to maintain the spaces between microtubules, to ensure the neuronal architecture and to provide the tracks for axonal transport; tau also serves as an anchor for other proteins or enzymes involved in cell signalling. Studies have shown that tau can actively regulate cell viability and activity [1,2], and it has been identified as an intrinsic acetyltransferase [3].

Under pathological conditions, tau proteins are abnormally modified and aggregated into intracellular filamentous inclusions in the form of NFTs (neurofibrillary tangles) in the brains of individuals with neurodegenerative disorders collectively known as tauopathies. Among various abnormal post-translational modifications of tau proteins, hyperphosphorylation has been identified in over 20 neurodegenerative diseases including AD (Alzheimer's disease), PSP (progressive supranuclear palsy), PiD (Pick's disease) and FTDP-17 (frontotemporal dementia with Parkinsonism-linked to chromosome-17). In AD patients, elevation of the abnormally hyperphosphorylated tau proteins has been detected in both the brain and CSF (cerebrospinal fluid) [4,5]. In patients with FTDP-17, tau gene mutation causes dissociation of the hyperphosphorylated tau from microtubules [6,7]. Several transgenic mouse models also show that overexpressing human mutant tau protein results in neuronal loss [8], whereas expression of normal human tau40, the longest isoform of tau, causes somatodendritic accumulation of hyperphosphorylated tau proteins [9].

Human tau gene: the transcripts and the proteins

Located on the chromosome 17q21, the human tau gene contains 16 exons. Exons 1, 4, 5, 7, 9, 11, 12 and 13 are constitutive exons and exon 1 is part of the promoter that is transcribed but not translated. Exons 2, 3 and 10 are alternatively spliced in adult human brains, of which exon 2 can appear alone, but exon 3 never appears independently of exon 2 [10] (Figure 1).

By alternative splicing of exons 2, 3 and 10, six isoforms of tau proteins (352–441 amino acid residues) differing in their affinity for microtubules are produced in adult human brains [11]. The alternative splicing of exon 2 and exon 3 generates tau with no N-terminal insert (0N), one insert (1N) or two inserts (2N), whereas the alternative splicing of exon 10 produces tau proteins with three (3R) or four (4R) microtubule-binding repeat domains. In fetal brain, only the 3R isoform is detected and the expression level is low, whereas both the level and the number of tau isoforms increase during brain development (Figure 1).

In normal human brain, the ratio of 4R to 3R tau is approximately 1:1, whereas alternative splicing of exon 10 changes the ratio of 4R to 3R tau. Therefore the alternative splicing of exon 10 has drawn significant attention. It has been found that some forms of FTDP-17 are caused by tau gene mutations that affect exon 10 splicing. Although RNA analysis indicates an elevation in exon 10-containing tau mRNA in AD patients, the molecular mechanism contributing

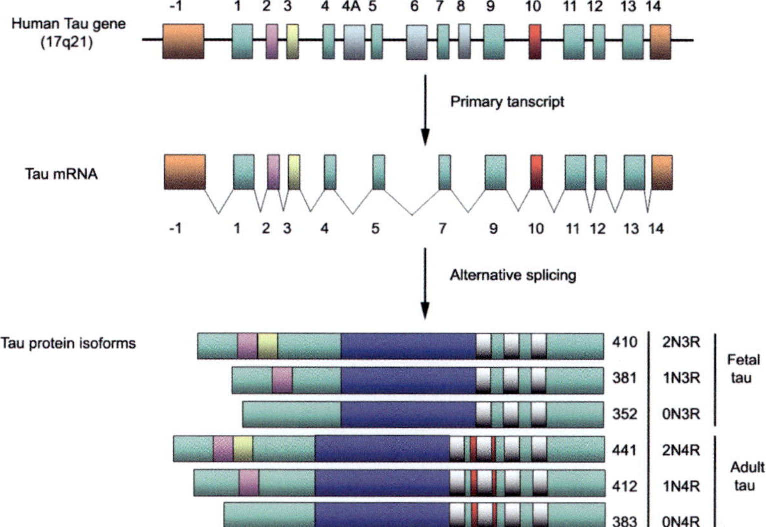

Figure 1. Schematic diagram of the tau gene and the protein isoforms in human brains

Exons 1, 4, 5, 7, 9, 11, 12 and 13 are constitutive exons, whereas exons 1, 4A, 6, 8 and 14 are not. Exons 2 (in purple), 3 (in yellow) and 10 (in red) are alternatively spliced to produce tau proteins with 3R (fetal) or 4R (adult) depending on the presence or absence of exon 10 (4R or 3R) and 0 (0N), 1 (1N) or 2 (2N) N-terminal inserts encoded by exons 2 and 3.

to the abnormal splicing of tau pre-mRNA is not understood because no tau mutations have been found to date in AD patients. Studies have shown that tau exon 10 splicing is regulated by several protein kinases, including GSK-3 (glycogen synthase kinase-3) and PKA (protein kinase A) [12]. Further studies to verify the effects of 4R and 3R on neuron activity and degeneration, as well as to identify the causative factors leading to the changed exon 10 splicing in AD will be important for disclosing the pathogenesis of neurodegeneration and for therapeutic intervention in sporadic AD.

To date, higher order structure in tau proteins has not been identified. The primary structure of tau proteins contains four regions: an N-terminal projection region, a proline-rich

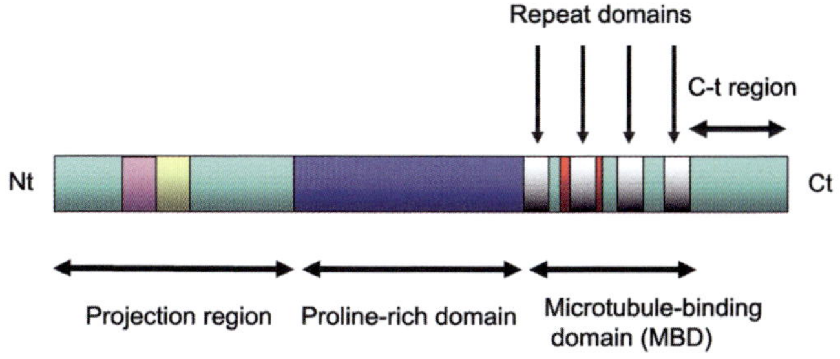

Figure 2. Schematic diagram showing the sub-regions of the longest tau protein

Tau is subdivided into four regions: the acidic region in the N-terminal (Nt) projection region, the proline-rich region, the region responsible for tau binding with microtubules that contains four repeat domains (MBD), namely R1, R3, R4 and R2 (in grey), and the C-terminal (Ct) region.

domain, an MBD (microtubule-binding domain) and a C-terminal region (Figure 2). The N-terminal projection of tau can associate with the cell membrane; this region of tau proteins may also interact with other cytoskeleton elements to regulate the spacing between microtubules. The proline-rich domain includes many phosphorylation sites and can bind to SH3 (Src homology 3) domains of other proteins, such as tyrosine kinase Fyn. The MBD of tau composed of four repeats (R1–R4 encoded by exons 9–12) and the adjacent regions determine the binding ability of tau to microtubules. The microtubules assembled with 3R tau and tubulin at the ratios that approximate those found in neurons glide faster than microtubules assembled with 4R tau, suggesting that 3R and 4R tau-assembled microtubules possess at least some isoform-specific features that affect kinesin translocation [13]. Phosphorylation of tau at Ser^{262} decreases the binding of tau to microtubules. Pseudophosphorylation of tau in its C-terminal region, particularly at Ser^{422}, preferentially promotes tau self-aggregation, whereas dephosphorylation of tau may facilitate tau cleavage at Lys^{421} by caspase and degradation by calpain into small fragments (17 kDa or 20 kDa), which have a high capacity to form fibrils.

Biological functions of tau proteins

Accounting for over 80% of the total microtubule-associated proteins, the primary function of tau is to promote microtubule assembly and to maintain the stability of microtubules, one of the major components of the neuronal cytoskeleton that defines the normal morphology/structure of the neurons and serves as tracks for axonal transport. It is well established that abnormally hyperphosphorylated tau detaches from the microtubule and thus causes disassembly of the microtubule, and dephosphorylation restores the microtubule binding and assembly of tau proteins [14]. Hyperphosphorylation also causes intracellular accumulation of tau proteins and thus reduces the anterograde and retrograde transport velocity of tau in axons [15]. Axoplasmic transport involves sophisticated machinery in addition to microtubules as a track. Currently, it is not fully understood whether and how abnormal tau may interact with molecular motors, such as KLC (kinesin light chain; responsible for binding of cargo during anterograde transport) and of DIC (dynein intermediate chain; a component of the dynein complex during retrograde transport), to cause impairment of axonal transport. *In vivo* time-lapse fluorescence imaging may shed light on how abnormal tau affects the cytoplasmic/axonal transport of tau itself and other vesicles, such as neurofilaments and mitochondria, and how abnormal tau-related transport deficits contribute to AD pathogenesis.

As a major microtubule-associated protein, most tau-related studies have been focused on its functions within the cytoskeleton. Recent studies demonstrate that tau protein is also actively involved in regulating cell viability and activity. As a competitive substrate of GSK-3β, tau phosphorylation can preserve survival factors, such as β-catenin, and thus protect cells from an acute apoptotic death [2].

Accumulating evidence also suggests that tau proteins are involved in multiple cell signalling pathways. The binding of tau to the SH3 domains of Src family tyrosine kinases may target tau to the plasma membrane where tau may play a role in membrane-associated signalling events. The dendritic location of tau mediates the synaptic impairment induced by Aβ (amyloid β-peptide), whereas knockout of tau in AD transgenic mice uncouples NMDAR (*N*-methyl-D-aspartate receptor)-mediated excitotoxicity and hence mitigates Aβ toxicity [16]. Tau can activate PLCγ (phospholipase-Cγ) by AA (arachidonic acid), which is involved in the pathogenesis of AD. Tau can also act as a direct enzyme inhibitor when it binds to HDAC6 (histone deacetylase 6), a unique cytoplasmic tubulin deacetylase, with a consequent increase in tubulin acetylation. Conversely, loss of HDAC6 can alleviate abnormal deposition of tau. Most recently, tau has been identified as an intrinsic acetyltransferase [3]. Similar to the prion protein, tau proteins seem transmissible between neurons and thus cause neurodegeneration. Overexpression of tau causes mitochondrial fusion with mitochondrial dysfunction.

Post-translational modifications of tau proteins

Tau proteins undergo various post-translational modifications including acetylation, glycation, glycosylation, methylation, nitration, oxidation, phosphorylation, polyamination, prolyl isomerization, SUMOylation, truncation and ubiquitination. Some of the post-translational modifications, such as phosphorylation, glycosylation and acetylation, are detected under both physiological (although at a lower level) and pathological conditions, whereas some of them are only observed under pathological conditions, such as glycation. Tau proteins prepared from normal adult brain show molecular masses in the range of ~37 to ~46 kDa, whereas due to different degrees of post-translational modification, heterogeneous tau species with a wide range of apparent molecular masses on SDS/PAGE (sodium dodecyl sulfate/polyacrylamide-gel electrophoresis) are produced.

Acetylation of tau proteins

Among the various post-translational modifications, acetylation of tau proteins is the most recently identified. It is found that the distribution pattern of acetylated tau is similar to hyperphosphorylated tau, which presents throughout all stages of AD pathology [3] and acetylation inhibits degradation of phosphorylated tau. Moreover, it has been demonstrated that tau proteins possess intrinsic acetyltransferase activity capable of catalysing self-acetylation. The discovery of tau enzymatic activity highlights tau as a potential therapeutic target.

Glycation of tau proteins

Glycation, which frequently occurs during aging, is a non-enzymatic reaction between a carbohydrate (such as glucose) and generally a lysine residue of a long-lived protein. On the tau protein, 12 glycation sites can be found, with seven of them located in the MBD (Figure 3). Glycation promotes formation of the AGEs (advanced glycation end products), which are preferentially found in PHF (paired helical filament)/NFT, and thus promote neuronal dysfunction and cell death [17]. Tau glycation prevents its degradation and promotes tau polymerization, but glycation alone does not seem to induce tau aggregation [18].

Glycosylation of tau proteins

Different from glycation, glycosylation is an enzyme-catalysed covalent attachment of oligosaccharides to the proteins. There are two types of glycosylation, namely N-glycosylation and O-glycosylation, resulting from the attachment of a sugar on the amine radical of an asparagine residue or on the hydroxyl radical of a serine or threonine residue. Tau proteins have 11

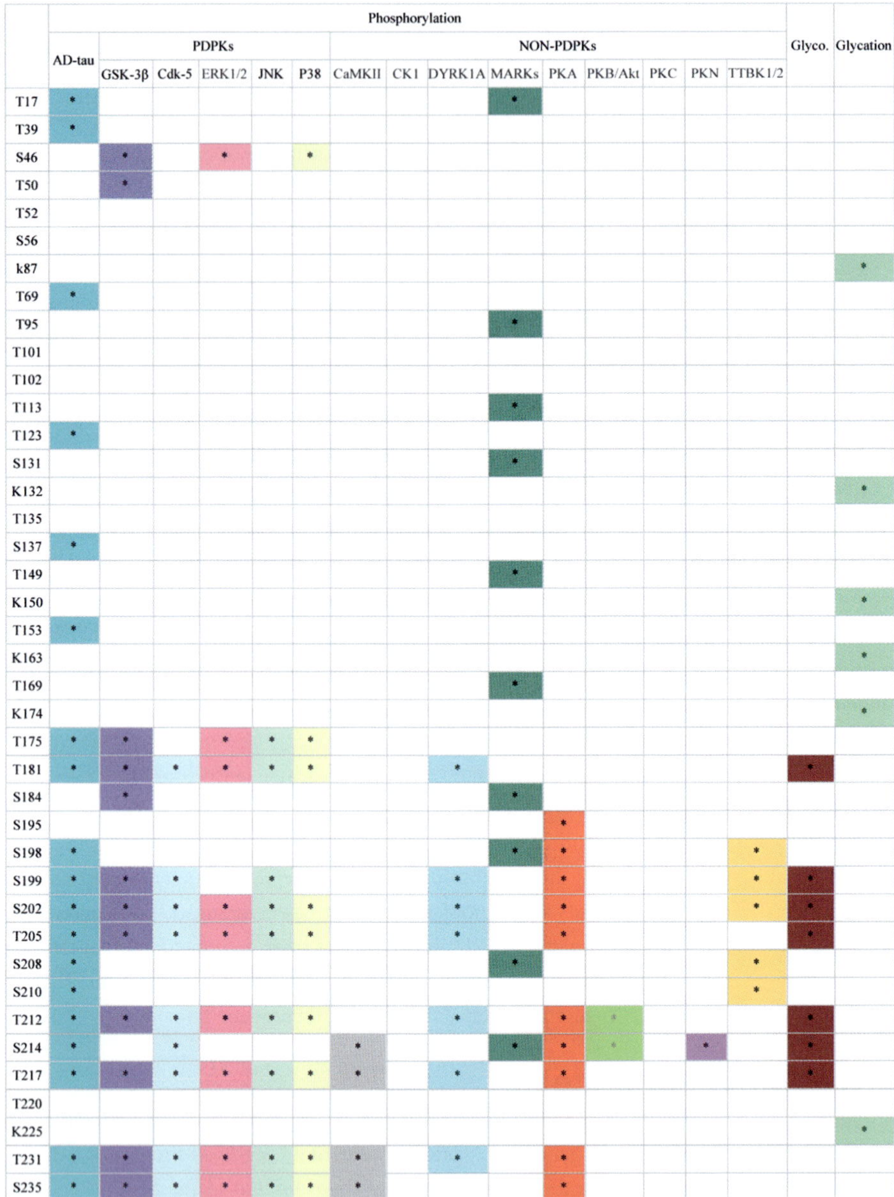

Figure 3. The post-translational modifications of tau proteins
AD-tau, abnormally hyperphosphorylated tau from AD brain; Glyco, glycosylation.

putative O-glycosylation sites, but only four sites in tau are O-glycosylated (Figure 3). A negative correlation has been observed between the O-glycosylation level and tau phosphorylation in AD and in a starved rat model, suggesting that O-glycosylation can protect tau from hyperphosphorylation [19]. The level of N-glycosylated tau is increased in AD patients. However, deglycosylation alone without dephosphorylation of the abnormally modified tau cannot restore the microtubule polymerization activity of tau [20].

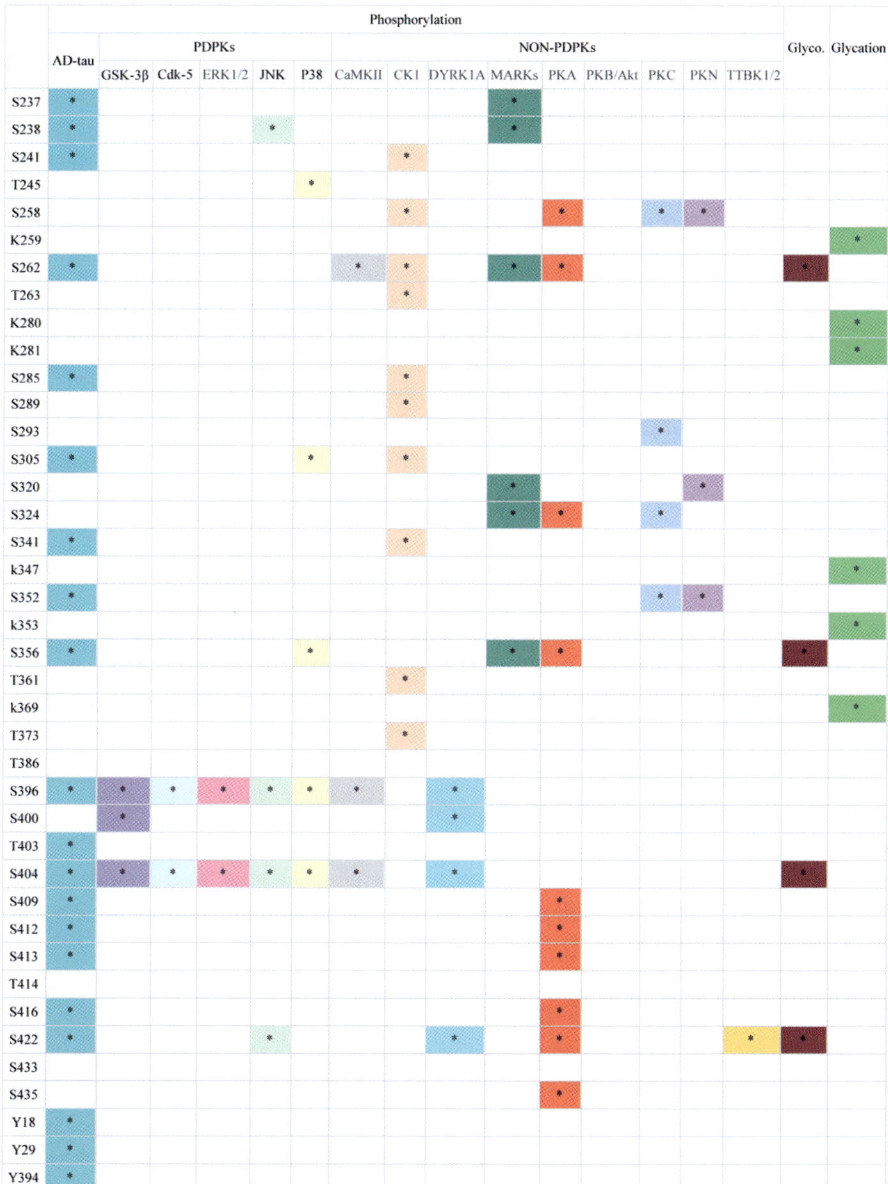

| | AD-tau | Phosphorylation | | | | | | | | | | | | | | Glyco. | Glycation |
| | | PDPKs | | | | | NON-PDPKs | | | | | | | | | | |
		GSK-3β	Cdk-5	ERK1/2	JNK	P38	CaMKII	CK1	DYRK1A	MARKs	PKA	PKB/Akt	PKC	PKN	TTBK1/2		
S237	*									*							
S238	*				*					*							
S241	*							*									
T245						*											
S258								*			*		*	*			
K259																	*
S262	*						*	*		*	*					*	
T263								*									
K280																	*
K281																	*
S285	*							*									
S289								*									
S293													*				
S305	*					*		*									
S320										*				*			
S324										*	*		*				
S341	*							*									
k347																	*
S352	*												*	*			
k353																	*
S356	*					*				*	*					*	
T361								*									
k369																	*
T373								*									
T386																	
S396	*	*	*	*	*	*	*		*								
S400		*							*								
T403	*																
S404	*	*	*	*	*	*	*		*							*	
S409	*										*						
S412	*										*						
S413	*										*						
T414																	
S416	*										*						
S422	*				*				*		*				*	*	
S433																	
S435											*						
Y18	*																
Y29	*																
Y394	*																

Figure 3. (*Continued*)

Nitration of tau proteins

Nitration is the addition of nitrogen dioxide on a tyrosine residue of an organic molecule. Four nitration sites have been identified in tau proteins, i.e. Tyr[18], Tyr[29], Tyr[197] and Tyr[394]. Nitration of Tyr[29] seems to be an AD-specific site [21], whereas Tyr[18] has been detected in both AD and age-matched controls, and Tyr[197] and Tyr[394] are observed in *in vitro* studies. The free radical peroxynitrite can induce tau nitration in rats with activation of GSK-3β and p38 kinases.

Similar to hyperphosphorylation, tau nitration facilitates tau aggregation. Therefore removing free radical peroxynitrite may prevent tau accumulation.

Polyamination of tau proteins

TG (transglutaminase)-catalysed polyamination involves a glutamine residue as acyl donor and a lysine residue as acyl acceptor, which provokes protein cross-linking. Eight acceptor sites and ten donor sites have been identified on tau proteins, in which the predominant donor site is Gln[424] and the principal acceptor region is located between residues Lys[163] and Lys[240]. TG levels are increased 5-fold in AD brains compared with control brains, with increased tau polyamination, and TG-catalysed cross-linking/polyamination stabilizes tau proteins and renders them resistant to proteolytic digestion [22].

Prolyl isomerization of tau proteins

Prolyl isomerization allows rearrangement of proline residues in proteins, which modifies the targeted protein from *cis* to *trans* conformation or vice versa. Pin1 (peptidylprolyl *cis–trans* isomerase NIMA-interacting 1) can specifically isomerize the proline residue in pS/T-P (phosphorylated-Ser/Thr-Pro) bonds and regulate the function of the phosphoproteins. Interestingly, Pin1 binds to only one pT-P motif in tau (i.e. Thr[231]/P) and changes tau to the *trans* conformation. *Trans*-tau is more accessible to dephosphorylation by PP2A (protein phosphatase 2A) [23]. This result suggests that Pin1 may be a potential target for arresting tau-related pathologies.

Truncation of tau proteins

Truncation of tau proteins at Asp[13], Asp[421] and Glu[391] has been observed in AD brains, and the truncation enhances tau aggregation and neuronal apoptosis. Caspase 3 can cleave tau at Asp[421], whereas calpain-mediated tau cleavage generates a product of 17 kDa that might involve residues 45 or 230. It is reported that tau phosphorylation at Ser[422] protects tau from caspase 3 cleavage at Asp[421] [24], suggesting that tau dephosphorylation at Ser[422] facilitates the proteolysis of tau by caspase 3.

Ubiquitination of tau proteins

Ubiquitination is the specific binding of one or more ubiquitin molecules to proteins as a signal for their degradation in the cytoplasm by the UPS (ubiquitin–proteasome system). Ubiquitination of tau can occur under both normal physiological and pathological conditions, at its C-terminal Lys[254], Lys[311] and Lys[353]. A high level of ubiquitinated tau proteins is detected in PHFs and cerebrospinal fluid of AD patients, and the accumulation of abnormally hyperphosphorylated tau precedes ubiquitination and formation of NFTs in AD brains. Accumulation of tau inhibits proteasome activity [25]. A recent study indicates that accumulation of hyperphosphorylated tau oligomers at human AD synapses is associated with an increase in ubiquitinated substrates that is consistent with dysfunction of the UPS [26,27]. These studies suggest that the UPS could play a role in tau accumulation.

Phosphorylation of tau proteins

Among the various post-translational modifications of tau, phosphorylation is the most extensively studied. Protein phosphorylation is the addition of a phosphate group by esterification at three types of amino acids: serine, threonine and tyrosine.

The longest tau isoform (namely tau40 or tau441) harbours 80 putative serine and threonine phosphorylation sites, and phosphorylation has been reported on approximately 30 of these sites in normal tau proteins, which are predominantly present in the proline-rich and the C-terminal regions flanking the MBDs and include Thr[181], Ser[198], Ser[199], Ser[202], Thr[217], Thr[231], Ser[235], Ser[396], Ser[400], Thr[403] and Ser[404] (Figure 3). In normal adult CNS, phosphorylation of tau generates a stoichiometry of 2–3 mol of phosphorous per mol of tau protein, which is required for the maintenance of the microtubule network. Five tyrosine residues have been identified in tau proteins and these sites can be phosphorylated by Src family kinases, such as Src, Lck, Syk, Fyn and by c-Abl kinase.

Abnormal hyperphosphorylation of tau in AD

Phosphorylation of tau is developmentally regulated. During embryonic and early postnatal periods, tau proteins (mainly 3R tau) are highly phosphorylated, whereas the phosphorylation level of tau decreases during the adult stage and increases again in the aged brain. In AD, tau is abnormally hyperphosphorylated at over 40 serine/threonine sites (Figure 3), which generates a stoichiometry of 5–9 mol of phosphorous per mol of tau protein. Besides the multiple putative phosphorylation sites harboured within the tau molecule, hyperphosphorylation could be considered as an increase in the number of sites phosphorylated in the same tau molecule and/or an increase in the number of tau molecules phosphorylated at the given sites, therefore, it is currently difficult to identify which site(s) may be the most critical pathological phosphorylation sites of tau in AD.

Effects of tau hyperphosphorylation on neuronal cell fate

An increasing number of studies has demonstrated that hyperphosphorylation of tau not only diminishes its biological activity, but also causes gain-of-toxic functions of tau. Hyperphosphorylated tau detaches from microtubules, sequesters normal microtubule-associated proteins [28], disrupts microtubule dynamics, causes somatodendritic accumulation of tau proteins, blocks axonal transport, damages synapses, promotes cell cycle re-entry, inhibits proteasome and AChT (acetylcholine transferase) activities, and facilitates tau aggregation. The unphosphorylated tau proteins (tau-1 positive) are normally distributed in neuronal axons, whereas abnormal hyperphosphorylation delocalizes tau proteins into the somatodendritic compartment of the neurons, and the post-synaptic location of tau mediates the toxicity of Aβ [16]. All of these can contribute to the neurotoxicity of tau. We have found recently that hyperphosphorylation of tau leads neurons to escape apoptosis [2]. Based on this finding and the fact that apoptosis is not the major mechanism of cell loss observed in AD, we have proposed that hyperphosphorylation of tau plays a dual role in leading neurons to abort acute apoptosis and simultaneously triggers chronic degeneration, and abortion of apoptosis may be the first step in neurodegeneration [1].

Imbalance in regulation of tau phosphorylation in AD

Tau phosphorylation has been mainly identified at serine and threonine residues, and is catalysed by protein kinases and protein phosphatases. Therefore activation of the protein kinases and/or inhibition of protein phosphatases are the direct cause of tau hyperphosphorylation.

Based on the kinase-recognized motifs, the serine/threonine kinases can be grouped into two classes: the PDPKs (proline-directed protein kinases) and the non-PDPKs. GSK-3β, CDK5 (cyclin-dependent kinase 5), CDK2 and the MAPK (mitogen-activated protein kinase) superfamily [MAPK/ERK (extracellular-signal-regulated kinase), SAPK (stress-activated protein kinase)/JNK (c-Jun N-terminal kinase) and p38] belong to the PDPKs. cAMP-dependent PKA, CaMKII (Ca^{2+}/calmodulin-dependent protein kinase II), PKB (protein kinase B; also known as Akt), PKC (protein kinase C), PKN (protein kinase N), CK1 (casein kinase 1), DYRK1A (dual-specificity tyrosine-phosphorylation-regulated kinase 1A), TTBK1/2 (tau-tubulin kinase 1/2) and MARKs (microtubule affinity-regulating kinases) belong to the non-PDPKs. The putative phosphorylation sites in tau by these kinases are listed in Figure 3. In AD brains, up-regulation of GSK-3β, CDK5, DYRK1A, p38 and CK1 have been reported. Among these kinases, GSK-3β is the first identified tau kinase and it is the most strongly implicated in AD-like tau hyperphosphorylation: GSK-3β catalyses tau phosphorylation with high stoichiometry. Activation of GSK-3β in primary neurons damages synaptic functions and causes cell death and memory deficits in rats [29]. In transgenic mice, inhibition of GSK-3β reduces tau phosphorylation and neurodegeneration, blocks formation of neurofibrillary tangles and rescues neuronal loss. These data suggest that inhibition of GSK-3β may be a promising therapeutic strategy for arresting tau pathologies.

The level of tau phosphorylation is also regulated by protein phosphatases, which dephosphorylate tau proteins. Among the currently identified serine/threonine phosphatases, PP2A, PP2B, PP1 and PP5, but not PP2C, can dephosphorylate tau at multiple AD-related sites both *in vitro* and *in vivo*, and PP2A is the most effective phosphatase in dephosphorylating hyperphosphorylated tau isolated from AD brains [14]. Inhibition of PP2A and PP1 by OA (okadaic acid) or CA (calyculin A) causes tau hyperphosphorylation and memory deficits in rats. Inhibition of PP2A and PP1 in neuroblastoma cells causes damage of axonal transport and significant retraction of the cell processes, which may partially explain the mechanisms underlying the impaired memory induced by inhibition of the phosphatases. PP2A accounts for approximately 71% of the total tau phosphatase activity in the human brain, and the activity of PP2A is significantly decreased in AD brains [30]. Therefore maintaining a normal level of PP2A may be a promising strategy in preventing AD-like tau pathology.

Other post-translational modifications of tau proteins

Tau proteins can also be oxidized at Cys^{322} and oxidation of tau promotes formation of PHFs *in vitro* and *in vivo* [31]. In immunopurified PHF samples isolated from AD brains, mono-methylation of tau at residue Lys^{254} was identified by nanoflow liquid chromatography-tandem mass spectrometry analysis, and the anti-methyl lysine antibody immunoreactivity was colocalized with ~78% of the tangles [32]. Tau proteins can also be SUMOylated at Lys^{340} by SUMO1 (small ubiquitin-like modifier protein 1), and to a lesser extent, by SUMO2 and SUMO3 *in vitro*, and SUMOylation can counteract tau ubiquitination [33]. However, the pathological role of oxidation at Cys^{322} and SUMOylation at Lys^{340} of tau has not been identified.

To date, it is difficult to define which of the described tau post-translational modifications are preferentially implicated in tau or AD pathologies. We believe that co-operation between different tau post-translational modifications must be involved.

Conclusions

Tau is an important microtubule-associated protein with normal function in maintaining neural structure and activity. The characteristics and biological function of tau proteins are regulated by alternative splicing and post-translational modifications, including phosphorylation, acetylation, glycation, glycosylation, methylation, nitration, oxidation, phosphorylation, polyamination, prolyl isomerization, SUMOylation, truncation and ubiquitination. Among the various abnormal post-translational modifications identified in AD brains, hyperphosphorylation is the most extensively studied. However, it is current not fully understood how abnormal hyperphosphorylation of tau leads to neurodegeneration. Furthermore, there are not many specific parameters applicable to define neurodegeneration in laboratory studies since the definition of neurodegeneration is not very clear. Based on our series of findings showing that tau hyperphosphorylation leads neurons to escape apoptosis, and at the same time, damages neuronal functions, we have proposed that neurodegeneration may represent a new type of chronic neuron death, which defines the nature or essence of neurodegeneration. We have also proposed that the tau hyperphosphorylation-induced abortion of apoptosis may be the first step in chronic neurodegeneration. In future studies, careful thought and powerful techniques, as well as appropriate animal models which allow longitudinal spatial/temporal observation, are needed because neural networks are so complex that focusing on a single point does not allow full understanding. According to a 2012 World Health Organization report, over 35 million people worldwide currently have dementia, a number that is expected to double by 2030 and triple by 2050. In light of those figures, new approaches should be developed to screen for potential treatments for AD and other neurodegenerative disorders.

Summary

- Tau is a major microtubule-associated protein that plays an important role in neuronal networks.
- Multiple abnormal post-translational modifications are involved in tau pathologies in AD patients.
- Abnormal hyperphosphorylation of tau plays a dual role in leading neurons to escape apoptosis and to enter chronic neurodegeneration.
- GSK-3β and PP2A play crucial roles in abnormal tau hyperphosphorylation.
- Being a critical factor in AD and other tauopathies, tau has been widely studied in the search for novel therapeutic targets to arrest neurodegeneration.

References

1. Wang, J.Z. and Liu, F. (2008) Microtubule-associated protein tau in development, degeneration and protection of neurons. Prog. Neurobiol. **85**, 148–175
2. Li, H.L., Wang, H.H., Liu, S.J., Deng, Y.Q., Zhang, Y.J., Tian, Q., Wang, X.C., Chen, X.Q., Yang, Y., Zhang, J.Y. et al. (2007) Phosphorylation of tau antagonizes apoptosis by stabilizing β-catenin, a mechanism involved in Alzheimer's neurodegeneration. Proc. Natl. Acad. Sci. U.S.A. **104**, 3591–3596
3. Cohen, T.J., Friedmann, D., Hwang, A.W., Marmorstein, R. and Lee, V.M. (2013) Microtubule-associated tau protein has intrinsic acetyltransferase activity. Nat. Struct. Mol. Biol. **20**, 756–762
4. Grundke-Iqbal, I., Iqbal, K., Tung, Y.C., Quinlan, M., Wisniewski, H.M. and Binder, L.I. (1986) Abnormal phosphorylation of the microtubule-associated protein tau in Alzheimer cytoskeletal pathology. Proc. Natl. Acad. Sci. U.S.A. **83**, 4913–4917

5. Hu, Y.Y., He, S.S., Wang, X., Duan, Q.H., Grundke-Iqbal, I., Iqbal, K. and Wang, J.Z. (2002) Levels of nonphosphorylated and phosphorylated tau in cerebrospinal fluid of Alzheimer's disease patients : an ultrasensitive bienzyme-substrate-recycle enzyme-linked immunosorbent assay. Am. J. Pathol. **160**, 1269–1278

6. Hutton, M., Lendon, C.L., Rizzu, P., Baker, M., Froelich, S., Houlden, H., Pickering-Brown, S., Chakraverty, S., Isaacs, A., Grover, A. et al. (1998) Association of missense and 5′-splice-site mutations in tau with the inherited dementia FTDP-17. Nature **393**, 702–705

7. Pérez, M., Lim, F., Arrasate, M. and Avila, J. (2000) The FTDP-17-linked mutation R406W abolishes the interaction of phosphorylated tau with microtubules. J. Neurochem. **4**, 2583–2589

8. Lewis, J., McGowan, E., Rockwood. J, Melrose, H., Nacharaju, P., Van Slegtenhorst, M., Gwinn-Hardy, K., Paul Murphy, M., Baker, M., Yu, X. et al. (2000) Neurofibrillary tangles, amyotrophy and progressive motor disturbance in mice expressing mutant (P301L) tau protein. Nat. Genet. **25**, 402–405

9. Götz, J., Probst, A., Spillantini, M.G., Schäfer, T., Jakes, R., Bürki, K. and Goedert, M. (1995) Somatodendritic localization and hyperphosphorylation of tau protein in transgenic mice expressing the longest human brain tau isoform. EMBO J. **14**, 1304–1313

10. Goedert, M., Spillantini, M.G., Potier, M.C., Ulrich, J. and Crowther, R.A. (1989) Cloning and sequencing of the cDNA encoding an isoform of microtubule-associated protein tau containing four tandem repeats: differential expression of tau protein mRNAs in human brain. EMBO J. **8**, 393–399

11. Andreadis, A., Brown, W.M. and Kosik, K.S. (1992) Structure and novel exons of the human tau gene. Biochemistry **31**, 10626–10633

12. Liu, F. and Gong, C.X. (2008) Tau exon 10 alternative splicing and tauopathies. Mol. Neurodegener. **3**, 8

13. Peck, A., Sargin, M.E., LaPointe, N.E., Rose, K., Manjunath, B.S., Feinstein, S.C. and Wilson, L. (2011) Tau isoform-specific modulation of kinesin-driven microtubule gliding rates and trajectories as determined with tau-stabilized microtubules. Cytoskeleton (Hoboken) **68**, 44–55

14. Wang, J.Z., Gong, C.X., Zaidi, T., Grundke-Iqbal, I. and Iqbal, K. (1995) Dephosphorylation of Alzheimer paired helical filaments by protein phosphatase-2A and -2B. J. Biol. Chem. **270**, 4854–4860

15. Yang, Y., Yang, X.F., Wang, Y.P., Tian, Q., Wang, X.C., Li, H.L., Wang, Q. and Wang, J.Z. (2007) Inhibition of protein phosphatases induces transport deficits and axonopathy. J. Neurochem. **102**, 878–886

16. Ittner, L.M., Ke, Y.D., Delerue, F., Bi, M., Gladbach, A., van Eersel, J., Wölfing, H., Chieng, B.C., Christie, M.J., Napier, I.A. et al. (2010) Dendritic function of tau mediates amyloid-beta toxicity in Alzheimer's disease mouse models. Cell **142**, 387–397

17. Smith, M.A., Taneda, S., Richey, P.L., Miyata, S., Yan, S.D., Stern, D., Sayre, L.M., Monnier, V.M. and Perry, G. (1994) Advanced Maillard reaction end products are associated with Alzheimer disease pathology. Proc. Natl. Acad. Sci. U.S.A. **91**, 5710–5714

18. Necula, M. and Kuret, J. (2004) Pseudophosphorylation and glycation of tau protein enhance but do not trigger fibrillization *in vitro*. J. Biol. Chem. **279**, 49694–49703

19. Liu, F., Shi, J., Tanimukai, H., Gu, J., Gu, J., Grundke-Iqbal, I., Iqbal, K. and Gong, C.X. (2009) Reduced O-GlcNAcylation links lower brain glucose metabolism and tau pathology in Alzheimer's disease. Brain **132**, 1820–1832

20. Wang, J.Z., Grundke-Iqbal, I. and Iqbal, K. (1996) Glycosylation of microtubule-associated protein tau: an abnormal posttranslational modification in Alzheimer's disease. Nat. Med. **2**, 871–875

21. Reynolds, M.R., Berry, R.W. and Binder, L.I. (2005) Site-specific nitration and oxidative dityrosine bridging of the tau protein by peroxynitrite: implications for Alzheimer's disease. Biochemistry **44**, 1690–1700

22. Zhang, Y.J., Xu, Y.F., Liu, Y.H., Yin, J., Li, H.L., Wang, Q. and Wang, J.Z. (2006) Peroxynitrite induces Alzheimer-like tau modifications and accumulation in rat brain and its underlying mechanisms. FASEB J. **20**, 1431–1442

23. Lu, P.J., Wulf, G., Zhou, X.Z., Davies, P. and Lu, K.P. (1999) The prolyl isomerase Pin1 restores the function of Alzheimer-associated phosphorylated tau protein. Nature **399**, 784–788

24. Gamblin, T.C., Chen, F., Zambrano, A., Abraha, A., Lagalwar, S., Guillozet, A.L., Lu, M., Fu, Y., Garcia-Sierra, F., LaPointe, N. et al. (2003) Caspase cleavage of tau: linking amyloid and neurofibrillary tangles in Alzheimer's disease. Proc. Natl. Acad. Sci. U.S.A. **100**, 10032–10037

25. Ren, Q.G., Liao, X.M., Chen, X.Q., Liu, G.P. and Wang, J.Z. (2007) Effects of tau phosphorylation on proteasome activity. FEBS Lett. **581**, 1521–1528

26. Iqbal, K. and Grundke-Iqbal, I. (1991) Ubiquitination and abnormal phosphorylation of paired helical filaments in Alzheimer's disease. Mol. Neurobiol. **5**, 399–410

27. Tai, H.C., Serrano-Pozo, A., Hashimoto, T., Frosch, M.P., Spires-Jones, T.L. and Hyman, B.T. (2012) The synaptic accumulation of hyperphosphorylated tau oligomers in Alzheimer disease is associated with dysfunction of the ubiquitin-proteasome system. Am. J. Pathol. **181**, 1426–1435

28. Alonso, A.D., Grundke-Iqbal, I., Barra, H.S. and Iqbal, K. (1997) Abnormal phosphorylation of tau and the mechanism of Alzheimer neurofibrillary degeneration: sequestration of microtubule-associated proteins 1 and 2 and the disassembly of microtubules by the abnormal tau. Proc. Natl. Acad. Sci. U.S.A. **94**, 298–303

29. Liu, S.J., Zhang, A.H., Li, H.L., Wang, Q., Deng, H.M., Netzer, W.J., Xu, H. and Wang, J.Z. (2003) Overactivation of glycogen synthase kinase-3 by inhibition of phosphoinositol-3 kinase and protein kinase C leads to hyperphosphorylation of tau and impairment of spatial memory. J. Neurochem. **87**, 1333–1344

30. Gong, C.X., Shaikh, S., Wang, J.Z., Zaidi, T. and Grundke-Iqbal, I. (1995) Phosphatase activity toward abnormally phosphorylated tau: decrease in Alzheimer disease brain. J. Neurochem. **65**, 732–738

31. Schweers, O., Mandelkow, E.M., Biernat, J. and Mandelkow, E. (1995) Oxidation of cysteine-322 in the repeat domain of microtubule-associated protein tau controls the *in vitro* assembly of paired helical filaments. Proc. Natl. Acad. Sci. U.S.A. **92**, 8463–8467

32. Thomas, S.N., Funk, K.E., Wan, Y., Liao, Z., Davies, P., Kuret, J. and Yang, A.J. (2012) Dual modification of Alzheimer's disease PHF-tau protein by lysine methylation and ubiquitylation: a mass spectrometry approach. Acta Neuropathol. **123**, 105–117

33. Dorval, V. and Fraser, P.E. (2006) Small ubiquitin-like modifier (SUMO) modification of natively unfolded proteins tau and α-synuclein. J. Biol. Chem. **281**, 9919–9924

Essays Biochem. (2014) 56, 125–135: doi: 10.1042/BSE0560125

9

Role of α-synuclein in neurodegeneration: implications for the pathogenesis of Parkinson's disease

Shun Yu and Piu Chan[1]

Department of Neurobiology, Beijing Institute of Geriatric Medical and Research Center, Xuanwu Hospital, Capital Medical University, Changchun Street 45, Xicheng District, Beijing 100053, China

Abstract

α-Syn (α-synuclein) is a small soluble acidic protein that is extensively expressed in the nervous system. Genetic, clinical and experimental studies demonstrate that α-syn is strongly implicated in the pathogenesis of PD (Parkinson's disease). However, the pathogenic mechanism remains elusive. In the present chapter, we first describe the normal expression and potential physiological functions of α-syn. Then, we introduce recent research progress related to the pathogenic role of α-syn in PD, with special emphasis on how α-syn oligomers cause the preferential degeneration of dopaminergic neurons in the substantia nigra and the spreading of α-syn pathology in the brain of PD patients.

Keywords:

autophagy, dopamine transporter, dopaminergic neuron, Lewy body, mitochondria, NMDA receptor, Parkinson's disease, substantia nigra, synaptic plasticity, vesicle recycling.

Introduction

α-Syn (α-synuclein) belongs to a multi-gene family of proteins, which also consists of β- and γ-synucleins [1]. Since the first mutation of the α-syn gene was reported to be linked to rare familial PD (Parkinson's disease) [2], there has been rising interest in the association of α-syn

[1]*To whom correspondence should be addressed (email pbchan90@gmail.com).*

with the pathogenesis of PD. In the present chapter, we first introduce the molecular structure, normal expression and potential physiological functions of α-syn. Then, we focus on the research progress regarding the pathogenic role of α-syn in PD. We specifically discuss how α-syn aggregation causes the preferential degeneration of dopaminergic neurons in the substantia nigra in PD patients.

Molecular structure and normal expression

Human α-syn is a soluble acidic protein of 140 amino acids, consisting of three distinct regions (Figure 1): the N-terminal amphipathic region (residues 1–65), the central hydrophobic NAC (non-amyloid β-peptide component) region (residues 66–95) and the C-terminal acidic region (residues 96–140) [3]. The N-terminal part of α-syn contains seven imperfect 11-mer repeats with a highly conserved hexamer motif KTKEGV, which make up a conserved apolipoprotein-like class-A2 helix that mediates the binding of α-syn to phospholipid vesicles. The NAC region is essential for the aggregation and toxicity of α-syn [3]. The C-terminal region is rich in acidic amino acids and appears to have chaperone activity, preventing α-syn from aggregating [3].

α-Syn is extensively expressed in the nervous system. In the brain, this protein is abundant in those areas that display synaptic plasticity such as the neocortex, hippocampus, striatum, thalamus and cerebellum. In the spinal cord, α-syn is mainly expressed in grey matter, with its levels most abundant in lamina 1 and 2. α-Syn is also abundant in the peripheral nervous system that innervates various organs, such as the digestive tract, heart, salivary gland, bladder, kidney and skin.

In both the central and peripheral nervous systems, α-syn is expressed specifically in neurons. Immunoelectron microscopy using ultra-small gold as a probe revealed extensive localization of α-syn in subcellular pools of neurons, including presynaptic terminals, axons, mitochondria, the Golgi complex, the ER (endoplasmic reticulum) and the nucleus [4].

Physiological functions

Data obtained so far suggest that α-syn is involved in many cellular processes, including neurotransmitter release, trafficking of transporters and receptors, and biosynthesis of DA (dopamine).

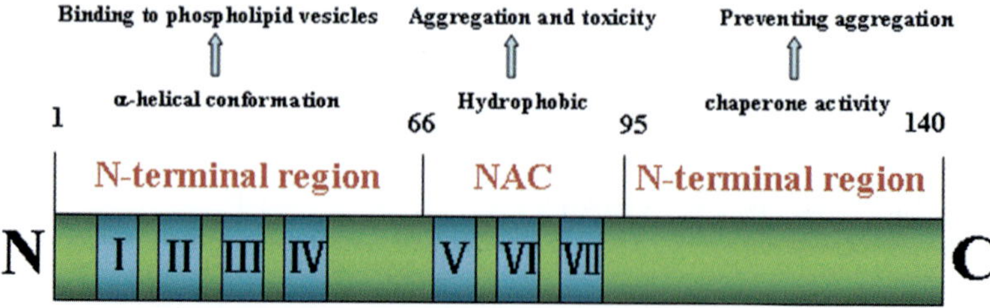

Figure 1. Structure of the α-syn molecule

Neurotransmitter release

Normally, α-syn is loosely associated with the distal reserve pool of synaptic vesicles [5], suggesting a role in synaptic vesicle trafficking or recycling. Indeed, the evidence obtained indicates that α-syn is involved in almost every step of synaptic vesicle recycling, including trafficking, docking, fusion and recycling after exocytosis [3] (Figure 2). The mechanisms may involve several aspects: (i) inhibition of the activity of PLD2 (phospholipase D2), an enzyme shown to participate in the regulation of vesicle trafficking and both endo- and exo-cytosis [6]; (ii) promotion of actin polymerization along which vesicles travel to reach their targets at the termini [7]; and (iii) regulation of synaptic vesicle recycling by assisting in the folding and refolding of synaptic proteins called SNAREs (soluble N-ethylmaleimide-sensitive fusion protein-attachment protein receptors), including synaptobrevin, syntaxin and SNAP-25 (25 kDa synaptosome-associated protein) which form a protein complex and play a role in vesicle priming, transfer of docked vesicles into an exocytosis-competent state, and vesicle fusion to the membrane [8]. By affecting synaptic vesicle trafficking and recycling, α-syn can modulate the release of neurotransmitters. For example, in dopaminergic neurons in the nigrostriatal pathway, α-syn has been shown to act as an essential presynaptic, activity-dependent negative regulator of DA release [9]. In contrast, in non-dopaminergic neurons in the Schaffer collaterals–CA1 pathway, α-syn has been demonstrated to promote the release of glutamate [10].

α-Syn can also regulate synaptic plasticity. In hippocampal neuronal cultures, α-syn has been shown to participate in the induction of long-lasting potentiation of synaptic transmission [11]. In corticostriatal pathways, however, high-frequency stimulation induces a presynaptic form of long-term depression solely in the mice overexpressing α-syn. In the dentate gyrus perforant pathway, α-syn accumulation in aged A30P transgenic mice causes a long-term depression of synaptic transmission after a stimulation protocol that normally induces long-term potentiation [12], although long-term potentiation was induced in the same transgenic adult mice in mossy fibres–CA3 synapses. The mechanism underlying the modulation of

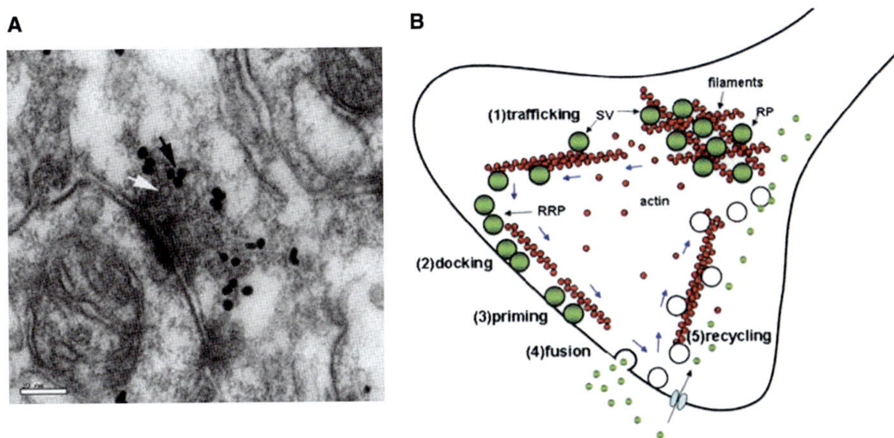

Figure 2. α-Syn in presynaptic termini
(A) The gold particles (black arrow) representing the localization of α-syn in the presynaptic zone are loosely associated with synaptic vesicles (white arrow). (B) The role of α-syn in the presynaptic terminal. α-Syn is involved in almost every step of synaptic vesicle recycling, including trafficking, docking, fusion and recycling after exocytosis.

α-syn in synaptic plasticity appears to be related to the altered release probability of neurotransmitters through regulation of synaptic vesicle mobilization or trafficking from the reserve pool to the readily releasable pool.

Trafficking of transporters and receptors

A body of evidence suggests that α-syn can modulate the trafficking of transporters between the cell surface and intracellular compartments. Data on this modulation have mainly been obtained from studies on MATs (monoamine transporters), the transmembrane proteins responsible for re-uptake of synaptic DA, NE (norepinephrine) and 5-HT (serotonin). These transporters, including the DAT (dopamine transporter), NET (norepinephrine transporter) and the SERT (serotonin transporter), play a central role in monoamine homoeostasis by rapidly removing their respective neurotransmitter substrates from the synaptic cleft. There is evidence that α-syn, together with β- and γ-synuclein, can influence MAT trafficking away from the cell surface. Clathrin-mediated endocytosis is shown to be involved in this modulation [13]. In addition, this modulation appears to be dependent on the interaction between α-syn, transporter proteins and some cytoskeletal proteins [14].

A few lines of evidence indicate that α-syn can also modulate the endocytic trafficking of membrane receptors. In cultured neuronal and non-neuronal cells, α-syn expression coupled with exposure to physiological levels of certain polyunsaturated fatty acids was shown to enhance the rate of internalization and recycling of transferrin receptors [15]. In cultured dopaminergic neuronal cells treated with exogenous α-syn or overexpressing α-syn, the cell surface NMDA (*N*-methyl-D-aspartate) receptors were found to decrease in number, with apparent reduction in Ca^{2+} influx and cell death rate upon NMDA stimulation, indicating enhanced internalization of NMDA receptors by α-syn [16]. Similar to the mechanism for the modulation of MAT, modulation of membrane receptors by α-syn is also mediated by clathrin-mediated endocytosis [16] (Figure 3).

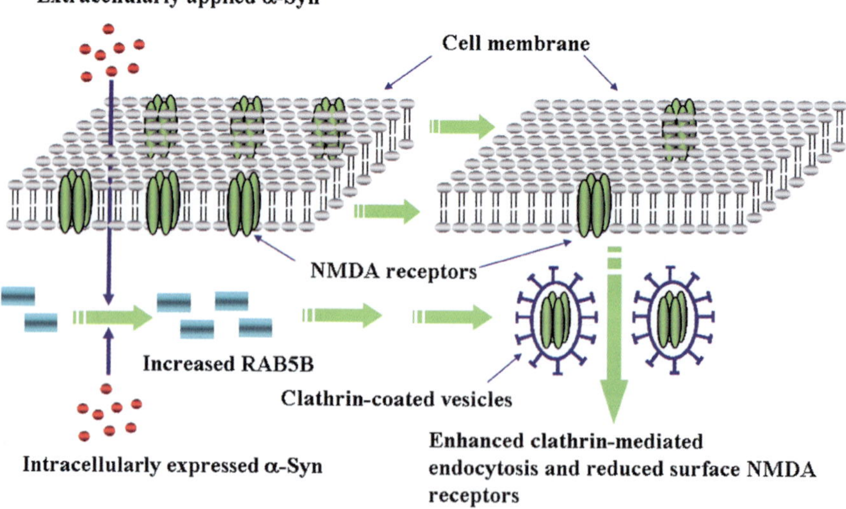

Figure 3. Regulation of surface NMDA receptors through clathrin-mediated endocytosis activated by either extracellularly applied or intracellularly expressed α-syn

DA biosynthesis

α-Syn regulates almost all steps of DA biosynthesis. The genes regulated by α-syn include GTP cyclohydrolase, SR (sepiapterin reductase), TH (tyrosine hydroxylase) and aromatic acid decarboxylase. TH is the rate-limiting enzyme for DA synthesis. Both the expression and activity of this enzyme are shown to be down-regulated in α-syn-transfected DA cells. α-Syn may down-regulate TH expression by reducing the activity of the TH gene promoter. In addition, α-syn may inhibit TH activity by preventing its phosphorylation [17]. Consistent with a role for α-syn in down-regulating DA biosynthesis in cell culture models, it was found in human and monkey brains that the age-related increases in nigral α-syn are strongly associated with age-related decreases in TH. Taken together, this evidence supports the idea that α-syn negatively regulates TH expression and activity.

Pathogenic role of α-syn

The link between genetic alterations and PD etiology

The link between genetic alterations of the α-syn gene (*SNCA*) and PD etiology is well established. Since the initial report of the link between a missense mutation (A53T) of *SNCA* and familial PD [2], several additional pathogenic point mutations (E46K, H50Q and G51D) have been identified [18]. These mutations induce early onset and autosomal dominantly inherited PD. Duplication and triplication of the wild-type *SNCA* are also reported to be associated with early onset familial PD. In addition, a dinucleotide repeat sequence (REP1) polymorphism in the *SNCA* promoter region has been shown to be associated with increased risk for PD [18].

Relevance of insoluble α-syn-containing inclusions to neurodegeneration

PD is morphologically characterized by accumulation of abnormal filamentous protein inclusions named LBs (Lewy bodies) and LNs (Lewy neurites). The major component of LBs and LNs is fibrillated α-syn [19]. Therefore LBs and LNs are also called α-syn pathology or Lewy pathology.

Although Lewy pathology is the characteristic pathological change in the substantia nigra where substantial loss of pigmented dopaminergic neurons induces typical PD symptoms, α-syn-related inclusions are demonstrated to be localized throughout the central nervous system, the peripheral nervous system and the autonomic nervous system.

The biological significance of Lewy pathology and its impact on neurodegeneration remain elusive. Most clinical PD cases correspond to LB pathology stages 3–6 based on Braak staging, when the subtantia nigra is severely affected. The cognitive decline in PD patients correlates well with Lewy pathology stages [20]. However, other evidence indicates that Lewy pathology may be a structural manifestation of a cytoprotective response or a failed cellular self-preservation mechanism to confine and eliminate cytotoxic proteins. For example, although iLBD (incidental LB disease) is often assumed to represent preclinical PD [21], in some PD patients, significant neurodegeneration and cellular dysfunction precedes Lewy pathology in the substantia nigra, challenging the pathogenic role of Lewy pathology in PD [22]. Moreover, post-mortem analysis of some PD patients with *LRRK2* mutations demonstrates neurodegeneration without Lewy pathology. The inconsistency between α-syn inclusion formation and cytotoxicity suggests that another form of the pathogenic proteins may be contributing to neurodegeneration.

Relevance of soluble oligomeric α-syn to neurodegeneration

Accumulating evidence supports that soluble α-syn, especially its oligomers or protofibrils, are toxic and pathogenic. For example, studies using protein-fragment complementation assays have demonstrated that α-syn oligomers are associated with enhanced cytotoxicity, which can be rescued by Hsp70 (heat-shock protein 70) in a process that reduces the formation of α-syn oligomers. Other convincing evidence comes from a study on α-syn-overexpressing cells, showing that the toxicity of α-syn was alleviated by a single-chain antibody (scFv; single-chain variable fragment) targeting the clearance of oligomeric, but not monomeric, α-syn. The neurotoxicity of α-syn oligomers has also been demonstrated in animal models using mutant forms of α-syn with decreased capacity to form fibrils, but increased propensity to form soluble oligomers [23]. Patients with parkinsonism and Gaucher's disease also have increased levels of α-syn oligomers compared with those without parkinsonism or to healthy controls [24]. These findings suggest a relationship between endogenous α-syn oligomers and neurodegeneration in PD.

Potential mechanisms of α-syn toxicity

How α-syn oligomers mediate cell death has not yet been fully elucidated, but likely involves a number of different intracellular and extracellular mechanisms. Although α-syn oligomers can destroy the cellular membrane system by forming pathologic pores, loss of normal function due to abnormal aggregation may constitute alternative mechanisms leading to neurodegeneration as outlined in the following sections.

DA and oxidative stress

One of the important reasons for preferential degeneration of the mesostriatal dopaminergic neurons is increased oxidative stress. These neurons synthesize DA, which easily undergoes oxidation to form reactive oxygen species and reactive quinones in the cytoplasm. DA is normally rapidly sequestered into vesicles by the action of VMAT2 (vesicular MAT 2) [25]. In addition, the high DAT/VMAT2 ratio characteristic of the DA neurons may allow DA to enter the presynaptic neurons at a higher rate than it is incorporated into vesicles, causing an increase in cytoplasmic DA concentration [26]. Therefore a defect in synaptic vesicle formation or function could predispose the DA neurons to, or even cause, some of the oxidative damage observed in PD. A direct connection between DA oxidation and increased α-syn aggregation has been observed in cellular and cell-free systems. In some studies, toxicity of α-syn has been shown to be higher in dopaminergic cells than in non-dopaminergic cells [27] and DA synthesis inhibitors can be neuroprotective *in vitro* [28]. It was demonstrated that DA and related auto-oxidation species can inhibit the final steps of α-syn aggregation (i.e. fibrillation). This promotes the accumulation of protofibrillar structures believed to be cytotoxic [29], possibly by causing perforation of the vesicular membranes [30], resulting in DA leakage and accumulation in the cytoplasm. This elevates the generation of reactive oxygen and nitrogen species [31], further enhancing the formation of DA reactive species and perpetuating a toxicity loop, which could eventually lead to neuronal cell degeneration.

Synaptic integrity

α-Syn oligomer formation may also lead to neurodegeneration by damaging synaptic integrity. α-Syn can act as a molecular chaperone, assisting in the folding and refolding of SNARE proteins [32]. It has been reported that up-regulation of α-syn can compensate for the loss of CSPα (cysteine string protein α) activity, restoring SNARE complexes to their correct levels and suppressing presynaptic degeneration, motor dysfunction and death of mice lacking CSPα [33]. It is possible that long-term alterations in α-syn, including expression, modification and aggregation, may cause first synaptic dysfunction and then gradual presynaptic degeneration. The latter possibility remains to be confirmed.

In addition, α-syn may affect postsynaptic function. α-Syn has been shown to regulate the density of cell-surface NMDA receptors by promoting the endocytosis of this receptor [16]. Alterations in α-syn may affect the density of cell-surface NMDA receptors, thereby impairing neurotransmission and synaptic plasticity. In support of this postulation, Diógenes et al. [34] demonstrated in hippocampal slices that prolonged exposure to α-syn oligomers, but not monomers or fibrils, increases basal synaptic transmission through NMDA receptor activation. However, slices treated with α-syn oligomers were unable to respond with further potentiation to theta-burst stimulation, leading to impaired LTP (long-term potentiation) [35]. The findings provide mechanistic insight into how α-syn oligomers may trigger neuronal dysfunction and toxicity associated with cognitive impairment in PD and other synucleinopathies.

Mitochondrial function

Several potential mechanisms have been implicated in mitochondrial dysfunction associated with α-syn. First, α-syn may destroy the integrity and permeability of mitochondrial membranes. Studies in cultured cells overexpressing α-syn presented mitochondrial depolarization, mitochondrial fragmentation and mitochondria-dependent cell death [36]. Secondly, α-syn may inhibit complex I activity. α-Syn was found to be localized in the mitochondria of brain neurons and down-regulates complex I activity in a dose-dependent manner. In accordance with this finding, mitochondria of the PD-vulnerable substantia nigra and striatum, but not the cerebellum from PD subjects, showed significant accumulation of α-syn and decreased complex I activity. These results provide evidence for mitochondrial complex I deficiency in the substantia nigra from PD patients. Thirdly, α-syn may impair the normal dynamics of mitochondria. In cultured cells, α-syn was demonstrated to impair the normal dynamics of mitochondria and this effect was particular prominent in the case of the A53T α-syn mutant.

Protein degradation system

In mammalian cells, most α-syn is degraded by lysosomal enzymes. It has been shown that CMA (chaperone-mediated autophagy), a protein degradation pathway that depends on lysosomal function, is affected by dominant α-syn mutations or modification by DA. Wild-type α-syn is degraded by CMA upon binding to the CMA-specific receptor Lamp-2a. However, the mutant and modified α-syn bind to Lamp-2a too strongly to be internalized, leading to inhibition of degradation of α-syn and other CMA substrates. This dysfunction can lead to alterations in macroautophagy and accumulation of autophagic vacuoles, which may result in neuronal death [34]. Aggregated α-syn may also impair the function of autophagy. α-Syn aggregates were shown to impair overall macroautophagy by reducing autophagosome clearance after they are internalized by cells [37]. This may contribute to the increased cell death that is observed in aggregate-bearing cells in the brain of PD patients. In patients with Gaucher's disease and in carriers of GBA mutations with synucleinopathies, activity of GCase is lowered, which can lead to lysosomal dysfunction and a consequent increase in α-syn accumulation. At the same time, glycosylceramide also accumulates, which increases oligomerization of α-syn. The increased concentrations of oligomerized α-syn might inhibit ER–Golgi trafficking of wild-type GCase, which leads to reduced GCase activity and, therefore, reduced degradation of α-syn.

Toxicity of extracellular α-syn and spreading of α-syn pathology

It has been found that a small proportion of α-syn is secreted into the extracellular medium via unconventional exocytosis, different to the classical exocytosis through the ER–Golgi. It is reported that α-syn has a higher aggregation rate into secretory vesicles compared with cytosolic α-syn. Data obtained to date suggest that extracellular α-syn may play a toxic role by inducing microglial activation and plasma membrane permeabilization.

The most important role of extracellular α-syn is probably spreading of α-syn pathology via a 'prion-like' mechanism. A prion-like spreading of α-syn pathology was observed in both animal models and PD patients. For instance, LB formation can be identified in grafted fetal dopaminergic neurons in the striatum of PD patients 10 years after they were transplanted, indicating a host-to-graft propagation of α-syn pathology [38]. In animal models, intracerebral injection of extracts from sick A53T human α-syn transgenic mice into younger healthy transgenic mice induced a late-onset severe motor phenotype and widespread formation of neuronal α-syn amyloidogenic inclusions. The pathological α-syn propagated along major central nervous system pathways to regions far beyond the injection sites, suggesting a transmission of α-syn pathology. In addition, fibrils of wild-type α-syn preformed *in vitro* are also able to induce the formation and transmission of α-syn inclusions in a healthy recipient brain [39].

Conclusions

α-Syn is a small soluble acidic protein extensively distributed in the central and peripheral nervous system. Although not fully understood, α-syn appears to participate in many cellular physiological processes such as neurotransmitter release, membrane receptor and transporter trafficking, and DA biosynthesis. Genetic, clinical, cellular and animal studies demonstrate that α-syn plays a central role in the pathogenesis of PD. Increasing evidence supports the idea that abnormal aggregation of α-syn is the main reason for the protein to induce neurodegeneration in disease conditions. Although a number of studies suggest that the toxicity of α-syn may result from its oligomers that damage the cell membrane system (toxic gain of function), loss of normal functions due to aggregation may be an alternative mechanism leading to neurodegeneration. In addition, although the spreading of α-syn pathology via a 'prion-like' mechanism may explain the extensive presence of α-syn-related pathology in the nervous system, the selective degeneration of DA neurons in the substantia nigra in PD may be determined by the link between DA metabolism and α-syn.

Summary

- α-Syn is a small soluble acidic protein extensively expressed in the nervous system.
- Normally, α-syn is involved in many physiological processes such as neurotransmitter release, DA biosynthesis and receptor and transporter trafficking.
- Alterations of α-syn, especially its oligomerization, are shown to be toxic to neurons, and are believed to play a central role in the pathogenesis of PD.
- Neurodegeneration induced by α-syn oligomers may involve both toxic-gain-of-function and loss-of-function mechanisms.
- The extensive presence of α-syn pathology in the nervous system in PD may result from the spreading of α-syn pathology via a 'prion-like' mechanism.
- The selective degeneration of DA neurons in the substantia nigra in PD may be determined by the link between DA metabolism and α-syn.

References

1. Clayton, D.F. and George, J.M. (1998) The synucleins: a family of proteins involved in synaptic function, plasticity, neurodegeneration and disease. Trends Neurosci. **21**, 249–254
2. Polymeropoulos, M.H., Lavedan, C., Leroy, E., Ide, S.E., Dehejia, A., Dutra, A., Pike, B., Root, H., Rubenstein, J., Boyer, R. et al. (1997) Mutation in the alpha-synuclein gene identified in families with Parkinson's disease. Science **276**, 2045–2047
3. Cheng, F., Vivacqua, G. and Yu, S. (2011) The role of α-synuclein in neurotransmission and synaptic plasticity. J. Chem. Neuroanat. **42**, 242–248
4. Zhang, L., Zhang, C., Zhu, Y., Cai, Q., Chan, P., Ueda, K., Yu, S. and Yang, H. (2008) Semi-quantitative analysis of alpha-synuclein in subcellular pools of rat brain neurons: an immunogold electron microscopic study using a C-terminal specific monoclonal antibody. Brain Res. **1244**, 40–52
5. Yu, S., Li, X., Liu, G., Han, J., Zhang, C., Li, Y., Xu, S., Liu, C., Gao, Y., Yang, H. et al. (2007) Extensive nuclear localization of α-synuclein in normal rat brain neurons revealed by a novel monoclonal antibody. Neuroscience **145**, 539–555
6. Cockcroft, S. (2001) Signalling roles of mammalian phospholipase D1 and D2. Cell. Mol. Life Sci. **58**, 1674–1687
7. Bellani, S., Sousa, V.L., Ronzitti, G., Valtorta, F., Meldolesi, J., and Chieregatti, E. (2010) The regulation of synaptic function by α-synuclein. Commun. Integr. Biol. **3**, 106–109
8. Goda, Y. (1997) SNAREs and regulated vesicle exocytosis. Proc. Natl. Acad. Sci. U.S.A. **94**, 769–772
9. Yavich, L., Tanila, H., Vepsalainen, S. and Jakala, P. (2004) Role of α-synuclein in presynaptic dopamine recruitment. J. Neurosci. **24**, 11165–11170
10. Gureviciene, I., Gurevicius, K., and Tanila, H. (2007) Role of α-synuclein in synaptic glutamate release. Neurobiol. Dis. **28**, 83–89
11. Liu, S., Fa, M., Ninan, I., Trinchese, F., Dauer, W. and Arancio, O. (2007) α-Synuclein involvement in hippocampal synaptic plasticity: role of NO, cGMP, cGK and CaMKII. Eur. J. Neurosci. **25**, 3583–3596
12. Gureviciene, I., Gurevicius, K. and Tanila, H. (2009) Aging and α-synuclein affect synaptic plasticity in the dentate gyrus. J. Neural Transm. **116**, 13–22

13. Kisos, H., Ben-Gedalya, T. and Sharon, R. (2013) The clathrin-dependent localization of dopamine transporter to surface membranes is affected by α-synuclein. J. Mol. Neurosci. **52**, 167–176

14. Oaks, A.W. and Sidhu, A. (2011) Synuclein modulation of monoamine transporters. FEBS Lett. **585**, 1001–1006

15. Ben, G.T., Loeb, V., Israeli, E., Altschuler, Y., Selkoe, D.J. and Sharon, R. (2009) α-Synuclein and polyunsaturated fatty acids promote clathrin-mediated endocytosis and synaptic vesicle recycling. Traffic **10**, 218–234

16. Cheng, F., Li, X., Li, Y., Wang, C., Wang, T., Liu, G., Baskys, A., Ueda, K., Chan, P. and Yu, S. (2011) α-Synuclein promotes clathrin-mediated NMDA receptor endocytosis and attenuates NMDA-induced dopaminergic cell death. J. Neurochem. **119**, 815–825

17. Wu, B., Liu, Q., Duan, C., Li, Y., Yu, S., Chan, P., Ueda, K. and Yang, H. (2011) Phosphorylation of α-synuclein upregulates tyrosine hydroxylase activity in MN9D cells. Acta Histochem. **113**, 32–35

18. Kruger, R., Kuhn, W., Muller, T., Woitalla, D., Graeber, M., Kosel, S., Przuntek, H., Epplen, J.T., Schols, L. and Riess, O. (1998) Ala30Pro mutation in the gene encoding α-synuclein in Parkinson's disease. Nat. Genet. **18**, 106–108

19. Appel-Cresswell, S., Vilarino-Guell, C., Encarnacion, M., Sherman, H., Yu, I., Shah, B., Weir, D., Thompson, C., Szu-Tu, C., Trinh, J. et al. (2013) α-Synuclein p.H50Q, a novel pathogenic mutation for Parkinson's disease. Mov. Disord. **28**, 811–813

20. Braak, H., Rüb, U. and Del Tredici, K. (2006) Cognitive decline correlates with neuropathological stage in Parkinson's disease. J. Neurol. Sci. **248**, 255–258

21. Maraganore, D.M., de Andrade, M., Elbaz, A., Farrer, M.J., Ioannidis, J.P., Kruger, R., Rocca, W.A., Schneider, N.K., Lesnick, T.G., Lincoln, S.J. et al. (2006) Collaborative analysis of α-synuclein gene promoter variability and Parkinson disease. JAMA **296**, 661–670

22. Baba, M., Nakajo, S., Tu, P.H., Tomita, T., Nakaya, K., Lee, V.M., Trojanowski, J.Q. and Iwatsubo, T. (1998) Aggregation of α-synuclein in Lewy bodies of sporadic Parkinson's disease and dementia with Lewy bodies. Am. J. Pathol. **152**, 879–884

23. Frigerio, R., Fujishiro, H., Ahn, T.B., Josephs, K.A., Maraganore, D.M., DelleDonne, A., Parisi, J.E., Klos, K.J., Boeve, B.F., Dickson, D.W. and Ahlskog, J.E. (2011) Incidental Lewy body disease: do some cases represent a preclinical stage of dementia with Lewy bodies? Neurobiol. Aging **32**, 857–863

24. Milber, J.M., Noorigian, J.V., Morley, J.F., Petrovitch, H., White, L., Ross, G.W. and Duda, J.E. (2012) Lewy pathology is not the first sign of degeneration in vulnerable neurons in Parkinson disease. Neurology **79**, 2307–2314

25. Karpinar, D.P., Balija, M.B., Kugler, S., Opazo, F., Rezaei-Ghaleh, N., Wender, N., Kim, H.Y., Taschenberger, G., Falkenburger, B.H., Heise, H. et al. (2009) Pre-fibrillar α-synuclein variants with impaired β-structure increase neurotoxicity in Parkinson's disease models. EMBO J. **28**, 3256–3268

26. Choi, J.H., Stubblefield, B., Cookson, M.R., Goldin, E., Velayati, A., Tayebi, N. and Sidransky, E. (2011) Aggregation of α-synuclein in brain samples from subjects with glucocerebrosidase mutations. Mol. Genet. Metab. **104**, 185–188

27. Yu, S., Ueda, K. and Chan, P. (2005) α-Synuclein and dopamine metabolism. Mol. Neurobiol. **31**, 243–254

28. Venda, L.L., Cragg, S.J., Buchman, V.L. and Wade-Martins, R. (2010) α-Synuclein and dopamine at the crossroads of Parkinson's disease. Trends Neurosci. **33**, 559–568

29. Petrucelli, L., O'Farrell, C., Lockhart, P.J., Baptista, M., Kehoe, K., Vink, L., Choi, P., Wolozin, B., Farrer, M., Hardy, J. and Cookson, M.R. (2002) Parkin protects against the toxicity associated with mutant α-synuclein: proteasome dysfunction selectively affects catecholaminergic neurons. Neuron **36**, 1007–1019

30. Xu, J., Kao, S.Y., Lee, F.J., Song, W., Jin, L.W. and Yankner, B.A. (2002) Dopamine-dependent neurotoxicity of α-synuclein: a mechanism for selective neurodegeneration in Parkinson disease. Nat. Med. **8**, 600–606

31. Conway, K.A., Rochet, J.C., Bieganski, R.M. and Lansbury, Jr, P.T. (2001) Kinetic stabilization of the α-synuclein protofibril by a dopamine–α-synuclein adduct. Science **294**, 1346–1349

32. Volles, M.J. and Lansbury, Jr, P.T. (2007) Relationships between the sequence of α-synuclein and its membrane affinity, fibrillization propensity, and yeast toxicity. J. Mol. Biol. **366**, 1510–1522

33. Jenner, P. (2003) Oxidative stress in Parkinson's disease. Ann. Neurol. **53**, S26–S36

34. Diógenes, M.J., Dias, R.B., Rombo, D.M., Vicente, M.H., Maiolino, F., Guerreiro, P., Nasstrom, T., Franquelim, H.G., Oliveira, L.M., Castanho, M.A. et al. (2012) Extracellular α-synuclein oligomers modulate synaptic transmission and impair LTP via NMDA-receptor activation. J. Neurosci. **32**, 11750–11762

35. Bonini, N.M. and Giasson, B.I. (2005) Snaring the function of α-synuclein. Cell **123**, 359–361

36. Chandra, S., Gallardo, G., Fernandez-Chacon, R., Schluter, O.M. and Sudhof, T.C. (2005) α-Synuclein cooperates with CSPα in preventing neurodegeneration. Cell **123**, 383–396

37. Nakamura, K., Nemani, V.M., Azarbal, F., Skibinski, G., Levy, J.M., Egami, K., Munishkina, L., Zhang, J., Gardner, B., Wakabayashi, J. et al. (2011) Direct membrane association drives mitochondrial fission by the Parkinson disease-associated protein α-synuclein. J. Biol. Chem. **286**, 20710–20726

38. Olanow, C.W. and Brundin, P. (2013) Parkinson's disease and α synuclein: is Parkinson's disease a prion-like disorder? Mov. Disord. **28**, 31–40

39. Vekrellis, K., Xilouri, M., Emmanouilidou, E., Rideout, H.J. and Stefanis, L. (2011) Pathological roles of α-synuclein in neurological disorders. Lancet Neurol. **10**, 1015–1025

© The Authors Journal compilation © 2014 Biochemical Society
Essays Biochem. (2014) 56, 137–148: doi: 10.1042/BSE0560137

10

Oligomers of α-synuclein: picking the culprit in the line-up

Nikolai Lorenzen[1] and Daniel E. Otzen[2]

Interdisciplinary Nanoscience Center (iNANO), Department of Molecular Biology, Center for Insoluble Protein Structures (inSPIN), Aarhus University, Gustav Wieds Vej 14, 8000 Aarhus C, Denmark

Abstract

In the present chapter, we discuss the key findings on αsyn (α-synuclein) oligomers from a biophysical point of view. Current structural methods cannot provide a high-resolution structure of αsyn oligomers due to their size, heterogeneity and tendency to aggregate. However, a low-resolution structure of a stable αsyn oligomer population is emerging based on compelling data from different research groups. αsyn oligomers are normally observed during the formation of amyloid fibrils and we discuss how they are connected to this process. Another important topic is the interaction of αsyn oligomers and membranes, and we will discuss the evidence which suggests that this interaction might be essential in the pathogenesis of Parkinson's disease and other neurodegenerative disorders. Finally, we present a remarkable example of how small molecules are able to stabilize non-amyloid oligomers and how this might be a potential strategy to inhibit the inherent toxicity of αsyn oligomers. A major challenge is to link the very complex oligomerization pathways seen in clever experiments *in vitro* with what actually happens in the cell. With the tremendous developments in optical microscopy in mind, we believe that it will be possible to make this link very soon.

Keywords:

epigallocatechin gallate (EGCG), membrane permeabilization, oligomer formation, oligomer–membrane interaction, oligomer structure, small molecule, toxicity.

[1]*Present address: Department of Protein Structure and Biophysics, Novo Nordisk A/S, 2760 Måløv, Denmark.*

[2]*To whom correspondence should be addressed (email dao@inano.au.dk).*

Introduction: the role of α-synuclein in Parkinson's disease

The interest in protein misfolding has increased spectacularly after it was established that the conversion of a range of soluble proteins into insoluble amyloid fibrils is linked to several diseases (see Chapter 1 by Louise Serpell). This link is direct in systemic amyloidosis, where excessive accumulation of amyloid fibrils in joints or organs leads to pathology. However, in neurodegenerative disorders such as PD (Parkinson's disease), the link is more indirect. In PD, amyloid fibrils consisting of the protein αsyn (α-synuclein) form intracellular deposits called LBs (Lewy bodies) and Lewy neurities, which appear to accompany the loss of dopaminergic neurons mainly in the part of the brain called the substantia nigra. Analogous observations have been made for Alzheimer's disease. Such observations initially led to the hypothesis that amyloid fibrils were responsible for the pathogenesis of PD and other neurodegenerative disorders. However, new observations have made a compelling case that pre-fibrillar oligomers, typically formed in the early stages of the fibril formation process, are the actual pathogenic culprits. This shift from amyloid fibrils to amyloid oligomers was inspired by the emergence of a similar oligomer hypothesis in Alzheimer's disease, where Aβ (amyloid β-peptide) was shown to form a range of oligomeric structures with cytotoxic properties [1]. Subsequently, Lansbury, Fink and co-workers demonstrated that αsyn oligomers, and not mature amyloid fibrils, have membrane-permeabilizing properties [2–5]. Their toxicity has been demonstrated *in vivo* [6], and elevated levels of αsyn oligomers have been found in cerebrospinal fluid from PD patients [7] and in post-mortem brain extracts from patients with LB dementia. Consequently, αsyn oligomers are now one of the primary targets in PD drug development. αsyn oligomers are included in a clinical trial as potential biomarkers for the neurodegenerative disorder multiple system atrophy, known as a Parkinson-plus syndrome (ClinicalTrials.gov, NCT01485549), whereas Aβ oligomers have been targeted by the compound scyllo-inositol (ClinicalTrials.gov, NCT00934050).

αsyn consists of 140 residues and is intrinsically disordered, i.e. it lacks persistent secondary and tertiary structure [8]. However, upon interaction with negatively charged membranes, residues 1–100 undergo a coil-helix conformational change [9]. Under these conditions αsyn can co-exist both as a single long helical chain (extended conformation) and as two helices in a hair-pin arrangement (horse shoe) [10]. This ability of αsyn to fold into membranes is believed to be essential for its physiological role. The basic N-terminal part (residues 1–60) initiates the interaction with membranes and leads to the subsequent folding of the NAC (non-amyloid β-peptide component) region (residues 61–95). The NAC region is hydrophobic and is known to constitute the core of amyloid fibrils [11]. The C-terminus is highly acidic and unstructured. Apart from possible electrostatic interactions between the YEMPS region (residues 125–129) and other regions of the polypeptide, the C-terminus is disordered in both the free monomer, the membrane-bound monomer, the oligomer and the fibril structure [11]. It has been suggested recently that αsyn could form a tetramer *in vivo* [12], but this remains a minority position, contradicted by a vast literature on the properties of natively unfolded αsyn as well as direct rebuttals which show αsyn to naturally form a disordered monomer [8].

Lashuel et al. [4] used EM (electron microscopy) to show that both αsyn and Aβ oligomers form annular ring-shaped oligomers (Figure 1). Combined with the observation that the oligomers were able to permeabilize synthetic membranes [3], this suggested that pore

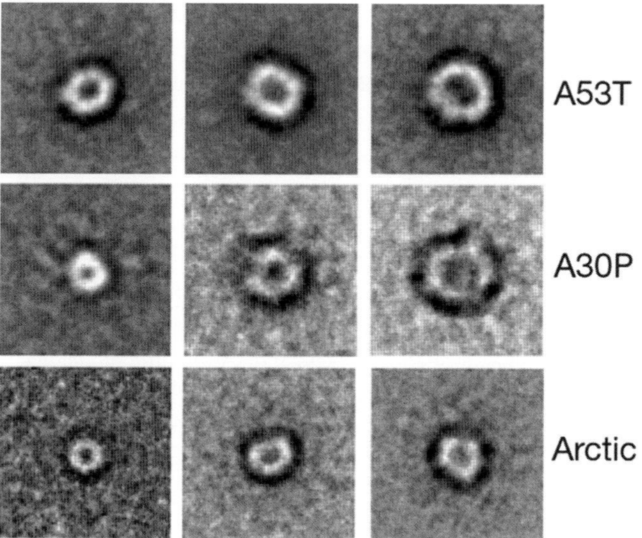

Figure 1. Amyloid oligomers of two disease-promoting mutations of αsyn (A30P and A53T), as well as the Arctic mutant of Aβ

The images are reconstructed from 5000 to 6000 individual particles, using the lowest-molecular-mass fraction of oligomer purified by SEC. Each picture has an area of 30.5 nm × 30.5 nm. Reprinted with permission from [4], Macmillan Publishers Ltd: *Nature* (Lashuel, H.A., Hartley, D., Petre, B.M., Walz, T. and Lansbury, Jr, P.T. (2002) Neurodegenerative disease: amyloid pores from pathogenic mutations. **418**, 291), copyright 2002.

formation in cell membranes led to oligomer toxicity. This pioneering finding has later been supported for amyloid oligomers formed by other peptides and proteins (ABri, ADan, serum amyloid A and amylin) which are ring formed and permeabilize membranes [13]. Note that sample preparation in EM and AFM (atomic force microscopy) involves drying which might induce structural artefacts. As discussed in the next section, solution studies suggest that the αsyn oligomer is ellipsoidal rather than ring shaped.

A low-resolution structure of αsyn oligomers: compact core with diffuse shell

In this section we discuss the structure of a type of αsyn oligomer which has been studied thoroughly by the Subramaniam group [11,14,15], and which is highly similar (if not identical) to the oligomers that are studied in our research group [16–19]. The Subramaniam group form stable αsyn oligomers by incubating αsyn at a concentration of 1 mM for 18 h at room temperature under vigorous shaking, followed by a 2 h incubation at 37°C without shaking. It is an open question to define the biologically most relevant conditions to prepare oligomers. Most researchers agree to use PBS buffer pH 7.4, but other conditions can vary. Oligomers form spontaneously when monomeric αsyn is dissolved at high concentrations and left on ice [20], but higher yields are obtained by shaking the sample at the more physiological temperature of 37°C. Although the biological relevance of shaking can be questioned, it certainly leads to more reproducible aggregation, particularly in combination with the use of glass beads [21,22].

Subsequently, oligomers are purified by SEC (size-exclusion chromatography), similar to other established protocols [4,16]. Subramaniam and co-workers elegantly used a combination of sub-stoichiometric labelling and single-molecule photobleaching to count the number of monomers per oligomer, arriving at a number of ~31 and at the same time showing the oligomer population to be monodisperse (i.e. only one type of oligomer) [14]. By labelling individual positions with the fluorescent residue tryptophan, they were able to conclude that the N-terminus and NAC region are part of the oligomer core, whereas the C-terminus remains disordered [11].

In 2010, we used SAXS (small-angle X-ray scattering) to resolve the structure of αsyn oligomers that accumulate during fibril formation [16]. We could resolve monomers, dimers, oligomers and fibrils in the fibril formation process and, by *ab initio* modelling, we determined the shape of the oligomers to be an ellipsoid with dimensions given in Figure 2 (left-hand panel). More recently, we have gone a step further. We purified the oligomers from samples with fibril formation, by incubating 840 µM αsyn for 5 h at 37°C with vigorous shaking and subsequent purification with SEC, similar to the approach of other groups [4,14,16]. This reasonably pure oligomer solution (<10% monomers) has provided a more detailed structural model. The oligomers consist of a rigid core with the same dimensions as our first SAXS model, but this core is covered by a 5 nm thick outer layer consisting of disordered polypeptides (Figure 2, right-hand panel) [18]. The SAXS analysis together with a complementary SEC-MALLS (multi-angle laser light scattering) analysis estimate that the average oligomer is built up of ~29 monomers [18], in strong agreement with the Subramaniam group [14]. All of these size-estimation methods are independent of the shape and conformation of the molecules, giving more reliable data on the oligomer structure than SEC, DLS (dynamic light scattering), EM and AFM which either report on hydrodynamic radius (SEC and DLS) or are

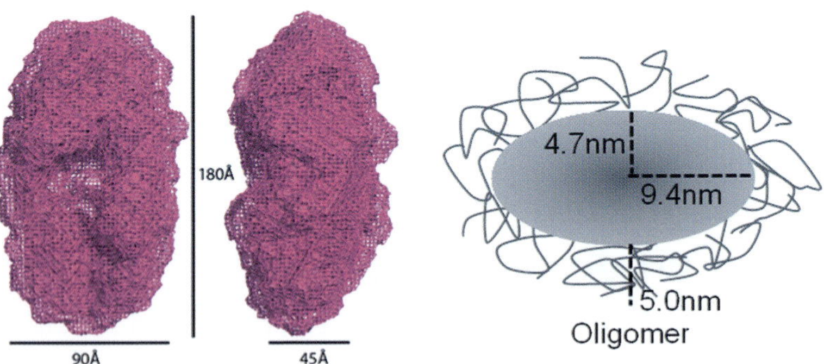

Figure 2. Ellipsoid structure of the αsyn oligomer
Left-hand panel, SAXS-based model of a αsyn oligomer which is populated during fibril formation. 1 Å = 0.1 nm. Reproduced with permission from [16]; Lise Giehm, Dmitri I. Svergun, Daniel E. Otzen and Bente Vestergaard (2011) Low-resolution structure of a vesicle disrupting α-synuclein oligomer that accumulates during fibrillation, PNAS, **108**, 3246–3251 copyright by National Academy of Sciences of the United States of America. Right-hand panel, schematic model of the structure of αsyn oligomers having a β-sheet core build up by the N-terminus and NAC region and a disordered brush shell outer layer consisting of the C-terminus. Reprinted with permission from [18]; Lorenzen, N., Nielsen, S.B., Buell, A.K., Kaspersen, J.D., Arosio, P., Vad, B.S., Paslawski, W., Christiansen, G. et al. (2014) The role of stable α-synuclein oligomers in the events underlying amyloid formation. J. Am. Chem. Soc. **136**, 3859–3868. Copyright © 2014 American Chemical Society

sensitive to drying artefacts (EM and AFM). Our revised structure of αsyn oligomers is in good agreement with the proposed micellar structure by the Subramaniam group where the less charged and more hydrophobic N-terminal and NAC regions forms the compact core, whereas the highly charged C-terminal forms a brush-like shell [23]. This compact organization might explain the monodispersity and the remarkable stability of the αsyn oligomers.

The oligomer core is most likely to be organized in β-sheets [5,24]. Fourier transform infrared spectroscopy suggests that both Aβ and αsyn oligomers contain β-sheet structure. Although mature amyloids of Aβ and αsyn fibrils consist of parallel β-strands, oligomers appear to contain anti-parallel β-strands [24]. This difference could arise in two ways. Either oligomers and fibrils belong to different aggregation pathways, or oligomers have to undergo structural rearrangements before they can become incorporated into fibril structures.

Note that there is not just *one* oligomer of αsyn. Different oligomers have been reported, containing different types of secondary structure, ranging from mainly α-helical to disordered, and of varying sizes, e.g. coexisting oligomers of ten and 15 monomers [25] (see below). Oligomers may also be induced by metal ions, lipids, alcohols and small molecules [26,27]. A tremendously important challenge is to determine which oligomer structures are relevant *in vivo*, and how they can be purified and stabilized for thorough analysis.

What is the role of αsyn oligomers in the process of fibril formation?

The amyloid fibril structure is a thermodynamically favourable state which has been suggested to be generic for all proteins. However, the mechanism of amyloid formation is not generic, but varies between proteins and is also highly dependent on solution conditions. A key question in this regard is whether oligomers, which are often observed during fibril formation, are compulsory precursors (on-pathway intermediates) for fibrils or rather dead-end species that are not incorporated into the fibrils. There is no simple answer to this; on- and off-pathway oligomers may co-exist and conflicting observations may also reflect different assembly processes under different conditions. However, it is generally believed that monomers are the elongating species in αsyn fibril formation, i.e. fibrils grow by addition of monomers to fibril ends (Figure 3).

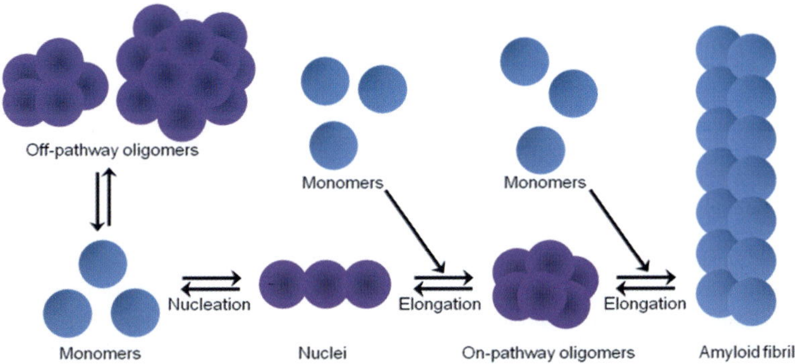

Figure 3. Schematic representation of the role of on- and off-pathway oligomers in the process of fibril formation
Oligomer structures are highlighted with purple colour.

On-pathway oligomers are formed at an early stage. They cover the whole range of species between monomers and fibrils and are also commonly known as fibril nuclei, pre-fibrillar oligomers and protofibrils. Off-pathway oligomers can also be observed under fibril forming conditions. These belong to a separate aggregation pathway and would have to dissociate into monomers, or possibly smaller oligomers, to be able to enter fibril formation.

On-pathway αsyn oligomers

Cremades et al. [25] have combined single-molecule techniques with kinetic analysis to monitor the development of different αsyn oligomers in the initial phases of the fibrillation process. Before making the oligomers, αsyn monomers were labelled with two different fluorophors. This made it possible to identify oligomers in solution as follows: when the oligomers were prepared from these labelled monomers and their fluorescence was measured under very dilute conditions (where one detects only one or a few molecules at a time), oligomers gave rise to co-incident bursts of light from both fluorophors (since they contained both types of labelled monomers), whereas monomers only gave bursts from one fluorophor at a time. The size of the burst provided an estimate of the oligomer size. In addition, the authors were also able to make a rough size classification of oligomers based on the level of FRET (Förster resonance energy transfer) between the two fluorophors in the oligomer. The higher the FRET values, the closer the fluorophors are to each other, although analysis is complicated by the fact that there are several fluorophors in each oligomer. FRET values were shown to follow a Gaussian distribution of values which was consistent with four different oligomer distributions, denoted as A_{small} (2–5-mers), A_{med} and B_{med} (both 5–15-mers, with the B oligomers being slightly larger) and B_{large} (~15–150-mers). A and B refer to mid- and high-FRET values respectively. The difference in FRET values of A and B oligomers suggest that they are of different structure. As shown in Figure 4, A oligomers are just as sensitive to protease degradation as the

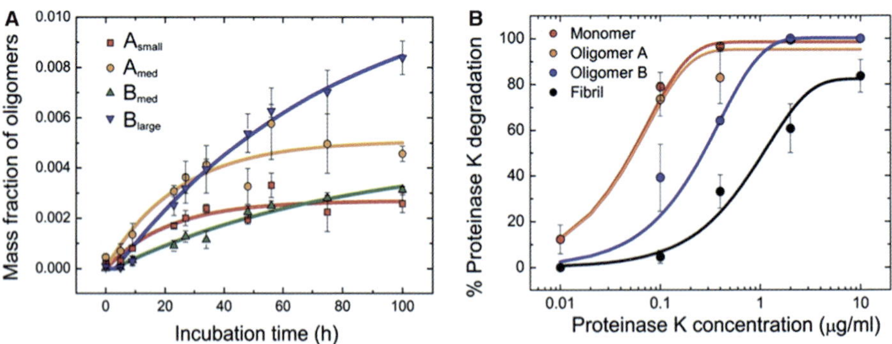

Figure 4. Size classification of oligomers using FRET values
(A) The time dependence of the mass fraction of the four oligomeric distributions A_{small} (red squares), A_{med} (orange circles), B_{med} (green triangles) and B_{large} (blue triangles). (B) Proteinase K degradation curves of the different protein species (monomer shown as red, type A oligomer shown as orange, type B oligomer shown as blue and fibrils shown as black). Reproduced with permission from [25]; Cremades N, Cohen SI, Deas E, Abramov AY, Chen AY, Orte A, Sandal M, Clarke RW, Dunne P, Aprile FA, Bertoncini CW, Wood NW, Knowles TP, Dobson CM, Klenerman D. (2012) Direct observation of the interconversion of normal and toxic forms of α-synuclein., Cell, **149**, 1048–1059 © 2012 Elsevier Inc. Published by Elsevier Inc. User rights governed by an Open Access license.

monomer, indicating a highly flexible structure; B oligomers were much more protease resistant, suggesting compact β-sheet structure (consistent with higher FRET values), whereas mature fibrils were the most resistant. A_{small} and A_{med} formed at similar rates and with hardly any lag time, whereas B_{med} and B_{large} showed a longer lag time. Thus B oligomers are likely to be formed from the A oligomers; A oligomers accumulate because they are formed more quickly from monomers (by nucleation) than they decay to B [25]. In this model, αsyn follows NCC (nucleated conformational conversion) where non-amyloid oligomers are readily formed by incorporation of monomers into the growing oligomer and accumulate until they undergo an internal structural rearrangement ('nucleated conversion' without the participation of monomers) to amyloid oligomers competent of being elongated into mature fibrils. Both types of oligomer can subsequently grow by incorporating more αsyn monomers. This NCC model has also been proposed as a nucleation mechanism for prions [28] and Aβ [29].

The experiments by Cremades et al. [25] provide the most detailed picture of the interconversion of different forms of αsyn oligomers under carefully controlled *in vitro* conditions. The obvious question is how this process occurs in the cell. Most likely, this question will be answered when we can apply fluorescence microscopy at single-molecule level in the cell using labelled αsyn, either prepared directly in the cell or introduced by e.g. electroporation [30].

Off-pathway αsyn oligomers

We have found that oligomers depicted in Figure 2 (right-hand panel) actually inhibit fibril formation and are unable to elongate into mature amyloid fibrils [18]. Thus although these oligomers accumulate during the fibril formation process, they appear to be unproductive in this process. These oligomers can aggregate further into non-fibrillar aggregates suggesting that they belong to an aggregation process distinct from fibril formation. However, it cannot be ruled out that these oligomers might also be connected to fibril formation by processes similar to NCC. Off-pathway oligomers have also been observed when stabilized by e.g. small molecules; an example is given in the final section.

The variety of oligomers is the natural consequence of a process which has not undergone biological evolution to optimize formation of the end product [5]. One current challenge is to understand to what extent off-pathway oligomers under different conditions might be able to undergo structural rearrangement and proceed in the process of fibril formation.

Oligomer–membrane interactions: the cause of toxicity?

Intriguingly, some conformational antibodies can recognize a range of different amyloid oligomers without recognizing the monomer or mature fibril form. This suggests that these oligomers have a common structure [31] which may be the basis for their cytotoxicity [32]. Several oligomers have exposed hydrophobic regions and bind the hydrophobic probe ANS (8-anilinonaphthalene-1-sulfonic acid) [33]. A common structural motif exposing 'sticky' surfaces may promote oligomer–membrane interactions and perturb the membrane [3,13,15,34,35]. It is possible that oligomer structural flexibility, leading to hydrophobic exposure and structural rearrangements following membrane interaction, is essential for toxicity.

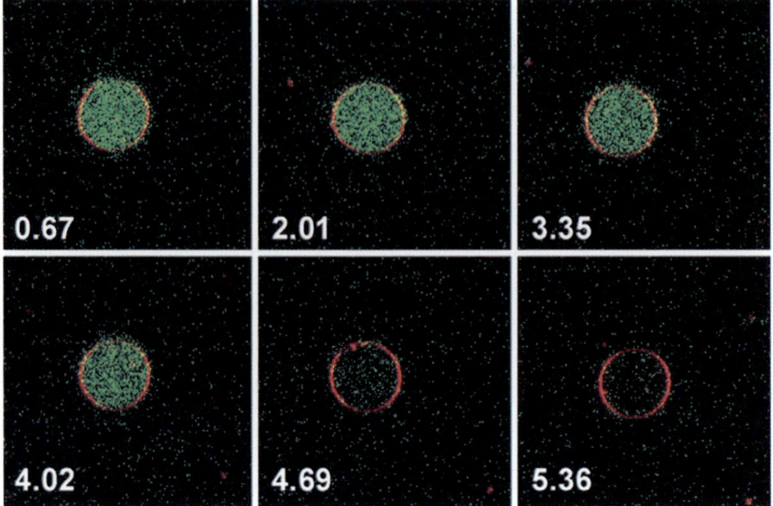

Figure 5. Confocal microscopy image of POPG giant unilamellar vesicles
The fluorophore HPTS (green) is entrapped inside the vesicle and the paired quencher, DPX, is present outside the vesicle. The membrane is stained with DOPE (1,2-dioleleoyl-sn-glycerol-3-phosphoethanolamine)-rhodamine (red). Time points are given in seconds. Reproduced with permission from [34]; van Rooijen BD, Claessens MM, Subramaniam V. (2010) Membrane Permeabilization by Oligomeric α-Synuclein: In Search of the Mechanism., PLoS ONE, **5**, e14292© 2010 van Rooijen et al.

The ability of αsyn oligomers to permeabilize membranes has been investigated intensely. An example of the permeabilization of synthetic membranes, composed of the anionic POPG lipid, by αsyn oligomers is shown in Figure 5. The degree of permeabilization is monitored by the fluorophore/quencher pair HPTS/DPX and the kinetics reveals that complete permeabilization (efflux/influx) is obtained within 5 s. Staining of the membrane shows that the form and size of the vesicles remains intact upon oligomer binding and permeabilization. The Subramaniam group has used single-tryptophan mutants to demonstrate that the N-terminus is involved in oligomer–membrane interactions, as is also the case for the monomer [11]. We have confirmed recently how the N-terminus is essential for oligomer–membrane interaction and membrane permeabilization [17]. The αsyn oligomer selectively binds to anionic lipids and preferentially to liquid-disordered-phase regions of the membranes [15] where the lipid bilayer is loosely packed and the hydrophobic membrane interior is more accessible [36]. Thus interaction of αsyn oligomers with membranes seems to be governed by electrostatic interactions of the N-terminus with the membrane, combined with hydrophobic interactions of accessible hydrophobic patches in the αsyn oligomer structure with the membrane interior.

Small molecules as potential drugs?

It is a tremendous challenge to develop drugs for neurodegenerative disorders due to the complex BBB (blood–brain barrier). The difficulty in delivering macromolecules such as antibodies and RNA aptamers has put focus on identifying small molecules which are able to cross the BBB and interact specifically with αsyn. Numerous small molecules with mono-, di- and tri-hydroxyphenyl groups inhibit protein aggregation while promoting oligomer formation.

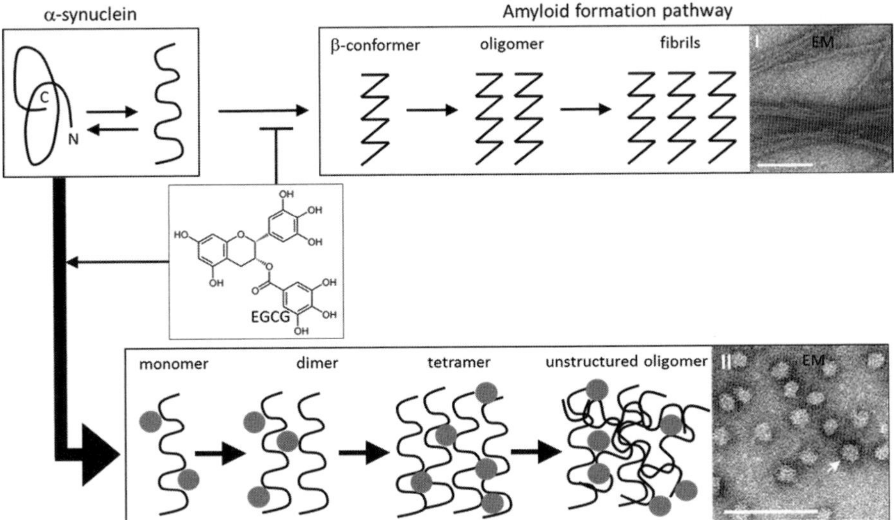

Figure 6. Schematic representation of the fibril formation pathway and the EGCG-directed aggregation pathway

αsyn monomers exist in equilibrium between disordered and partially folded conformations. Fibril formation occurs through the development of on-pathway oligomers by nucleation events and subsequent addition of monomers leads to mature fibrils. EGCG binds αsyn monomers and leads to stepwise aggregation into disordered non-toxic and off-pathway oligomers. Scale bars, 100 nm. Reproduced with permission from [39]; Lorenzen, N., Wanker, E. and Otzen, D.E. (2013) Inhibitors of amyloid and oligomer formation in: Amyloid Fibrils and Prefibrillar Aggregates: Molecular and Biological Properties, Otzen, D.E (ed.), Wiley, UK Copyright © 2013, John Wiley and Sons.

Examples include the neurotransmitter dopamine [26], the flavonoid baicalein obtained from herbal medicine [37] and the catechin EGCG (epigallocatechin gallate) from green tea [27]. The effect of EGCG on αsyn oligomerization and fibril formation is a remarkable example of how small molecules can redirect aggregation pathways.

EGCG binds preferentially to disordered polypeptides, but also to structured regions at high concentrations. Wanker and co-workers have proposed a model where EGCG binds the αsyn monomer and redirects the protein from the process of fibril formation into sequential aggregation, leading to stable non-toxic oligomers [27] (Figure 6). These off-pathway oligomers are amorphous and show no β-sheet content. Moreover, EGCG is able to reorganize mature amyloid fibrils of αsyn and Aβ into amorphous and non-toxic oligomers [27].

The effect of EGCG on the aggregation of αsyn and Aβ is only one of many possible strategies to prevent the formation of toxic amyloid oligomers. Another strategy is to use small molecules to stabilize the protein in the monomeric form; at the other extreme, pro-aggregators can shift the equilibrium towards the amyloid fibrils, which are believed to be less toxic [38].

Conclusions

To clarify the role of αsyn oligomers in the amyloid fibril formation process and their potential role in the pathogenesis of PD will be important for the understanding and treatment of not only PD, but also other related neurodegenerative disorders such as Alzheimer's disease and

Huntington's disease. The major hurdle here is to define the cytotoxic species. Current research points towards oligomers as the prime suspects. Therefore it is crucial to establish which oligomers are relevant in the amyloid process *in vivo*, and whether it is a defined oligomer or rather a whole spectrum of different pre-fibrillar oligomers that are cytotoxic. Until then, it will be difficult to rationally design drug discovery programmes towards oligomers. For now, an alternative strategy might be the development of small molecules or nanoparticles that are specific towards αsyn, and which stabilize the monomer form in such a way that amyloid formation is completely inhibited without compromising the protein's underlying biological function. This, on the other hand, will not be trivial to accomplish.

Summary

- αsyn oligomers are likely to be the cytotoxic species in the pathogenesis of PD.
- A low-resolution structure is emerging for stable αsyn oligomers.
- αsyn oligomers are observed as both on- and off-pathway in the fibril formation process.
- Oligomers interact strongly with membranes and this is possibly the cause of neuronal damage in PD and other neurodegenerative disorders.
- Small molecules, such as EGCG, redirect the aggregation pathway of αsyn.

We apologize to the many authors whose work we could not include because of limitations in the number of references. We thank Jørn Døvling Kaspersen and Jan Skov Pedersen for very fruitful collaborations on SAXS analysis of the αsyn oligomers. We are supported by the Michael J. Fox Foundation and the Danish Research Foundation (inSPIN).

References

1. Walsh, D.M. and Selkoe, D.J. (2007) Aβ oligomers: a decade of discovery. J. Neurochem. **101**, 1172–1184
2. Conway, K.A., Lee, S.J., Rochet, J.C., Ding, T.T., Williamson, R.E. and Lansbury, Jr, P.T. (2000) Acceleration of oligomerization, not fibrillization, is a shared property of both α-synuclein mutations linked to early-onset Parkinson's disease: implications for pathogenesis and therapy. Proc. Natl. Acad. Sci. U.S.A. **97**, 571–576
3. Volles, M.J., Lee, S.J., Rochet, J.C., Shtilerman, M.D., Ding, T.T., Kessler, J.C. and Lansbury, Jr, P.T. (2001) Vesicle permeabilization by protofibrillar alpha-synuclein: implications for the pathogenesis and treatment of Parkinson's disease. Biochemistry **40**, 7812–7819
4. Lashuel, H.A., Hartley, D., Petre, B.M., Walz, T. and Lansbury, Jr, P.T. (2002) Neurodegenerative disease: amyloid pores from pathogenic mutations. Nature **418**, 291
5. Kaylor, J., Bodner, N., Edridge, S., Yamin, G., Hong, D.P. and Fink, A.L. (2005) Characterization of oligomeric intermediates in α-synuclein fibrillation: FRET studies of Y125W/Y133F/Y136F α-synuclein. J. Mol. Biol. **353**, 357–372
6. Winner, B., Jappelli, R., Maji, S.K., Desplats, P.A., Boyer, L., Aigner, S., Hetzer, C., Loher, T., Vilar, M., Campioni, S. et al. (2011) *In vivo* demonstration that alpha-synuclein oligomers are toxic. Proc. Natl. Acad. Sci. U.S.A. **108**, 4194–4199

7. Tokuda, T., Qureshi, M.M., Ardah, M.T., Varghese, S., Shehab, S.A., Kasai, T., Ishigami, N., Tamaoka, A., Nakagawa, M. and El-Agnaf, O.M. (2010) Detection of elevated levels of alpha-synuclein oligomers in CSF from patients with Parkinson disease. Neurology **75**, 1766–1772

8. Fauvet, B., Mbefo, M.K., Fares, M.B., Desobry, C., Michael, S., Ardah, M.T., Tsika, E., Coune, P., Prudent, M., Lion, N. et al. (2012) α-Synuclein in central nervous system and from erythrocytes, mammalian cells, and *Escherichia coli* exists predominantly as disordered monomer. J. Biol. Chem. **287**, 15345–15364

9. Ulmer, T.S., Bax, A., Cole, N.B. and Nussbaum, R.L. (2005) Structure and dynamics of micelle-bound human α-synuclein. J. Biol. Chem. **280**, 9595–9603

10. Robotta, M., Braun, P., van Rooijen, B., Subramaniam, V., Huber, M. and Drescher, M. (2011) Direct evidence of coexisting horseshoe and extended helix conformations of membrane-bound α-synuclein. Chemphyschem **12**, 267–269

11. van Rooijen, B.D., van Leijenhorst-Groener, K.A., Claessens, M.M. and Subramaniam, V. (2009) Tryptophan fluorescence reveals structural features of α-synuclein oligomers. J. Mol. Biol. **394**, 826–833

12. Bartels, T., Choi, J.G. and Selkoe, D.J. (2011) α-Synuclein occurs physiologically as a helically folded tetramer that resists aggregation. Nature **477**, 107–110

13. Quist, A., Doudevski, I., Lin, H., Azimova, R., Ng, D., Frangione, B., Kagan, B., Ghiso, J. and Lal, R. (2005) Amyloid ion channels: a common structural link for protein-misfolding disease. Proc. Natl. Acad. Sci. U.S.A. **102**, 10427–10432

14. Zijlstra, N., Blum, C., Segers-Nolten, I.M., Claessens, M.M. and Subramaniam, V. (2012) Molecular composition of sub-stoichiometrically labeled α-synuclein oligomers determined by single-molecule photobleaching. Angew. Chem. Int. Ed. Engl. **51**, 8821–8824

15. van Rooijen, B.D., Claessens, M.M. and Subramaniam, V. (2008) Membrane binding of oligomeric α-synuclein depends on bilayer charge and packing. FEBS Lett. **582**, 3788–3792

16. Giehm, L., Svergun, D.I., Otzen, D.E. and Vestergaard, B. (2011) Low-resolution structure of a vesicle disrupting α-synuclein oligomer that accumulates during fibrillation. Proc. Natl. Acad. Sci. U.S.A. **108**, 3246–3251

17. Lorenzen, N., Lemminger, L., Pedersen, J.N., Nielsen, S.B. and Otzen, D.E. (2014) The N-terminus of α-synuclein is essential for both monomeric and oligomeric interactions with membranes. FEBS Lett. **588**, 497–502

18. Lorenzen, N., Nielsen, S.B., Buell, A.K., Kaspersen, J.D., Arosio, P., Vad, B.S., Paslawski, W., Christiansen, G. et al. (2014) The role of stable α-synuclein oligomers in the events underlying amyloid formation. J. Am. Chem. Soc. **136**, 3859–3868

19. Paslawski, W., Mysling, S., Thomsen, K., Jørgensen, T.J.D. and Otzen, D.E. (2014) Co-existence of two different α-synuclein oligomers with different core structures determined by hydrogen/deuterium exchange mass spectrometry. Angew. Chem. Int. Ed. Engl., doi: 10.1002/ange.201400491

20. Lashuel, H.A., Petre, B.M., Wall, J., Simon, M., Nowak, R.J., Walz, T. and Lansbury, P.T. (2002) α-Synuclein, especially the Parkinson's disease-associated mutants, forms pore-like annular and tubular protofibrils. J. Mol. Biol. **322**, 1089–1102

21. Giehm, L. and Otzen, D.E. (2013) Experimental approaches to inducing amyloid aggregates. In Amyloid Fibrils and Prefibrillar Aggregates: Molecular and Biological Properties (Otzen, D.E., ed.), pp. 295–320, Wiley, Weinheim

22. Giehm, L. and Otzen, D.E. (2010) Strategies to increase the reproducibility of α-synuclein fibrillation in plate reader assays. Anal. Biochem. **400**, 270–281

23. Stöckl, M.T., Zijlstra, N. and Subramaniam, V. (2013) α-Synuclein oligomers: an amyloid pore? Insights into mechanisms of α-synuclein oligomer-lipid interactions. Mol. Neurobiol. **47**, 613–621

24. Celej, M.S., Sarroukh, R., Goormaghtigh, E., Fidelio, G.D., Ruysschaert, J.M. and Raussens, V. (2012) Toxic prefibrillar α-synuclein amyloid oligomers adopt a distinctive antiparallel β-sheet structure. Biochem. J. **443**, 719–726

25. Cremades, N., Cohen, S.I., Deas, E., Abramov, A.Y., Chen, A.Y., Orte, A., Sandal, M., Clarke, R.W., Dunne, P., Aprile, F.A. et al. (2012) Direct observation of the interconversion of normal and toxic forms of α-synuclein. Cell **149**, 1048–1059

26. Conway, K.A., Rochet, J.C., Bieganski, R.M. and Lansbury, Jr, P.T. (2001) Kinetic stabilization of the α-synuclein protofibril by a dopamine–α-synuclein adduct. Science **294**, 1346–1349

27. Bieschke, J., Russ, J., Friedrich, R.P., Ehrnhoefer, D.E., Wobst, H., Neugebauer, K. and Wanker, E.E. (2010) EGCG remodels mature α-synuclein and amyloid-β fibrils and reduces cellular toxicity. Proc. Natl. Acad. Sci. U.S.A. **107**, 7710–7715

28. Serio, T.R., Cashikar, A., Kowal, A.S., Sawicki, G.J., Moslehi, J.J., Serpell, L., Arnsdorf, M.F. and Lindquist, S. (2000) Nucleated conformational conversion and the replication of conformational information by a prion determinany. Science **289**, 1317–1321

29. Lee, J., Culyba, E.K., Powers, E.T. and Kelly, J.W. (2011) Amyloid-β forms fibrils by nucleated conformational conversion of oligomers. Nat. Chem. Biol. **7**, 602–609

30. Bekei, B., Rose, H.M., Herzig, M., Dose, A., Schwarzer, D. and Selenko, P. (2012) In-cell NMR in mammalian cells: part 1. Methods Mol. Biol. **895**, 43–54

31. Kayed, R., Head, E., Thompson, J.L., McIntire, T.M., Milton, S.C., Cotman, C.W. and Glabe, C.G. (2003) Common structure of soluble amyloid oligomers implies common mechanism of pathogenesis. Science **300**, 486–489

32. Bucciantini, M., Giannoni, E., Chiti, F., Baroni, F., Formigli, L., Zurdo, J., Taddei, N., Ramponi, G., Dobson, C.M. and Stefani, M. (2002) Inherent toxicity of aggregates implies a common mechanism for protein misfolding diseases. Nature **416**, 507–511

33. Bolognesi, B., Kumita, J.R., Barros, T.P., Esbjorner, E.K., Luheshi, L.M., Crowther, D.C., Wilson, M.R., Dobson, C.M., Favrin, G. and Yerbury, J.J. (2010) ANS binding reveals common features of cytotoxic amyloid species. ACS Chem. Biol. **5**, 735–740

34. van Rooijen, B.D., Claessens, M.M. and Subramaniam, V. (2010) Membrane permeabilization by oligomeric α-synuclein: in search of the mechanism. PLoS One **5**, e14292

35. Campioni, S., Mannini, B., Zampagni, M., Pensalfini, A., Parrini, C., Evangelisti, E., Relini, A., Stefani, M., Dobson, C.M., Cecchi, C. and Chiti, F. (2010) A causative link between the structure of aberrant protein oligomers and their toxicity. Nat. Chem. Biol. **6**, 140–147

36. van Rooijen, B.D., Claessens, M.M. and Subramaniam, V. (2009) Lipid bilayer disruption by oligomeric α-synuclein depends on bilayer charge and accessibility of the hydrophobic core. Biochim. Biophys. Acta **1788**, 1271–1278

37. Hong, D.P., Fink, A.L. and Uversky, V.N. (2008) Structural characteristics of α-synuclein oligomers stabilized by the flavonoid baicalein. J. Mol. Biol. **383**, 214–223

38. Bieschke, J., Herbst, M., Wiglenda, T., Friedrich, R.P., Boeddrich, A., Schiele, F., Kleckers, D., Lopez Del Amo, J.M., Gruning, B.A., Wang, Q. et al. (2011) Small-molecule conversion of toxic oligomers to nontoxic β-sheet-rich amyloid fibrils. Nat. Chem. Biol. **8**, 93–101

39. Lorenzen, N., Wanker, E. and Otzen, D.E. (2013) Inhibitors of amyloid and oligomer formation. In Amyloid Fibrils and Prefibrillar Aggregates: Molecular and Biological Properties (Otzen, D.E., ed.), pp. 345–372, Wiley, Weinheim

© The Authors Journal compilation © 2014 Biochemical Society
Essays Biochem. (2014) 56, 149–165: doi: 10.1042/BSE0560149

11

Many roads lead to Rome? Multiple modes of Cu,Zn superoxide dismutase destabilization, misfolding and aggregation in amyotrophic lateral sclerosis

Helen R. Broom, Jessica A.O. Rumfeldt and Elizabeth M. Meiering[1]

Guelph-Waterloo Centre for Graduate Studies in Chemistry and Biochemistry, and Department of Chemistry, University of Waterloo, 200 University Avenue West, Waterloo, ON, Canada, N2L 3G1

Abstract

ALS (amyotrophic lateral sclerosis) is a fatal neurodegenerative syndrome characterized by progressive paralysis and motor neuron death. Although the pathological mechanisms that cause ALS remain unclear, accumulating evidence supports that ALS is a protein misfolding disorder. Mutations in Cu,Zn-SOD1 (copper/zinc superoxide dismutase 1) are a common cause of familial ALS. They have complex effects on different forms of SOD1, but generally destabilize the protein and enhance various modes of misfolding and aggregation. In addition, there is some evidence that destabilized covalently modified wild-type SOD1 may be involved in disease. Among the multitude of misfolded/aggregated species observed for SOD1, multiple species may impair various cellular components at different disease stages. Newly developed antibodies that recognize different structural features of SOD1 represent a powerful tool for further unravelling the roles of different SOD1 structures in disease. Evidence for similar cellular targets of misfolded/aggregated proteins, loss of cellular proteostasis and cell–cell transmission of aggregates point to common pathological mechanisms

[1]*To whom correspondence should be addressed (email meiering@uwaterloo.ca).*

between ALS and other misfolding diseases, such as Alzheimer's, Parkinson's and prion diseases, as well as serpinopathies. The recent progress in understanding the molecular basis for these devastating diseases provides numerous avenues for developing urgently needed therapeutics.

Keywords:

amyotrophic lateral sclerosis (ALS), Cu,Zn superoxide dismutase (SOD1), misfolding, protein aggregation, protein stability.

Introduction

ALS (amyotrophic lateral sclerosis) is a devastating and fatal neurodegenerative syndrome characterized by the rapid progressive death of motor neurons exhibiting hallmark clumps of proteins, referred to as aggregates. Mutant SOD1s (Cu,Zn superoxide dismutases) (Figure 1) are among the most common causes of fALS (familial ALS), and form granule-coated fibrillar structures in patients. Recent studies by our own group and others have characterized the folding, misfolding and aggregation of diverse forms of SOD1, and have provided insights into possible disease mechanisms. In the present chapter, we focus on recent advances in the molecular biophysical characterization of SOD1 mutants, and the possible mechanisms of damage to cells caused by SOD1 misfolding. SOD1-linked ALS is considered in the broader context of other protein misfolding diseases, including amyloidoses such as Alzheimer's, Parkinson's, Huntington's and prion diseases, and other non-amyloid diseases such as serpinopathies. In these diseases, protein misfolding results in the formation of intracellular and/or extracellular protein aggregates. The structures of these protein aggregates can vary depending on the aggregating protein and disease differences, which are not well understood. Uncovering the cause of protein aggregation is of critical importance for understanding these devastating diseases.

Amyotrophic lateral sclerosis

ALS is a very heterogeneous disorder (reviewed in [1]). As with many other neurodegenerative diseases, the majority of ALS cases are sporadic (sALS), i.e. of unknown cause, and a small proportion (~10%) are familial (fALS). ALS-linked mutations have been found in more than 20 genes affecting many different aspects of cellular function. The onset and duration of disease within a given family are highly variable, indicating that multiple factors may modulate disease. ALS is associated with aging, with the onset of symptoms typically from the fourth decade of life. The disease duration is usually 2–5 years, and ALS accounts for ~1 in 1000 adult deaths. Recent research has increasingly recognized distinguishing pathological features among subsets of patients, but also overlapping symptoms (e.g. dementia) with other neurodegenerative disorders as disease progresses [1,2]. Although the cause of ALS remains unknown, a leading hypothesis is that it is caused by toxic protein misfolding, similar to many other neurodegenerative and amyloid diseases.

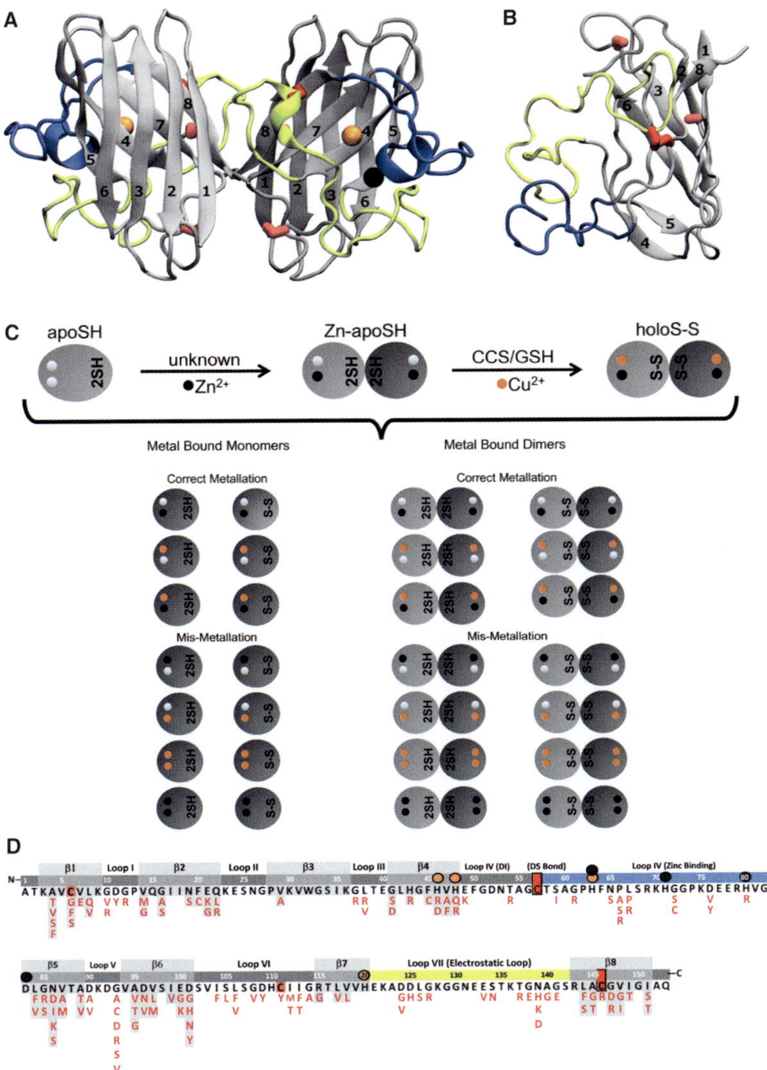

Figure 1. Structures of human SOD1 and variants associated with ALS

The structures of two different forms of SOD1 highlight how post-translational modifications have major effects on the structure of the protein. fALS-associated mutations are located throughout the protein and may promote misfolding in different ways. (**A**) Crystal structure of holoSS SOD1 (PDB code 1HL5) with the protein backbone represented as a ribbon. HoloSS is a homodimer of 153 amino acid subunits, which adopt a Greek key β-barrel structure consisting of eight β-strands and connecting loops. Each subunit binds one Zn (black sphere) and one Cu (orange sphere), contains a highly conserved intramolecular disulfide bond between Cys[57] and Cys[146] (red ball and stick), and is naturally N-acetylated (not shown). SOD1 also contains two free cysteine residues at positions 6 and 111 (pink ball and stick). The longest loops are the Zn-binding loop (Loop IV, yellow) and the electrostatic loop (Loop VII, blue). The Zn-binding loop contains residues that form the Zn-binding site, as well as one of the cysteine residues involved in the intrasubunit disulfide bond, which attaches this loop to β-strand 8. In addition, the Zn-binding loop contains residues involved in forming the dimer interface. Zn binding, disulfide bond formation and dimerization constrain the flexibility of the Zn-binding loop and markedly increase protein stability. (**B**) Solution structure of apoSS monomer variant of SOD1 (PDB code 1RK7). The colour scheme is identical to (**A**).

Although many misfolding diseases involve the formation of a particular type of fibrillar aggregate known as amyloid, it is not clear to what extent protein aggregation in ALS resembles amyloid formation [3]. Amyloidoses are characterized histopathologically using the dye Congo Red, which exhibits green–gold birefringence upon binding to unbranched amyloid fibres containing a highly protease-resistant core cross-β-structure, with β-strands oriented perpendicular to the fibre axis [4]. Congo Red birefringence is not observed in ALS [3]; nevertheless, the observations of fibrillar aggregates and a proximal pattern of cell death [1,5] suggest that ALS has similar disease mechanisms to amyloidoses. These diseases may also have similarities to serpinopathies, which include diverse disorders such as dementia and cirrhosis [6]. The serpinopathies arise from mutations in serpins (serine protease inhibitors), which destabilize the protein and promote its polymerization into non-amyloid fibres. These various diseases are often associated with autosomal dominant mutations in different proteins, which confer a toxic gain-of-function that may involve a range of toxic effects of misfolded/aggregated protein, such as loss of membrane integrity, oxidative stress, mitochondrial dysfunction, chronic inflammation, and impairment of cellular proteostasis, and ultimately results in cell death [1,5].

Superoxide dismutase 1

SOD1 is a paradigm for understanding protein structure and function as well as folding and misfolding in disease, as it has been studied in great detail, both experimentally and using modelling [7,8]. The human protein (hSOD1) (Figure 1) is a homodimeric metalloenzyme, it plays an important role in protecting cells from oxidative damage by catalysing the dismutation of O_2^- radical to O_2 and H_2O_2. Each Greek key subunit contains a catalytic Cu ion, a structural Zn ion, a disulfide bond, two free cysteine residues and two relatively long functional loops. The Zn-binding loop stabilizes the protein through Zn binding and forming part of the dimer interface, whereas the electrostatic loop helps attract O_2^-. Over 150, predominantly missense, mutations are associated with ALS, giving rise to ~20% of fALS cases (Figure 1) (see ALSoD at http://alsod.iop.kcl.ac.uk/). The mutations are associated with characteristic average disease durations, which vary greatly, for example from ~1 year for the dimer interface mutation A4V, the most common mutation in North America, to ~18 years for H46R, a metal-binding mutant.

The most abundant form of SOD1 *in vivo* is generally holoSS, the mature, fully metallated and disulfide-intact dimer; however, conditions such as mutation or aging may promote

---

Figure 1. (*Continued*)
The structure of the monomer is less defined than in mature holoSS. (**C**) Different forms of SOD1 involved in natural maturation or misfolding. Predominantly folded SOD1 monomers are depicted as grey spheres, which are smaller when metals are bound and/or the disulfide is formed to indicate a more compact structure. Bound Cu and Zn are shown by orange and black spheres respectively. SS refers to disulfide intact (i.e. oxidized) forms and 2SH refers to disulfide reduced forms. When the protein is initially synthesized in the reducing environment of the cytosol it is thought to exist in the reduced apo form (apoSH). The mechanism of Zn (black sphere) acquisition is unknown; Cu (orange sphere) can be acquired by interaction with CCS (copper chaperone for SOD1) or by a CCS-independent mechanism involving glutathione. CCS also catalyses intrasubunit disulfide bond formation. Varying levels of many natural or aberrant species differing in metal and disulfide bonding, as well as other covalent modifications, may be formed due to maturation, mutation and aging [7,9–11]. (**D**) The primary sequence of the SOD1 monomer and missense mutations associated with ALS (adapted from [7]). The secondary structural elements are listed above the primary sequence and coloured as in (**A**) and (**B**). fALS-associated mutations are listed vertically in red below the WT amino acid in black. The black and orange spheres indicate Zn and Cu-co-ordinating residues respectively.

increased population of various immature less stable forms of the protein (Figure 1). The form(s) of SOD1 most relevant to pathology remains unknown. The effects of fALS-associated mutations and aberrant covalent modifications associated with aging and disease [1,9–11] on folding and misfolding have been characterized in detail for different forms of SOD1, in particular, holoSS, apoSS (metal-free disulfide-intact dimer) and apoSH (metal-free disulfide-reduced monomer). Misfolded SOD1 is defined in the present chapter as any conformation of SOD1 that has increased population in ALS, arising from mutation, covalent modification or deviation from normal maturation (e.g. under- or mis-metallation, lack of or aberrant intra- or inter-molecular disulfide bond, disrupted dimerization, partial unfolding of loops or strands). Aggregated refers to larger, insoluble, fibrillar or amorphous assemblies of SOD1.

SOD1 folding

A central aspect in understanding protein misfolding diseases is knowledge of the protein structural states that are relevant to pathology and their respective stabilities and mechanisms of formation. The populations of protein in different states are determined by their relative

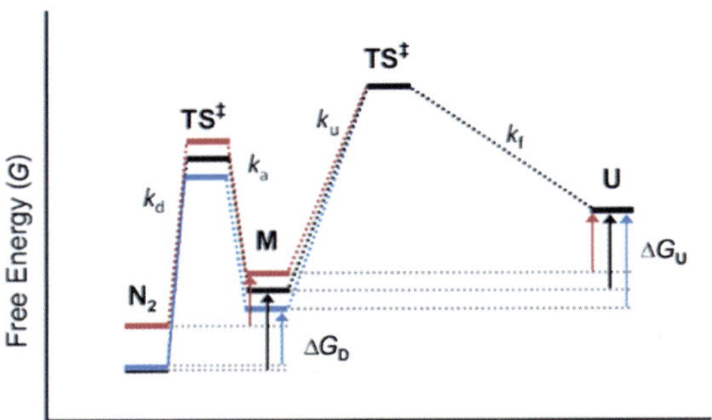

Figure 2. Thermodynamic and kinetic stability of SOD1
The equilibrium population of different thermodynamic states of a protein, and the rates of interconversion between these states, is illustrated using a Gibbs free energy diagram. The Gibbs free energy profile is shown for apoSS for conditions that favour folding, with energy levels for different states approximated based on experimental data [25]. Native dimer (N_2) is more stable (lower energy) than folded monomer (M), which is more stable than unfolded monomer (U). The change in free energy for dimer dissociation, ΔG_D ($=2G_M - G_{N2}$), and monomer unfolding, ΔG_U ($=G_M - G_U$), are indicated by arrows. The total free energy of unfolding is $\Delta G_{U,tot}$ ($=2\Delta G_U + \Delta G_D$). The free energy of the two transitions in the diagram, monomer folding and association, are scaled according to their different molecularities. The values of ΔG determine the population of each species at equilibrium: for the WT protein (black bars) at a total protein concentration of 10 μM dimer equivalents, the population of each state is 99.6% N_2, 0.4% M and 0.0001% U. Mutations and/or oxidative damage can change the relative stabilities of different states. For example, the fALS A4V mutation (red bars) in the dimer interface destabilizes both the dimer interface and the folded monomer (i.e. decreases both ΔG_D and ΔG_U), altering the equilibrium populations to 94.5% N_2, 5.4% M and 0.04% U at 10 μM dimer. On the other hand, the fALS H46R (blue bars) metal-binding site mutation destabilizes the dimer interface, but stabilizes the folded monomer (i.e. decreases ΔG_D and increases ΔG_U), resulting in 98.8% N_2, 1.2% M and 0.0002% U. The rates of interconversion between different species are determined by the rate constants for dimer dissociation (k_d), monomer association (k_a), monomer unfolding (k_u) and monomer folding (k_f). The magnitudes of the rate constants are determined by the heights of the transition state (TS) barriers from different ground states, and govern kinetic stability. For additional details, see reviews [7,26].

stabilities (Figure 2). Thermodynamic stability defines the populations of different states at equilibrium, whereas kinetic stability describes the rates of interconversion between states [12,13]. Thus thermodynamic and kinetic measurements provide complementary approaches for determining the conformations that a protein is likely to adopt. Decreased protein stability is associated with increased unfolding, either from the folded state to less folded states, or local unfolding or misfolding within the ensemble of conformers that comprise a given state. Different conformers can vary greatly in their propensity to form aggregates [14–16].

In general, protein folding can depend very strongly on solution conditions, such as protein concentration, denaturant concentration and temperature, and these can be varied in order to characterize different structural transitions [16–18] (Figure 3). Most proteins in Nature, including SOD1, consist of more than one polypeptide chain, and as a consequence, their folding inherently depends on protein concentration [18]. The denaturant- and temperature-induced unfolding of SOD1 have been fit to two- or three-state mechanisms (Figure 3). For monomeric apoSH, reversible unfolding fits a two-state transition between M (folded monomer) and U (unfolded monomer) ($M \leftrightarrow U$). At low protein concentrations, monomers are more highly populated and dimeric apoSS and holoSS exhibit three-state equilibrium transitions between N_2 (folded dimer), M and U ($N_2 \leftrightarrow 2M \leftrightarrow 2U$). Increasing protein concentrations decrease the proportion of M such that only a net two-state process ($N_2 \leftrightarrow 2U$) is observed at equilibrium, although interconversion among all three states may still be observed kinetically (Figure 4). In the following sections, we describe studies on different forms of the SOD1, which highlight the complex effects of mutations on structural transitions.

Metal-free disulfide-reduced SOD1 (apoSH)

In its most immature form, apoSH, WT (wild-type) SOD1 adopts a folded, but highly dynamic monomeric structure [19,20] (Figure 1B). This form of SOD1 has marginal stability, with ~95% of the protein being folded at physiological temperature and pH. Kinetic studies further show that disulfide reduction decreases stability by increasing the rate of unfolding [21]. Accordingly, the stability of apoSH is relatively low compared with other globular proteins [7], and far lower than more mature forms of SOD1 (Figure 3). In general, mutations have the largest effects on the stability of the apoSH form, ranging from slightly increasing to, more often, greatly decreasing its melting temperature to below physiological temperature (37°C). Thus mutations can markedly alter the populations of folded and unfolded conformations [20].

Metal-free disulfide-oxidized SOD1 (apoSS)

Disulfide bond formation stabilizes both the folded monomer and the dimer interface of SOD1, such that three-state folding can be analysed by equilibrium chemical [22] and in some cases thermal [17] denaturation, as well as by kinetics (Figures 3 and 4). In contrast with apoSH, WT and mutant apoSS are predominantly folded under physiological conditions [20,22]. Nevertheless, based on equilibrium denaturation and molecular dynamics simulations, the effects of mutations tend to propagate extensively through the protein structure and disrupt the dimer interface [22,23]. Kinetic experiments have shown that mutations can increase the rate of dissociation and/or monomer unfolding (Figure 4B) [24,25]. Thus, in apoSS, mutations generally have destabilizing effects, resulting in increased native-state structural fluctuations and small increases in the population of folded and unfolded monomers.

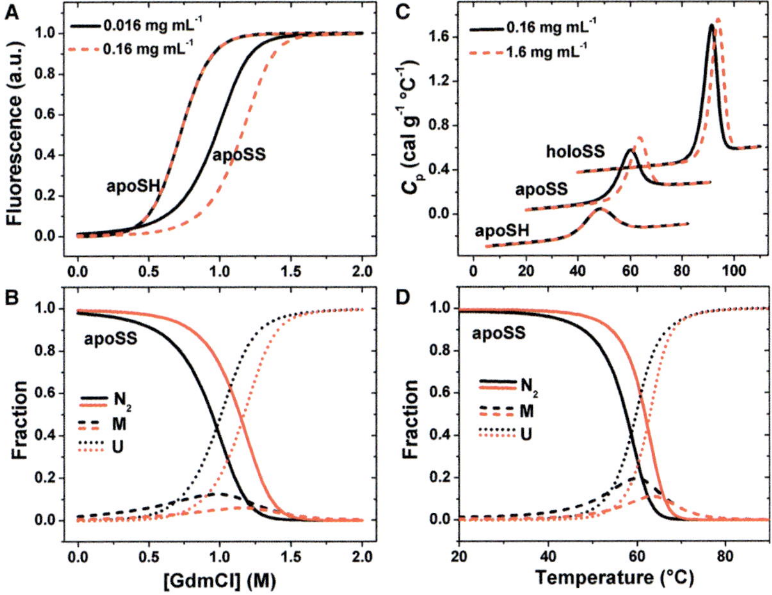

Figure 3. Equilibrium chemical and thermal denaturation measurements of monomeric apo (SH) and dimeric (SS) SOD1 stability

Chemical and thermal denaturation are common methods for measuring equilibrium stability of proteins [12]. The equilibrium is dependent on protein concentration for oligomeric proteins, including dimeric SOD1 (lower concentration is shown as black, higher is shown as red) [17,18]. (**A**) Chemical denaturation simulated based on experimental data for apoSH and apoSS [18,20]. Normalized fluorescence values are plotted: fluorescence is low when the protein is folded (low denaturant) and high when the protein is unfolded (high denaturant). Monomeric apoSH undergoes a protein concentration-independent two-state transition, $M \leftrightarrow U$. Dimeric apoSS undergoes a three-state transition, $N_2 \leftrightarrow 2M \leftrightarrow 2U$. Owing to mass action, increasing protein concentration shifts the equilibrium towards N_2, with the transition appearing more two-state due to lower population of M. Denaturation of holoSS has similar protein concentration dependence as apoSS, with additional complexities due to metal dissociation at low concentrations [27]. (**B**) The fractional populations of N_2 (solid lines), M (dashed lines) and U (dotted lines) corresponding to apoSS in panel (**A**). (**C**) DSC (differential scanning calorimetry) thermograms illustrating an endothermic peak in heat capacity upon protein unfolding with increasing temperatures. Traces are simulated based on experimental data [17,20,28] (H.R. Broom, J.A.O. Rumfeldt and E.M. Meiering, unpublished work) for apoSH, apoSS and holoSS, as described elsewhere [17]. Heat capacities are normalized per gram of protein and offset for clarity. As for chemical denaturation, monomeric apoSH undergoes a two-state transition ($M \leftrightarrow U$) that is independent of protein concentration. The holoSS dimer undergoes a two-state dimer transition ($N_2 \leftrightarrow 2U$) that shifts to higher temperatures with increasing protein concentration. The moderately stable apoSS dimer undergoes a three-state transition ($N_2 \leftrightarrow 2M \leftrightarrow 2U$). (**D**) The fractional population of N_2 (solid lines), M (dashed lines) and U (dotted lines) corresponding to apoSS in panel (**C**). Typically, DSC requires much higher protein concentrations than chemical denaturation, such that two-state behaviour is more commonly observed, whereas more complex transitions are characterized more readily using chemical denaturation.

Metal-bound disulfide-oxidized SOD1 (holoSS)

Metal binding strongly stabilizes SOD1 and reduces its dynamics. All mutations characterized to date decrease the stability of holoSS [7,26–28], but because the folded dimer is extremely stable, the absolute increases in the amounts of unfolded species (M and U) are extremely

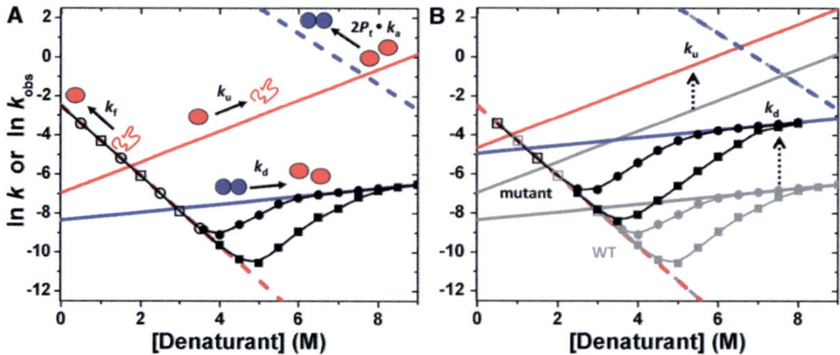

Figure 4. Folding and unfolding kinetics of dimeric apoSS SOD1

Folding and unfolding kinetics of monomeric proteins can often be analysed with a simple protein-concentration-independent two-state folding mechanism ($M \leftrightarrow U$) resulting in a classic V-shaped chevron plot [12]. For oligomeric proteins, additional steps involving subunit association are protein concentration-dependent, as occurs for dimeric apoSS SOD1. The k_{obs} for folding (open symbols) and unfolding (closed symbols) are a denaturant and protein concentration-dependent combination of the microscopic rate constants for different transitions. (**A**) Microscopic rate constants (k, coloured lines, symbols for transitions as in Figure 2) and observed rate constants (k_{obs}, black symbols and lines) for reversible three-state transitions between N_2, M and U (Figure 2), as a function of denaturant concentration. The rate constants are based on values measured for SOD1 [18,52]. Microscopic rate constants associated with unfolding (dimer dissociation k_d, blue; monomer unfolding k_u, red) are shown in solid lines, and those associated with folding are shown as dashed lines (monomer folding k_f, red; the apparent monomer association rate constant is $2P_t^* k_a$, the total protein concentration in monomer equivalents multiplied by the rate constant for dimer association, blue). In low [denaturant] where folding is favoured, k_{obs} coincides with k_f, which is the rate-determining step, whereas subsequent monomer association is fast and not observed. Similarly, at very high [denaturant] where unfolding is favoured, k_{obs} coincides with the rate-determining k_d since subsequent monomer unfolding is much faster and not observed. As [denaturant] decreases, k_u becomes lower, whereas k_a becomes faster and acts in opposition to k_u so that ln k_{obs} curves downwards; the contribution of k_a is increased with increasing protein concentration, illustrated for 300 µM dimer (squares) and 1 µM dimer (circles). The k_{obs} in this region is significantly affected by k_d, k_u, k_a and P_t, and does not coincide with any microscopic rate constant. (**B**) Kinetics for a hypothetical mutant SOD1 (coloured as in **A**) compared with WT (grey). The k_a and k_f for mutant are the same as for WT, k_d is 30-fold faster and k_u is 10-fold faster at all denaturant concentrations. The increase in these two rate constants is similar to the destabilizing effects of the A4V mutation (illustrated with the red bars in Figure 2), which decreases both ΔG_D and ΔG_U and results in an increased population of both M and U.

small, and hence are unlikely to directly affect aggregation. Rather, increased local structural fluctuations tend to promote metal loss and/or disruption of the dimer interface, and so expose regions that are normally buried [29]. Various covalent modifications have similar destabilizing effects (Figure 1). For example, oxidation of active site histidine residues destabilizes holoSS, promotes monomerization, increases exposure of hydrophobic residues and leads to metal loss [11]. Similarly, glutathionylation of free cysteine residues, a modification that may occur under oxidative stress, has been shown to destabilize the dimer interface of WT holoSS [30].

Metal binding also increases the kinetic stability of SOD1. WT holoSS unfolds extremely slowly via formation of a folded monomer which has weakened metal binding compared with the dimer [26]. Various mutations increase the unfolding rates of holoSS, and increase the accessibility of misfolded species, notably mis-metallated monomers. Collectively, these studies have revealed that mutations and covalent modifications provide multiple avenues to increase structural fluctuations and misfolding in the otherwise extremely stable holoSS.

Modes of aggregation

A key theme emerging from the above-described studies of SOD1 is that mutations have differing effects on the amounts of unfolded and misfolded species that may be populated in disease. This suggests that aggregation may arise from multiple and very different initial conformations. Enhanced aggregation has been reported for many species of SOD1, including mutant and/or modified protein, with formation of diverse structures, ranging from amorphous to various kinds of fibrils. Varying experimental conditions (e.g. temperature and agitation) strongly influence observed aggregation mechanisms and structures, which have different aberrant interactions, for example, between the edges of the β-barrel, exposed hydrophobic groups, improper loop interactions, domain swapping and disulfide-bonding residues. Collectively, experimental findings provide support for the possible contribution of many SOD1 species to aggregation in ALS, as outlined below.

Metal-free SOD1

In recent years, there has been extensive research on the aggregation of apoSH, as this unstable form of SOD1 has been proposed to be particularly likely to aggregate in disease [7,19,20]. *In vitro*, the extent and type of aggregation for apoSH varies greatly with experimental conditions (Figure 5). Thermal denaturation has been shown to be highly reversible for apoSH WT and some mutants, suggesting resistance to aggregation from partially or fully unfolded states, although other mutations show evidence of misfolding [20]. In contrast, other conditions strongly enhance aggregation of even WT apoSH. Agitation of both WT and mutant apoSH can cause formation of various amyloid-like fibres [19] (Figure 5). Mutations modulate the structural features of the fibres, resulting in distinct, or common, protease-resistant cores under different conditions [31,32]. Intriguingly, such structural polymorphisms may be analogous to different 'strains' observed in prion aggregation [4]. Furthermore, under agitation conditions, small amounts of apoSH can seed the aggregation of more stable forms of SOD1 [32,33]. It is well established that amyloid can form quite readily from highly unfolded sections of proteins. Also, agitation induces aggregation of many proteins through mechanisms that are not well understood, but may involve unfolding at air–water or water–solid interfaces and/or disulfide shuffling. Recent studies showed that various forms of metal-free SOD1 can make amyloid-like fibres with smooth unbranched morphologies under agitation conditions, and this occurs from the globally unfolded rather than the folded state [34]. In contrast, under quiescent solution conditions, WT apoSH shows little tendency to aggregate, and different apoSH mutants form different sizes of amorphous aggregates at different rates [20] (Figure 5). These varying results suggest that the mode(s) of apoSH aggregation are particularly diverse, and sensitive to varying conditions, due to the marginal stability, and hence, easily altered conformational properties, of apoSH.

Owing to the higher stability of apoSS compared with apoSH, more strongly destabilizing and/or disulfide oxidizing/shuffling conditions are generally required to induce its aggregation on an experimentally tractable time scale [35–38]. For apoSS, different destabilizing conditions result in multiple aggregate structures, ranging from amorphous to non-amyloid and amyloid

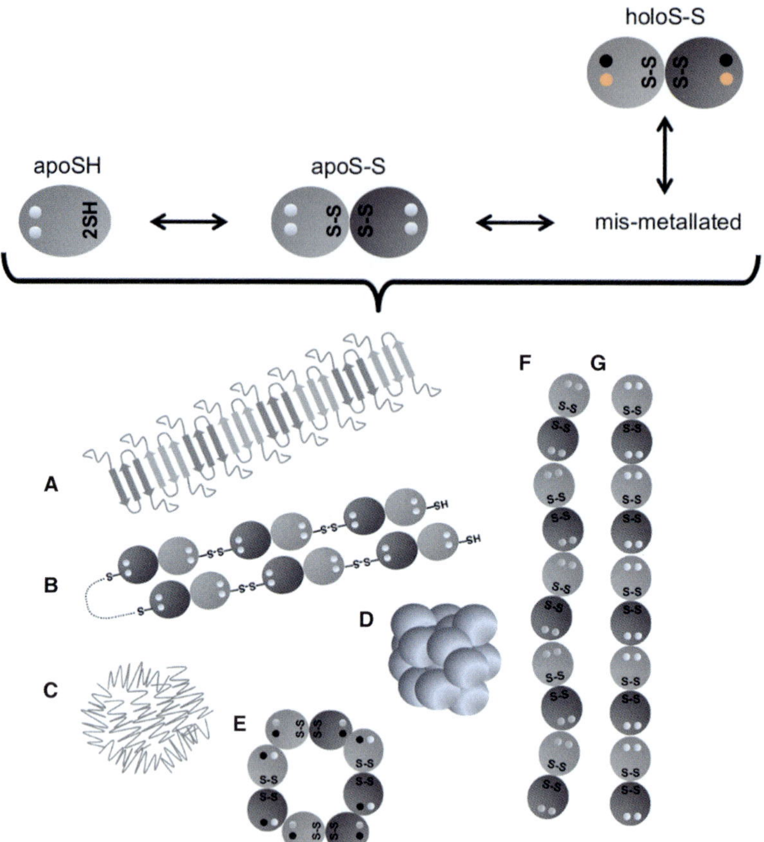

Figure 5. Diverse structures of SOD1 aggregates

Some of the many reported misfolded/aggregated structures of SOD1 are illustrated schematically (**A–J**). The type of structures observed can depend strongly on the conformation of various possible precursor SOD1 species. Soluble natively folded SOD1 is represented by spheres as in Figure 1. (**A**) SOD1 can form amyloid fibrils under certain conditions. Agitation of apoSH promotes formation of a nucleus containing intermolecular disulfide bonds involving Cys[57] and Cys[146], which can then recruit additional apoSH or more stable apo and part metallated SS forms of SOD1. The resulting fibres bind the fluorescent dye ThT (Thioflavin T) and exhibit twisted morphologies by AFM (atomic force microscopy) [33]. In addition, various destabilizing conditions result in formation of fibres with features of classic amyloid [34,36,39], as has often been observed for proteins aggregating from a globally unfolded state [34]. Such 'classic' fibrils have a protease-resistant cross-β-spine, cause large enhancements in ThT fluorescence, exhibit green–gold birefringence upon binding the dye Congo Red, and have fibril diameters of ~5–20 nm [34,39]. Other amyloid-like SOD1 aggregates exhibit polymorphisms due to a protease-resistant fibril core being formed by different segments of intact SOD1 [31]. (**B**) Intact dimers of apoSS linked via disulfide linkages, which requires the normally reduced Cys[6] and Cys[111] [35,53]. (**C** and **D**) Different amorphous aggregates formed by structured (**C**) or unstructured (**D**) protein [11,20,29]. (**E**) Amyloid pores formed by Zn-bound SS SOD1 dimers. The Zn-binding loop of one dimer interacts with the β-barrel of another dimer at an angle. The Zn-binding loop forms an additional β-strand, giving rise to an extended β-sheet that spirals around the long axis [40]. (**F** and **G**) Amyloid-like fibrils formed as a result of non-native interactions between apoSS dimers [40]. Exposure of the edge of the β-barrel in apoSS due to disorder in the Zn-binding and electrostatic loops results in a zig-zag packing of dimers when the edge is partially exposed (**F**) or linear packing when the edge is fully exposed (**G**).

fibrils, in varying proportions [37,39]. Destabilization of apoSS can also cause misfolding involving disulfide shuffling between the normally reduced free cysteine residues (Cys^6 and Cys^{111}) and those normally forming the disulfide bond (Cys^{57} and Cys^{146}) [38] (Figure 1). Furthermore, under non-destabilizing oxidizing conditions, aberrant disulfide bonding involving the free cysteine residues is required for the formation of amyloid-like fibrils [35] (Figure 5B). The roles of aberrant disulfide bonding for misfolding and aggregation are complex and not fully clear in both *in vitro* and *in vivo* studies; in disease models, early roles are uncertain, but they are likely to be significant as disease progresses due to increasingly oxidizing cellular conditions [10]. Alternatively, apoSS can form other amyloid-like fibres, without aberrant disulfide bonds. These fibres are composed of native-like dimers undergoing local unfolding, forming non-native intermolecular interactions involving the Zn binding and electrostatic loops and exposed β-barrel edge strands [40,41] (Figure 5F and 5G). Thus aggregation of apoSS may proceed from various locally or globally unfolded conformations, with or without aberrant disulfide linkages.

Metallated SOD1

The very stable holoSS form of SOD1 is generally thought to be highly resistant to aggregation [11,33,37,42]. Nevertheless, agitation of holoSS, in combination with strongly destabilizing solution conditions results in fibril formation [33,36], and prolonged quiescent incubation of both WT and mutant holoSS under physiological temperature and pH eventually results in formation of amorphous aggregates [29]. Lag phases are characteristic of unfavourable nucleation–rapid elongation aggregation mechanisms, and have been observed for many disease-linked amyloid-forming proteins (Figure 6). Similar to these proteins, for SOD1 various mutations may decrease the length of the lag phase, possibly due to enhanced metal loss and/or dimer dissociation [29,43]. In cells, this may, in turn, promote disulfide reduction [44]. Increased population of various misfolded forms of SOD1 due to these changes could also contribute to aggregation in ALS. Of note, loss of all bound metals is not required for amorphous aggregation [29], and crystallographic studies found that part-metallated SS SOD1 can form helical fibrils via non-native loop and β-barrel interactions [40] (Figure 5E). In addition, the oxidation of various residues has been implicated in misfolding/aggregation. For example, oxidation of active site histidine residues promotes amorphous aggregation of metallated SS SOD1 [11]. Thus mutation and/or other covalent changes to holoSS can also give rise to misfolded aggregation-prone species. Taken together, the above-described findings provide evidence for multiple possible aggregation processes, which may play various roles in disease, that are considered further below.

Targets and toxic effects of aggregates

There is extensive evidence that misfolded/aggregated SOD1 may have altered interactions with many cellular components. Such components include the specific copper chaperone for SOD1 [45], other protein folding chaperones such as Hsp70 [46], proteasomal machinery, axonal transport components [1], membranes, e.g. mitochondrial [47,48] and endoplasmic reticulum, and RNA (disrupting expression, e.g. of neurofilament proteins which also form fibrillar aggregates in ALS [1,2]). Many of these cellular components have likewise been implicated as targets for other misfolded proteins associated with disease [4]. Cells have very extensive and

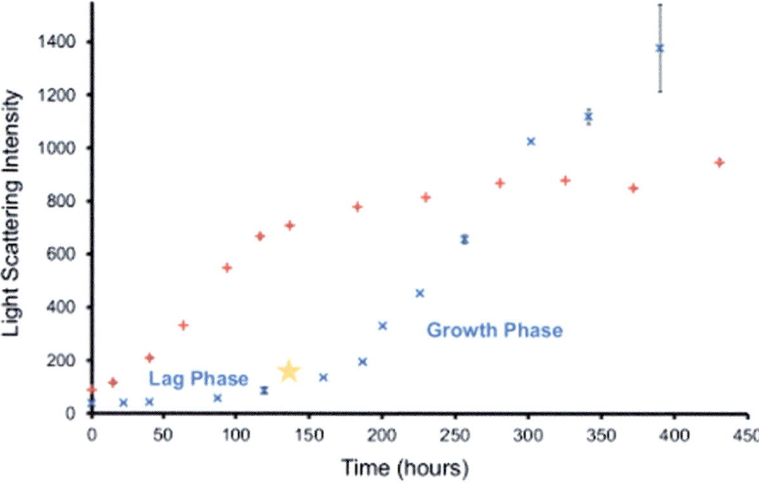

Figure 6. Different mechanisms of aggregation monitored by light scattering
Light scattering increases with the concentration and size of different species in solution, and so can be used to characterize differences in aggregation mechanisms. Illustrative data are for aggregation of apoSH under quiescent conditions [20]. Aggregation with no lag time (red +), suggests that the protein is initially in an aggregation-ready conformation, as observed for apoSH A4V SOD1. Alternatively, aggregation may proceed only after a lag time, which occurs due to an unfavourable nucleation event (yellow star), and is followed by rapid aggregate growth (blue ×), as observed for apoSH H43R SOD1. Nucleation may involve a protein conformational change and/or intermolecular association. Adding pre-aggregated 'seeds' can abolish the lag time by providing sites for aggregate growth through recruitment of soluble protein. Nucleation-dependent aggregation is very commonly observed for misfolded proteins associated with disease. Different time courses and sizes of aggregates formed by mutant apo SOD1s suggests they may have varying modes of aggregation [20].

sophisticated mechanisms for eliminating misfolded proteins, presumably owing to the toxicity of misfolded protein. The failure of these mechanisms in misfolding diseases, often described as a loss of proteostasis, results in impairment of critical cellular processes, with accelerating and increasing pathological consequences as disease progresses. Mutations in different proteins may impair specific different targets early in disease, but then converge to common pathology, ultimately resulting in the formation of large protein aggregates and cell death.

A key question in ALS is, what is the role of SOD1 at different stages of disease? Generally, smaller misfolded protein species appear to be particularly cytotoxic, and may be pathogenic. Large aggregates become prominent after the onset of disease symptoms, and may be a source of smaller species while also having their own distinct toxic effects, for example in causing inflammation [1,6]. In addition, loss of functional SOD1 due to misfolding/aggregation may contribute to the observed increased oxidative stress and cellular damage as disease progresses. Thus, both gain and loss of SOD1 function may be important in ALS [1], as has also been suggested for serpinopathies [35].

Beyond the above-described intracellular effects, there is striking new evidence that cell-to-cell propagation of SOD1 aggregates, and the recruitment by these aggregates of soluble SOD1 occur in a cell culture model [49]. This propagation or seeding behaviour is 'prion-like', and increasing evidence suggests it may also occur in other neurodegenerative diseases, e.g. for Aβ (amyloid β-peptide) and tau in Alzheimer's disease, and α-synuclein in Parkinson's disease

[1,5]. These findings are of tremendous significance for understanding disease progression. It should be noted, however, that infectivity of protein aggregates has only been demonstrated for prion diseases, and the disease relevance of such 'transmissible proteins' has yet to be demonstrated in other diseases [5].

Antibody studies

Recently, important progress has been made in characterizing the structures and targets of misfolded SOD1 using antibodies; these specifically recognize many different, including conformation-specific, epitopes in SOD1 [1,3,9,48], and have shown protective effects in mouse ALS models [50]. Interestingly, some studies have reported antibody evidence for misfolded SOD1 in both sALS and fALS, implicating misfolded WT SOD1 in disease pathology [9,48]. Others, however, observed binding only in mutant SOD1-linked fALS [3]. The different results may be caused by the presence of different conformations of SOD1 in different cases, and/or methodological differences. Intriguingly, antibodies have provided evidence for distinct mutant SOD1 conformers bound to mitochondrial membranes, providing clues to unravelling differences in disease progression [47]. Antibody experiments on serpins have shown that aggregates formed in model systems are often, and unexpectedly, different from those in patients [6]. Thus antibody studies may be critical for determining the roles in disease of different misfolded/aggregated species.

Future prospects

The findings described above represent major progress in characterizing the molecular mechanisms of pathology in ALS. They have also opened important avenues for future research, including development of new therapies. Key outstanding, and experimentally accessible, questions to address include: (i) what is the role of WT SOD1, and its many possible covalent modifications, in fALS and in sALS; (ii) how are different forms of SOD1 (apoSH, apoSS, holoSS, mismetallated, monomer, dimer and covalently modified) and mechanisms of aggregation involved in early- and late-stage misfolding and aggregation; (iii) how and why do pathologies differ for mutant SOD1s, and can differences in mutant aggregated structures be considered as prion-like conformational strains; (iv) can disease features in ALS be further classified as common or subtypes; (v) what is the molecular basis for cellular transmission of aggregated SOD1; and (vi) can misfolding be effectively targeted for disease diagnosis and treatment?

The advances in understanding disease mechanisms have provided new avenues for developing therapies. One approach may be the rational design of small molecules to stabilize the folded state(s) of SOD1. This approach has proved successful recently for inhibiting native tetramer dissociation and subsequent monomer misfolding of transthyretin in the amyloidosis familial amyloid polyneuropathy [51]. Another approach may be development of small molecules or peptides to specifically interfere with the formation of toxic SOD1 conformations [6]. Also, vaccination or antibodies against SOD1 may be developed further for ALS diagnosis, prevention or treatment. More generally, the common cellular pathways that are disrupted in different neurodegenerative diseases and overlapping symptoms suggest that common treatments may ultimately be possible [4]. Although there is much work still to be done in order to achieve these goals, the prospects for further advances are promising.

Summary

- ALS is a heterogeneous motor neuron disorder in which misfolded and/or aggregated proteins such as SOD1 may impair a range of cellular components at different stages of disease, giving rise to a complex cascade of pathological effects that ultimately result in motor neuron death.

- SOD1 mutations have complex, usually destabilizing, effects that promote local or global unfolding or misfolding to varying extents for different forms of SOD1. Mutations tend mainly to increase local unfolding for more mature and stable forms (holoSS and apoSS), but, in addition, can markedly increase the population of globally unfolded protein in the most immature and least stable form (apoSH).

- Different forms of SOD1 have varying propensities to form a wide range of misfolded/aggregated structures, which are promoted to varying degrees by mutation, covalent modification and solution conditions. Multiple misfolded and aggregated structures of SOD1 have been observed and may modulate disease characteristics.

- The development of antibodies to detect different structural features of SOD1 provide a powerful tool for assessing the conformation of misfolded/aggregated SOD1 *in vitro* and *in vivo*, and so provide a means for unravelling biological effects of different misfolded/aggregated SOD1 structures.

- Knowledge of the molecular mechanisms of SOD1 folding, misfolding and aggregation have opened new avenues for developing therapeutic strategies to combat ALS and related neurodegenerative and other common protein misfolding diseases.

This chapter is dedicated to the late James R. Lepock, for convincing us to tackle this fascinating and complex protein, and for his great inspiration and wisdom. We apologize that many important references have been omitted, which is due to limitations on the number of citations. Work discussed in the present chapter was supported by grants from the Canadian Institutes of Health Research and the Natural Sciences and Engineering Research Council.

References

1. Robberecht, W. and Philips, T. (2013) The changing scene of amyotrophic lateral sclerosis. Nat. Rev. Neurosci. **14**, 248–264
2. Keller, B.A., Volkening, K., Droppelmann, C.A., Ang, L.C., Rademakers, R. and Strong, M.J. (2012) Co-aggregation of RNA binding proteins in ALS spinal motor neurons: evidence of a common pathogenic mechanism. Acta Neuropathol. **124**, 733–747
3. Kerman, A., Liu, H.N., Croul, S., Bilbao, J., Rogaeva, E., Zinman, L., Robertson, J. and Chakrabartty, A. (2010) Amyotrophic lateral sclerosis is a non-amyloid disease in which extensive misfolding of SOD1 is unique to the familial form, Acta Neuropathol. **119**, 335–344

4.   Eisenberg, D. and Jucker, M. (2012) The amyloid state of proteins in human diseases. Cell **148**, 1188–1203

5.   Soto, C. (2012) Transmissible proteins: expanding the prion heresy. Cell **149**, 968–977

6.   Lomas, D.A. (2013) Twenty years of polymers: a personal perspective on alpha-1 antitrypsin deficiency. COPD **10**, 17–25

7.   Broom, H.R., Primmer, H.A., Rumfeldt, J.A.O., Stathopulos, P.B., Vassall, K.A., Hwang, Y.M. and Meiering, E.M. (2012) Folding and aggregation of Cu, Zn-superoxide dismutase. In Amyotrophic Lateral Sclerosis (Maurer, M.H., ed.), doi:10.5772/31629, InTech, Rijeka

8.   Valentine, J.S., Doucette, P.A. and Zittin Potter, S. (2005) Copper-zinc superoxide dismutase and amyotrophic lateral sclerosis. Annu. Rev. Biochem. **74**, 563–593

9.   Bosco, D.A., Morfini, G., Karabacak, N.M., Song, Y., Gros-Louis, F., Pasinelli, P., Goolsby, H., Fontaine, B.A., Lemay, N., McKenna-Yasek, D. et al. (2010) Wild-type and mutant SOD1 share an aberrant conformation and a common pathogenic pathway in ALS. Nat. Neurosci. **13**, 1396–1403

10. Karch, C.M., Prudencio, M., Winkler, D.D., Hart, P.J. and Borchelt, D.R. (2009) Role of mutant SOD1 disulfide oxidation and aggregation in the pathogenesis of familial ALS, Proc. Natl. Acad. Sci. U.S.A. **106**, 7774–7779

11. Mulligan, V.K., Kerman, A., Laister, R.C., Sharda, P.R., Arslan, P.E. and Chakrabartty, A. (2012) Early steps in oxidation-induced SOD1 misfolding: implications for non-amyloid protein aggregation in familial ALS. J. Mol. Biol. **421**, 631–652

12. Fersht, A. (1999) Structure and Mechanism in Protein Science: a Guide to Enzyme Catalysis and Protein Folding, W.H. Freeman and Company, New York

13. Jackson, S.E. (1998) How do small single-domain proteins fold? Fold Des. **3**, R81–R91

14. Chiti, F. and Dobson, C.M. (2009) Amyloid formation by globular proteins under native conditions. Nat. Chem. Biol. **5**, 15–22

15. Jahn, T.R. and Radford, S.E. (2005) The Yin and Yang of protein folding. FEBS J. **272**, 5962–5970

16. Wang, W., Nema, S. and Teagarden, D. (2010) Protein aggregation: pathways and influencing factors. Int. J. Pharm. **390**, 89–99

17. Doyle, C.M., Rumfeldt, J.A., Broom, H.R., Broom, A., Stathopulos, P.B., Vassall, K.A., Almey, J.J. and Meiering, E.M. (2013) Energetics of oligomeric protein folding and association. Arch. Biochem. Biophys. **531**, 44–64

18. Rumfeldt, J.A., Galvagnion, C., Vassall, K.A. and Meiering, E.M. (2008) Conformational stability and folding mechanisms of dimeric proteins. Prog. Biophys. Mol. Biol. **98**, 61–84

19. Furukawa, Y. and O'Halloran, T.V. (2005) Amyotrophic lateral sclerosis mutations have the greatest destabilizing effect on the apo- and reduced form of SOD1, leading to unfolding and oxidative aggregation. J. Biol. Chem. **280**, 17266–17274

20. Vassall, K.A., Stubbs, H.R., Primmer, H.A., Tong, M.S., Sullivan, S.M., Sobering, R., Srinivasan, S., Briere, L.A., Dunn, S.D., Colon, W. and Meiering, E.M. (2011) Decreased stability and increased formation of soluble aggregates by immature superoxide dismutase do not account for disease severity in ALS. Proc. Natl. Acad. Sci. U.S.A. **108**, 2210–2215

21. Lindberg, M.J., Normark, J., Holmgren, A. and Oliveberg, M. (2004) Folding of human superoxide dismutase: disulfide reduction prevents dimerization and produces marginally stable monomers. Proc. Natl. Acad. Sci. U.S.A. **101**, 15893–15898

22. Vassall, K.A., Stathopulos, P.B., Rumfeldt, J.A., Lepock, J.R. and Meiering, E.M. (2006) Equilibrium thermodynamic analysis of amyotrophic lateral sclerosis-associated mutant apo Cu,Zn superoxide dismutases. Biochemistry **45**, 7366–7379

23. Khare, S.D. and Dokholyan, N.V. (2006) Common dynamical signatures of familial amyotrophic lateral sclerosis-associated structurally diverse Cu, Zn superoxide dismutase mutants. Proc. Natl. Acad. Sci. U.S.A. **103**, 3147–3152

24. Lindberg, M.J., Bystrom, R., Boknas, N., Andersen, P.M. and Oliveberg, M. (2005) Systematically perturbed folding patterns of amyotrophic lateral sclerosis (ALS)-associated SOD1 mutants. Proc. Natl. Acad. Sci. U.S.A. **102**, 9754–9759

25. Svensson, A.K., Bilsel, O., Kayatekin, C., Adefusika, J.A., Zitzewitz, J.A. and Matthews, C.R. (2010) Metal-free ALS variants of dimeric human Cu,Zn-superoxide dismutase have enhanced populations of monomeric species. PLoS ONE **5**, e10064

26. Rumfeldt, J.A., Lepock, J.R. and Meiering, E.M. (2009) Unfolding and folding kinetics of amyotrophic lateral sclerosis-associated mutant Cu,Zn superoxide dismutases. J. Mol. Biol. **385**, 278–298

27. Rumfeldt, J.A., Stathopulos, P.B., Chakrabarrty, A., Lepock, J.R. and Meiering, E.M. (2006) Mechanism and thermodynamics of guanidinium chloride-induced denaturation of ALS-associated mutant Cu,Zn superoxide dismutases. J. Mol. Biol. **355**, 106–123

28. Stathopulos, P.B., Rumfeldt, J.A., Karbassi, F., Siddall, C.A., Lepock, J.R. and Meiering, E.M. (2006) Calorimetric analysis of thermodynamic stability and aggregation for apo and holo amyotrophic lateral sclerosis-associated Gly-93 mutants of superoxide dismutase. J. Biol. Chem. **281**, 6184–6193

29. Hwang, Y.M., Stathopulos, P.B., Dimmick, K., Yang, H., Badiei, H.R., Tong, M.S., Rumfeldt, J.A., Chen, P., Karanassios, V. and Meiering, E.M. (2010) Nonamyloid aggregates arising from mature copper/zinc superoxide dismutases resemble those observed in amyotrophic lateral sclerosis. J. Biol. Chem. **285**, 41701–41711

30. Redler, R.L., Wilcox, K.C., Proctor, E.A., Fee, L., Caplow, M. and Dokholyan, N.V. (2011) Glutathionylation at Cys-111 induces dissociation of wild type and fALS mutant SOD1 dimers. Biochemistry **50**, 7057–7066

31. Furukawa, Y., Kaneko, K., Yamanaka, K. and Nukina, N. (2010) Mutation-dependent polymorphism of Cu,Zn-superoxide dismutase aggregates in the familial form of amyotrophic lateral sclerosis. J. Biol. Chem. **285**, 22221–22231

32. Chan, P.K., Chattopadhyay, M., Sharma, S., Souda, P., Gralla, E.B., Borchelt, D.R., Whitelegge, J.P. and Valentine, J.S. (2013) Structural similarity of wild-type and ALS-mutant superoxide dismutase-1 fibrils using limited proteolysis and atomic force microscopy. Proc. Natl. Acad. Sci. U.S.A. **110**, 10934–10939

33. Chattopadhyay, M., Durazo, A., Sohn, S.H., Strong, C.D., Gralla, E.B., Whitelegge, J.P. and Valentine, J.S. (2008) Initiation and elongation in fibrillation of ALS-linked superoxide dismutase. Proc. Natl. Acad. Sci. U.S.A. **105**, 18663–18668

34. Lang, L., Kurnik, M., Danielsson, J. and Oliveberg, M. (2012) Fibrillation precursor of superoxide dismutase 1 revealed by gradual tuning of the protein-folding equilibrium. Proc. Natl. Acad. Sci. U.S.A. **109**, 17868–17873

35. Banci, L., Bertini, I., Boca, M., Girotto, S., Martinelli, M., Valentine, J.S. and Vieru, M. (2008) SOD1 and amyotrophic lateral sclerosis: mutations and oligomerization. PLoS ONE **3**, e1677

36. Oztug Durer, Z.A., Cohlberg, J.A., Dinh, P., Padua, S., Ehrenclou, K., Downes, S., Tan, J.K., Nakano, Y., Bowman, C.J., Hoskins et al. (2009) Loss of metal ions, disulfide reduction and mutations related to familial ALS promote formation of amyloid-like aggregates from superoxide dismutase. PLoS ONE **4**, e5004

37. Stathopulos, P.B., Rumfeldt, J.A., Scholz, G.A., Irani, R.A., Frey, H.E., Hallewell, R.A., Lepock, J.R. and Meiering, E.M. (2003) Cu/Zn superoxide dismutase mutants associated with amyotrophic lateral sclerosis show enhanced formation of aggregates *in vitro*. Proc. Natl. Acad. Sci. U.S.A. **100**, 7021–7026

38. Toichi, K., Yamanaka, K. and Furukawa, Y. (2013) Disulfide scrambling describes the oligomer formation of superoxide dismutase (SOD1) proteins in the familial form of amyotrophic lateral sclerosis. J. Biol. Chem. **288**, 4970–4980

39. Stathopulos, P.B., Scholz, G.A., Hwang, Y.M., Rumfeldt, J.A., Lepock, J.R. and Meiering, E.M. (2004) Sonication of proteins causes formation of aggregates that resemble amyloid. Protein Sci. **13**, 3017–3027

40. Elam, J.S., Taylor, A.B., Strange, R., Antonyuk, S., Doucette, P.A., Rodriguez, J.A., Hasnain, S.S., Hayward, L.J., Valentine, J.S., Yeates, T.O. and Hart, P.J. (2003) Amyloid-like filaments and water-filled nanotubes formed by SOD1 mutant proteins linked to familial ALS. Nat. Struct. Biol. **10**, 461–467

41. Strange, R.W., Yong, C.W., Smith, W. and Hasnain, S.S. (2007) Molecular dynamics using atomic-resolution structure reveal structural fluctuations that may lead to polymerization of human Cu-Zn superoxide dismutase. Proc. Natl. Acad. Sci. U.S.A. **104**, 10040–10044

42. Rousseau, F., Schymkowitz, J. and Oliveberg, M. (2008) ALS precursor finally shaken into fibrils. Proc. Natl. Acad. Sci. U.S.A. **105**, 18649–18650

43. Khare, S.D., Caplow, M. and Dokholyan, N.V. (2004) The rate and equilibrium constants for a multistep reaction sequence for the aggregation of superoxide dismutase in amyotrophic lateral sclerosis. Proc. Natl. Acad. Sci. U.S.A. **101**, 15094–15099

44. Tiwari, A. and Hayward, L.J. (2003) Familial amyotrophic lateral sclerosis mutants of copper/zinc superoxide dismutase are susceptible to disulfide reduction. J. Biol. Chem. **278**, 5984–5992

45. Seetharaman, S.V., Prudencio, M., Karch, C., Holloway, S.P., Borchelt, D.R. and Hart, P.J. (2009) Immature copper-zinc superoxide dismutase and familial amyotrophic lateral sclerosis. Exp Biol Med (Maywood) **234**, 1140–1154

46. Taylor, D.M., Tradewell, M.L., Minotti, S. and Durham, H.D. (2007) Characterizing the role of Hsp90 in production of heat shock proteins in motor neurons reveals a suppressive effect of wild-type Hsf1. Cell Stress Chaperones **12**, 151–162

47. Pickles, S., Destroismaisons, L., Peyrard, S.L., Cadot, S., Rouleau, G.A., Brown, Jr, R.H., Julien, J.P., Arbour, N. and Vande Velde, C. (2013) Mitochondrial damage revealed by immunoselection for ALS-linked misfolded SOD1. Hum. Mol. Genet. **22**, 3947–3959

48. Pickles, S. and Vande Velde, C. (2013) Misfolded SOD1 and ALS: zeroing in on mitochondria. Amyotroph Lateral Scler. **13**, 333–340

49. Munch, C., O'Brien, J. and Bertolotti, A. (2011) Prion-like propagation of mutant superoxide dismutase-1 misfolding in neuronal cells. Proc. Natl. Acad. Sci. U.S.A. **108**, 3548–3553

50. Urushitani, M., Ezzi, S.A. and Julien, J.P. (2007) Therapeutic effects of immunization with mutant superoxide dismutase in mice models of amyotrophic lateral sclerosis. Proc. Natl. Acad. Sci. U.S.A. **104**, 2495–2500

51. Johnson, S.M., Connelly, S., Fearns, C., Powers, E.T. and Kelly, J.W. (2012) The transthyretin amyloidoses: from delineating the molecular mechanism of aggregation linked to pathology to a regulatory-agency-approved drug. J. Mol. Biol. **421**, 185–203

52. Svensson, A.K., Bilsel, O., Kondrashkina, E., Zitzewitz, J.A. and Matthews, C.R. (2006) Mapping the folding free energy surface for metal-free human Cu,Zn superoxide dismutase. J. Mol. Biol. **364**, 1084–1102

53. Banci, L., Bertini, I., Durazo, A., Girotto, S., Gralla, E.B., Martinelli, M., Valentine, J.S., Vieru, M. and Whitelegge, J.P. (2007) Metal-free superoxide dismutase forms soluble oligomers under physiological conditions: a possible general mechanism for familial ALS. Proc. Natl. Acad. Sci. U.S.A. **104**, 11263–11267

© The Authors Journal compilation © 2014 Biochemical Society
Essays Biochem. (2014) 56, 167–180: doi: 10.1042/BSE0560167

12

Spontaneous self-assembly of pathogenic huntingtin exon 1 protein into amyloid structures

Philipp Trepte, Nadine Strempel and Erich E. Wanker[1]

Neuroproteomics, Max Delbrueck Center for Molecular Medicine, Robert-Roessle-Str. 10, 13125 Berlin, Germany

Abstract

PolyQ (polyglutamine) diseases such as HD (Huntington's disease) or SCA1 (spinocerebellar ataxia type 1) are neurodegenerative disorders caused by abnormally elongated polyQ tracts in human proteins. PolyQ expansions promote misfolding and aggregation of disease-causing proteins, leading to the appearance of nuclear and cytoplasmic inclusion bodies in patient neurons. Several lines of experimental evidence indicate that this process is critical for disease pathogenesis. However, the molecular mechanisms underlying spontaneous polyQ-containing aggregate formation and the perturbation of neuronal processes are still largely unclear. The present chapter reviews the current literature regarding misfolding and aggregation of polyQ-containing disease proteins. We specifically focus on studies that have investigated the amyloidogenesis of polyQ-containing HTTex1 (huntingtin exon 1) fragments. These protein fragments are disease-relevant and play a critical role in HD pathogenesis. We outline potential mechanisms behind mutant HTTex1 aggregation and toxicity, as well as proteins and small molecules that can modify HTTex1 amyloidogenesis *in vitro* and *in vivo*. The potential implications of such studies for the development of novel therapeutic strategies are discussed.

Keywords:

chaperone, (–)-epigallocatechin gallate (EGCG), Huntington's disease, inclusion body, nucleation-dependent polymerization, polyglutamine disease, protein aggregation.

[1]*To whom correspondence should be addressed (email ewanker@mdc-berlin.de).*

Introduction

PolyQ (polyglutamine) tracts with lengths of between five and 30 glutamine residues are conserved and found in 0.34% of all human proteins, indicating that they play an important functional role [1]. This view is supported by systematic computational and experimental investigations of polyQ-containing proteins, which suggest that polyQ domains mediate protein–protein interactions [1]. For example, polyQ sequences in transcription factors can influence gene expression in yeast and mammalian cells by promoting the formation of regulatory protein complexes that facilitate transcriptional activation [2–4]. Thus polyQ sequences form functionally relevant protein domains that play a critical role in the assembly and disassembly of protein complexes.

However, substantial experimental evidence demonstrates that abnormally expanded polyQ tracts in proteins are toxic for cells and can cause severe inherited human diseases [4]. Such polyQ expansions are the result of rare genetic mutations, which were identified in patient families through positional cloning approaches [5]. The neurodegenerative disease HD (Huntington's disease) is caused by a CAG trinucleotide expansion in the *HTT* gene, which leads to the synthesis of an elongated polyQ tract within the corresponding HTT (huntingtin) protein [6]. Wild-type non-pathogenic HTT contains six to 35 glutamine residues, whereas the mutant pathogenic protein in patients harbours more than 40 glutamine residues [6]. The polyQ tract in HTT is located at the N-terminus, followed by a proline-rich region and three conserved HEAT repeats, which have a typical α-helical solenoid structure [7]. Both the proline-rich and the HEAT repeat regions in HTT are critical for the assembly of protein complexes in neuronal cells [7,8]. HTT is a large protein with a predicted molecular mass of approximately 350 kDa. Currently, its normal function in cells is not fully understood. However, studies in cell models and transgenic animals indicate that wild-type HTT plays a functional role in vesicle transport processes, cell signalling and transcriptional gene regulation, suggesting that it is a multifunctional scaffold protein that influences various cellular processes [9].

HD is the most frequent form of the hereditary choreas. It has a multifaceted phenotype, including cognitive, psychiatric and motor impairments [6]. Symptoms of HD commonly become noticeable between the ages of 35 and 50 years; however, they can begin at any age from childhood to old age. HD affects the whole brain, but certain areas such as the caudate nucleus and the putamen are most vulnerable. In these areas predominantly striatal medium spiny neurons are degraded, which play a key role in the control of movement and behaviour [10].

To date, ten inherited polyQ expansion diseases have been reported, as summarized in Table 1. Although cellular dysfunction and toxicity are predominantly observed in neurons of the central nervous system (Table 1), the disease-causing proteins are ubiquitously expressed in all human tissues. Differentiated post-mitotic neurons seem significantly more vulnerable to proteins with pathogenic polyQ tracts than fast-dividing mitotic cells. The molecular basis for the selective degeneration of neuronal cells in polyQ diseases, however, is still unclear [11].

Neurodegenerative polyQ expansion diseases are characterized by the accumulation of insoluble protein aggregates in neuronal cells (Table 1). These aggregates, which are often concentrated in large IBs (inclusion bodies), are observed in brain regions that display massive neurodegeneration, suggesting that the process of polyQ-mediated protein misfolding and aggregation drives pathogenesis [10]. This hypothesis is supported by investigations in transgenic mouse, fly and worm models, which indicate that toxicity in neuronal cells correlates

Table 1. Overview of the ten known polyQ diseases

CACNA1A, voltage-dependent P/Q-type calcium channel subunit α-1A; DRPLA, dentatorubropallidoluysian atrophy; MJD, Machado–Joseph disease; PPP2R2B, serine/threonine-protein phosphatase 2A 55 kDa regulatory subunit B β isoform; SBMA, spinal and bulbar muscular atrophy; SCA, spinocerebellar ataxia. Reprinted from [4]; Biochim. Biophys. Acta, **1779**, Hands, S., Sinadinos, C. and Wyttenbach, A., Polyglutamine gene function and dysfunction in the ageing brain, 507–521., Copyright (2008), with permission from Elsevier.

Disease	Protein	Pathological repeat length	Affected brain region
DRPLA	Atropin-1	49–88	Cerebral cortex
HD	HTT	40–121	Striatum and cortex
SBMA	Androgen receptor	38–62	Motor neurons, brain stem and spinal cord
SCA1	Ataxin-1	39–82	Cerebellum
SCA2	Ataxin-2	32–200	Cerebellar Purkinje cells
MJD	Ataxin-3	61–84	Ventral pons and substantia nigra
SCA6	CACNA1A	10–33	Cerebellar Purkinje cells
SCA7	Ataxin-7	37–306	Cerebellar Purkinje cells, brain stem and spinal cord
SCA12	PPP2R2B	66–78	Cerebral and cerebellar cortex
SCA17	TATA-binding protein	47–63	Cerebellar Purkinje cells

with the formation of polyQ-containing protein aggregates [12]. Moreover, *in vitro* studies with polyQ disease proteins have demonstrated that both spontaneous protein aggregation and toxicity are dependent on polyQ length. Proteins with short non-pathogenic polyQ tracts remain soluble, whereas proteins with long pathogenic polyQ tracts self-assemble into insoluble fibrillar protein aggregates or amyloids [13,14]. Hence the formation of amyloidogenic protein aggregates is likely to be an important pathobiological process.

In the present chapter, we will mainly review protein aggregation studies that focus on polyQ-containing disease-relevant N-terminal HTTex1 (HTT exon 1) fragments. Such protein fragments are generated in HD patients through the aberrant splicing of *HTT* mRNA [15]. HTTex1 rapidly self-assembles into protein aggregates in cell-free, as well as cell-based, assays and induces toxicity in various *in vivo* disease model systems [12,13]. A better understanding of the mechanism of HTTex1 aggregation and its impact on biological systems is critical for a better understanding of pathogenesis in HD and other polyQ disorders.

Pathogenic polyQ-containing protein aggregates in patients and disease models

The deposition of N-terminal HTT protein fragments with expanded polyQ sequences in neuronal IBs is one pathological characteristic of HD brains [10,12]. IBs, which generally have a diameter of 1–5 μm, are predominantly detected in cortical and striatal neurons [14,16].

Immunohistological studies revealed that IBs are exclusively detected with anti-HTT antibodies raised against N-terminal HTT regions [17], suggesting that truncated fragments, rather than full-length protein, form insoluble disease-relevant protein aggregates in patient brains. Strikingly, such IBs are predominantly detected in the nuclei of neuronal cells, implying that the nuclear environment promotes the aggregation of the pathogenic protein [10] (Figure 1A). It is currently assumed that the misfolding and aggregation of mHTT (mutant HTT) recruits cellular proteins such as ubiquitin, molecular chaperones or components of the ubiquitin-proteasome system into IBs and thereby causes a redistribution of important functional proteins [16]. This might lead to the loss of function of multiple cellular pathways that depend on low-abundance proteins, such as transcription factors or molecular chaperones. Accordingly, neuronal IBs consisting of truncated aggregated HTT fragments and multiple other cellular proteins are distinct subcellular structures that are exclusively detectable in the brains of patients and HD models with disease phenotypes.

Aggregation-prone HTT fragments also form soluble protein aggregates in neuronal cells [18]. These fibrillar oligomers, or protofibrils, are diffusible structures (Figure 1B) that can cause abnormal protein–protein interactions with other cellular proteins or lipids [19,20]. This may result in the co-precipitation of metastable natively unfolded proteins and perturb the membrane integrity of cells or transport vesicles [19,21].

In vitro and cell-based studies with polyQ-containing N-terminal HTT fragments showed that HTTex1 fragments with pathogenic polyQ tracts spontaneously self-assemble into insoluble protein aggregates with a β-sheet-rich fibrillar morphology [13,14] (Figures 1B and 1C). Therefore HTT aggregation is reminiscent of the Aβ (amyloid β-peptide) and α-synuclein fibrillogenesis observed in the brains of patients with Alzheimer's and Parkinson's disease respectively [22]. Strikingly, detailed investigations of HTTex1 fragments with different polyQ tracts have revealed that spontaneous HTTex1 fibrillogenesis is a polyQ-length-dependent

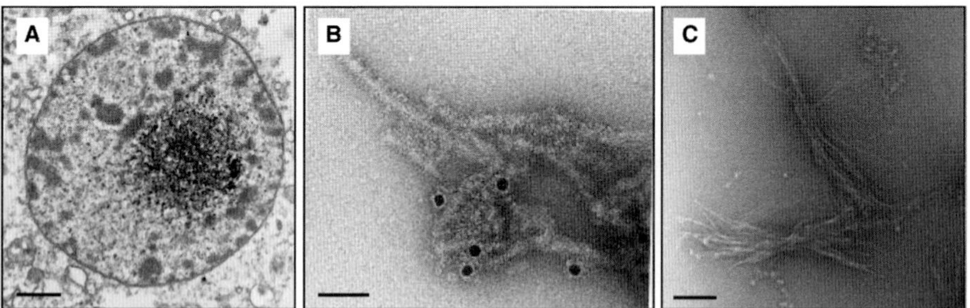

Figure 1. Electron microscopy of *in vivo* human nuclear inclusions and *in vitro* HTTex1 aggregates

(**A**) Nuclear inclusion in cortical neurons from an HD patient. Scale bar, 1 μm. From [10], DiFiglia, M., Sapp, E., Chase, K.O., Davies, S.W., Bates, G.P., Vonsattel, J.P. and Aronin, N. (1997) Aggregation of huntingtin in neuronal intranuclear inclusions and dystrophic neurites in brain. Science **277**, 1990–1993. Reprinted with permission from AAAS. (**B**) HTTex1 fibrillar structures isolated from COS-1 cells and immunogold labelled. Scale bar, 50 nm. Reproduced from [13]; Scherzinger, E., Sittler, A., Schweiger, K., Heiser, V., Lurz, R., Hasenbank, R., Bates, G.P., Lehrach, H. and Wanker, E.E. (1999) Self-assembly of polyglutamine-containing huntingtin fragments into amyloid-like fibrils: implications for Huntington's disease pathology. Proc. Natl. Acad. Sci. U.S.A. **96**, 4604–4609, Copyright (1999) National Academy of Sciences, U.S.A. (**C**) *In vitro* generated fibrillar HTTex1 aggregates show morphological similarity. Scale bar, 100 nm.

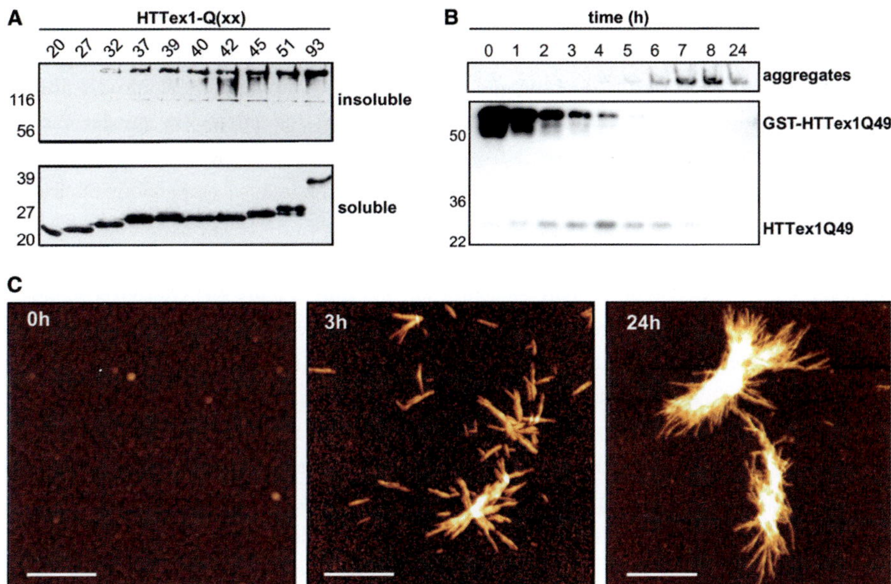

Figure 2. Spontaneous HTTex1 aggregation is polyQ- and time-dependent
(**A**) COS-1 cells expressing HTTex1 fragments with different polyQ lengths form aggregates in a polyQ-length-dependent manner. Cell lysates were separated into insoluble (pellet) and soluble (supernatant) fractions by centrifugation. Reproduced from [13]; Scherzinger, E., Sittler, A., Schweiger, K., Heiser, V., Lurz, R., Hasenbank, R., Bates, G.P., Lehrach, H. and Wanker, E.E. (1999) Self-assembly of polyglutamine-containing huntingtin fragments into amyloid-like fibrils: implications for Huntington's disease pathology. Proc. Natl. Acad. Sci. U.S.A. **96**, 4604–4609, Copyright (1999) National Academy of Sciences, U.S.A. (**B**) Proteolytic cleavage of GST–HTTex1Q49 fusion protein results in the release of HTTex1Q49 fragments, which form insoluble aggregates *in vitro* in a time-dependent manner. (**C**) The HTTex1Q49 fragment forms bundles of amyloid-like aggregates with a fibrillar morphology in a time-dependent manner. Aggregation was monitored by AFM. Scale bar, 500 nm.

process [13]. HTTex1 fragments with non-pathogenic polyQ tracts are soluble, but large aggregate structures are detected in association with pathogenic HTTex1 fragments (Figure 2A). Thus the polyQ-length-dependent aggregation of HTTex1 *in vitro* mirrors observations in patients and in transgenic model systems [10,12].

Mechanism of polyQ-mediated HTTex1 protein aggregation

Studies with amyloidogenic polypeptides and proteins such as IAPP (islet amyloid polypeptide), Aβ, α-synuclein or PrP (prion protein) have demonstrated that the process of fibril self-assembly is generic and can be divided in two phases: (i) a lag phase where few or no fibrils form and (ii) a fibril growth phase where a dramatic exponential increase in fibril mass is observed [23]. Usually, such spontaneous amyloid polymerization reactions have been explained with nucleation-dependent polymerization models [13,14,23]. These theoretical models assume that the rate-limiting step in the amyloidogenic pathway is the formation of a 'nucleus', which develops slowly during the lag phase of the fibril assembly cascade. The 'nucleus' is an oligomeric aggregate species of low abundance that is kinetically unstable and assembles with low propensity. Once formed, however, it rapidly grows into larger amyloid fibrils through an addition of monomers [13,23]. Thus the characteristic sigmoidal fibrillar growth profile observed for many amyloidogenic polypeptides reflects the greater ease by which monomers are added on to existing aggregates compared with the *de novo* formation of amyloidogenic oligomers (nuclei) from monomers through primary homogenous nucleation [23].

Spontaneous HTTex1 fibrillogenesis *in vitro* critically depends on the length of the polyQ tract (Figure 2A), as well as on protein concentration and time (Figure 2B). Moreover, aggregation can be stimulated by preformed fibrils, indicating that HTTex1 fibrillogenesis is dominated by a nucleation-dependent mechanism similar to that of other amyloidogenic polypeptides [13,14]. However, the details of the molecular mechanisms by which disease-relevant polyQ-containing HTTex1 fragments self-assemble into amyloid structures are currently not very well understood. Biochemical and biophysical studies hint that HTTex1 fragments with pathological polyQ tracts are converted into mature amyloid fibrils via spherical oligomers and/or protofibrils [18,24]. These structures were indeed detected in cell-free aggregation reactions by AFM (atomic force microscopy) [24]. However, these studies also provided experimental evidence that the vast majority of spontaneously forming HTTex1 fibrils are obtained through addition of monomers rather than through precursor oligomers [24]. Further studies are necessary to elucidate the critical steps in the HTTex1 polymerization cascade.

Proteotoxicity of polyQ-containing protein aggregates

Neurodegenerative disorders caused by CAG repeat expansions share two main characteristics: the deposition of protein aggregates and neuronal cell death. However, the identification of a defined neurotoxic aggregate species and the mechanism by which it ultimately causes toxicity is challenging and remains elusive.

Different types of mHTT aggregates such as oligomers, fibrils and IBs have been identified in neuronal cells [13,18,24,25]. IBs composed of mHTT fragments trap multiple proteins such as ubiquitin and chaperones, thereby exerting constant stress on the cellular environment [16,21]. Nevertheless, a number of studies indicate that IBs are less toxic for mammalian cells than small soluble HTT protein aggregates. According to the evidence provided, mHTT fragments are transported into distinct IB-like quality control compartments that accumulate the misfolded polyQ protein. Such compartments include structures such as the aggresome, the IPOD (insoluble protein deposit), the JUNQ (juxta-nuclear quality control) or the StiF (Sti1-inducible foci) [16,26,27]. Interestingly, the maturation of these IB-like compartments is regulated by cytosolic chaperones and their co-chaperones, suggesting that chaperone pathways control the toxic effects of misfolded proteins in mammalian cells. Therefore improving the capacity of the cells to deal with misfolded proteins by increasing the levels of molecular chaperones should reduce mHTT-induced toxicity. Indeed, observations in mammalian and yeast cells have been made that the molecular chaperones Hsc70 (heat-shock cognate 70 stress protein) and Sti1p promote the accumulation of mHTT fragments into IB-like compartments [25,27]. This ultimately leads to reduced toxicity, suggesting that the process of the chaperone-induced formation of IBs is a strategy to protect cells against misfolded proteotoxic polyQ proteins. Taken together, these studies imply that IBs, at least in rapidly dividing cells, have a protective role by serving as compartments for misfolded aggregation-prone proteins. Even though IBs containing insoluble HTT aggregates are considered less harmful than soluble aggregate species by some investigators, they still exert a constant stress on protein homoeostasis in mammalian cells. Recently, an artificial β-sheet-rich polypeptide, which forms typical amyloid fibrils in *in vitro* aggregation assays, was shown to be highly toxic for mammalian cells [25]. This polypeptide is thought to cause cellular toxicity through the formation of stable β-sheet-rich protein aggregates that can sequester several important metastable proteins. PolyQ aggregates in cells potentially cause dysfunction and toxicity by binding essential cellular proteins, thereby preventing their ability to perform their normal cellular tasks [25]. However, the relevance of different aggregate species to pathogenesis needs further elucidation.

Mitotic cells have the ability to asymmetrically distribute IBs to only one of the daughter cells, allowing the other to develop free of aggregates. Cells left with IBs show a reduced capacity for reproduction, suggesting that they experience increased cellular stress [11]. As neurons are post-mitotic cells, they are constantly exposed to IBs and thus to proteotoxic stress. This is likely to lead to the dysfunction of key cellular pathways and the accumulation of additional misfolded proteins in a process that may last for decades. Numerous studies have analysed the effects of polyQ-containing HTT fragments on a range of distinct cellular pathways (reviewed in [4]). For example, mHTT fragments disrupt autophagy and the UPS (ubiquitin–proteasome system) in cells, indicating that components of the cell's protein degradation machinery are specifically vulnerable to polyQ aggregates [16,28,29]. In human HD brains, neuronal autophagosomes are enlarged and accumulate, supporting the view that mHTT aggregates perturb protein degradation pathways. In addition, reduced cytosolic turnover of mHTT aggregates has been observed in cell models. This phenomenon is thought to be the result of the defective recognition of HTT aggregates rather than of impaired autophagosome–lysosome fusion [28]. Interestingly, mHTT fragments are also present in synaptic terminals in neurons, where they form aggregates and cause an impairment of the local UPS [29]. As the UPS is a critical modulator of synaptic plasticity and function, this highlights the importance of synaptic pathology in HD. Additionally, pathogenic HTT fragments disrupt axonal transport in neuronal cells. Under pathological conditions, the transport protein kinesin binds to microtubules with reduced affinity [30]. This is due to increased phosphorylation by the axonal JNK3 (c-Jun N-terminal kinase 3), which is hyperactivated by mHTT in neuronal cells. This disruption of the axonal transport machinery ultimately leads to an undersupply of synapses with essential membrane-bound cargos and thus to an impairment of synaptic function [30].

Previous studies have also suggested that mHTT aggregates are toxic to cells because they directly produce reactive oxygen species [31]. Similar results have also been reported for Aβ aggregation reactions, supporting the observations with aggregation-prone HTTex1 fragments [32]. Intriguingly, experimental evidence suggests that aggregates formed of simple polyQ peptides are cytotoxic to mammalian cells when transported into the nucleus [33]. This suggests that the nuclear environment is especially vulnerable to polyQ protein aggregates. This could be due to the fact that polyQ aggregates recruit other polyQ or Q-rich proteins such as the TBP (TATA-binding protein), which subsequently lose their normal cellular functions [34]. Finally, there is evidence that *in vitro*-produced fibrillar HTTex1 aggregates, rather than oligomers or monomers, are toxic to mammalian cells [19]. One potential mechanism for this behaviour is that amyloid-like polyQ-containing protein aggregates can disrupt cellular membranes, potentially resulting in an uncontrolled breakage of cells or subcellular compartments [19]. These findings suggest that both small diffusible mHTT aggregates and large IBs containing insoluble protein aggregates are harmful for cells. However, additional studies with disease-relevant model systems such as iPS (induced pluripotent stem) cell-derived neurons from HD patients need to be performed in order to elucidate the details of the molecular mechanisms by which polyQ protein aggregates perturb cellular systems.

Modulation of polyQ-mediated protein aggregation by distinct cellular pathways and proteins

Numerous proteins that modulate mHTT aggregation and toxicity in cell-free or cell-based assays have been identified [35,36]. Molecular chaperones and chaperone-associated proteins can directly bind to polyQ proteins. They can either stabilize the conformation and prevent the conversion of polyQ sequences from a random coil into an aggregation-prone β-sheet-rich structure [35], or induce the degradation of the polyQ protein [36]. The chaperone CHIP (C-terminus of the Hsc70-interacting protein), which possesses E3 ubiquitin ligase activity, binds to proteins with expanded polyQ tracts including mHTT, which leads to an increased ubiquitination and degradation of the targeted protein [36]. Protein aggregates can also be cleared from cells via macroautophagy or CMA (chaperone-mediated autophagy). Selective catabolism in CMA is conferred by the presence of a KFERQ-like targeting motif in polyQ proteins, by which molecular chaperones recognize the hydrophobic surfaces of the misfolded substrates and transfer them to the lysosomal membrane protein LAMP-2A. They are then taken up into lysosomes, where they are degraded by lysosomal enzymes [37]. A synthetic fusion peptide consisting of an Hsc70-binding motif and two polyQ-binding sequences can promote the degradation of mHTT through CMA [37]. The peptide activates CMA by stimulating the association of mHTT with the chaperone machinery. Enhanced clearance of mHTT fragments through treatment with this construct was observed in cell models as well as transgenic mice [37]. A similar strategy was applied to promote the degradation of polyQ aggregates through macroautophagy. In this case, a synthetic peptide derived from the key autophagy protein beclin1 was used to induce protein degradation [38]. Thus the development of autophagy-stimulating peptides is a powerful strategy to promote the clearance of polyQ-containing protein aggregates from mammalian cells.

For the sake of completeness, it should be stated that post-translational modifications such as phosphorylation, acetylation or SUMOylation influence the aggregation propensity of polyQ-containing HTT fragments in various model systems. Acetylation at Lys[444] increases the clearance of mHTT through macroautophagy. Expression of an acetylation-resistant mHTT fragment led to a dramatic increase in aggregation and neurodegeneration in primary cortical neurons and mouse brain [39]. Taken together, autophagy, chaperones and post-translational modifications dramatically influence the biological activity of mHTT and its aggregation propensity in cells.

Identification of small molecules that influence polyQ-mediated protein aggregation

Cellular processes that maintain proteostasis are of critical importance with regard to aggregation of polyQ-containing disease proteins. Proteostasis is maintained and regulated by molecular chaperones, autophagy, the UPS and stress signalling pathways that sense the accumulation of abnormally folded proteins in cells [4,35–37,39]. Modulation of proteostasis is believed to have a powerful influence on misfolding and proteotoxicity of aggregation-prone disease proteins. Studies with the small molecule GA (geldanamycin), a potent inhibitor of Hsp90 (heat-shock protein 90) ATPase activity, have revealed that increases in the levels of molecular chaperones such as Hsp70 or Hsp40 are associated with reduced aggregation and toxicity of mutant HTTex1 fragments in cells and flies [40]. The importance of chaperone networks in managing misfolded proteins in cells is also supported by the effect of the compound YM-1, which increases the binding affinity of Hsp70 for polyQ disease proteins, leading to an increased efficiency of their ubiquitination and degradation [41]. High-throughput screens have led to the identification of numerous novel small molecules that influence the expression of molecular chaperones in mammalian cells [42]. The mechanism of action of these compounds needs to be further investigated, however, to develop new therapeutic strategies.

Small molecules that induce autophagy might also be of therapeutic value in the treatment of polyQ diseases. The well-known inducer rapamycin, an inhibitor of the mTOR pathway, potently decreases the abundance of insoluble polyQ HTT aggregates in cell models of HD and transgenic flies [43]. Rapamycin has only a mild effect in neurons, whereas the compound NCP {10-[4′-(N-diethylamino)butyl]-2-chlorophenoxazine}, an Akt inhibitor, was found to induce autophagy in neuronal cells more potently, suggesting that different classes of compound may be required to promote the degradation of polyQ aggregates in different cell types [44]. Besides small molecule promoters of functional proteostasis, compounds that directly target the aggregation process have been identified. They include substances such as Congo Red, Thioflavin S, PGL-135 and EGCG [(−)-epigallocatechin gallate], which reduce the formation of polyQ-containing HTTex1 aggregates [45–47]. To date, the mode of action of EGCG has been studied most extensively (Figure 3A). It directly binds to soluble HTTex1 fragments, reducing their propensity to spontaneously convert into β-sheet-rich fibrillar protein aggregates. Interestingly, EGCG does not block HTTex1 aggregation in cell-free assays. Rather, it promotes the formation of amorphous HTTex1 protein aggregates which are not observed in the absence of the substance [47]. This indicates that EGCG redirects the polyQ-mediated HTTex1 aggregation pathway, leading to the formation of a new type of aggregate structure. Studies in cells have revealed that this new type of HTTex1 protein aggregate can be degraded more efficiently than β-sheet-rich fibrillar aggregates, resulting in decreased toxicity for mammalian cells.

Several studies indicate that critical features of neurodegenerative diseases such as protein misfolding, aggregation and neurotoxicty can be reproduced in transgenic fly models [48].

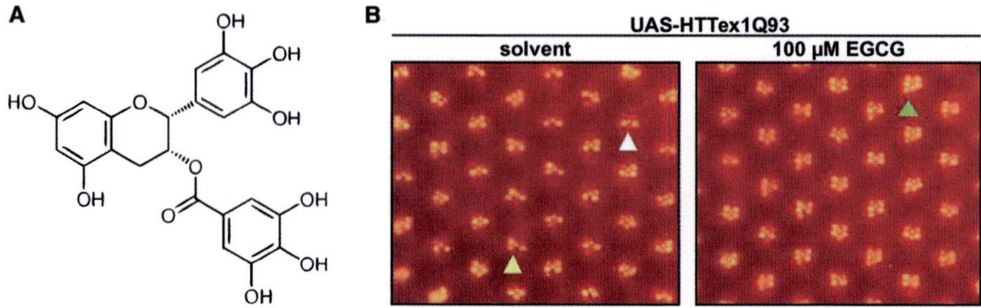

Figure 3. EGCG protects against HTTex1Q93-induced photoreceptor degeneration in *Drosophila melanogaster*
(**A**) Chemical structure of EGCG. (**B**) *D. melanogaster* flies (7 days old) expressing HTTex1Q93 show extensive photoreceptor degeneration. When treated with solvent the ommatidia contain three (white arrowhead) or four (yellow arrowhead) rhabdomers. Flies fed on 100 µM EGCG show reduced degeneration, with up to seven rhabdomers (green arrow). Reproduced with permission from [47]; Ehrnhoefer, D.E., Duennwald, M., Markovic, P., Wacker, J.L., Engemann, S., Roark, M., Legleiter, J., Marsh, J.L., Thompson, L.M. and Lindquist, S. et al. (2006) Green tea (–)-epigallocatechin-gallate modulates early events in huntingtin misfolding and reduces toxicity in Huntington's disease models. Hum. Mol. Genet. **15**, 2743–2751.

These investigations motivated us to assess the effect of EGCG on photoreceptor neurodegeneration in HD transgenic flies, overproducing an aggregation-prone HTTex1 protein with a pathogenic polyQ tract of 93 glutamine residues (HTTex1Q93). In this model, the expression of HTTex1Q93 causes the progressive disruption of the regular trapezoidal arrangement of seven visible photoreceptor neurons (rhabdomers) that can be monitored by light microscopy. We found that in the absence of EGCG, HTTex1Q93-expressing neurons deteriorate until on average ~3.5 photoreceptors per ommatidium remain after 7 days (Figure 3B). In EGCG-treated flies, however, neurodegeneraton was significantly diminished, indicating that the compound has a protective effect on neurotoxicity in transgenic flies [47]. Intriguingly, EGCG is also a potent inhibitor of α-synuclein and Aβ fibrillogenesis, suggesting that it is a generic modulator of protein misfolding and aggregation [49]. We propose that EGCG functions as a chemical chaperone that can target multiple aggregation-prone proteins in a way similar to that of protein chaperones. In summary, targeting aggregation-prone proteins directly with small molecules might be an avenue for therapeutic interventions in polyQ and, more broadly, in protein misfolding diseases.

Conclusions

PolyQ diseases are caused by a CAG-expansion mutation in a disease gene, which leads to an elongated polyQ sequence in the protein product. HTTex1 containing a pathogenic polyQ stretch self-assembles and forms aggregates of different morphologies *in vitro* and *in vivo*. Similar to other amyloidogenic proteins, HTTex1 fibrillogenesis follows a polyQ-length-dependent nucleation and polymerization pathway. Controlled by the proteostasis network, cells have developed defence mechanisms which inhibit misfolding and facilitate aggregate clearance. A better understanding of the basic principles of protein misfolding and aggregation will be the basis for the identification of small molecules which may be applicable as therapeutic agents.

Summary

- PolyQ diseases are neurological disorders that are caused by a polyQ expansion mutation.
- The expansion of the polyQ tract in the disease protein leads to misfolding and intracellular aggregate formation associated with cell-type-specific neurotoxicity and brain-region-specific atrophy.
- HTTex1 spontaneously self-assembles into amyloid structures.
- The aggregation reaction follows a nucleation-dependent mechanism.
- PolyQ aggregates are β-sheet-rich structures.
- Intracellular IBs sequester a wide variety of cellular proteins leading to a disturbance of proteostasis.
- Small diffusible mHTT aggregates as well as large IBs are harmful for cells.
- There is no effective treatment for any of the polyQ diseases.

References

1. Schaefer, M.H., Wanker, E.E. and Andrade-Navarro, M.A. (2012) Evolution and function of CAG/polyglutamine repeats in protein-protein interaction networks. Nucleic Acids Res. **40**, 4273–4287

2. Atanesyan, L., Günther, V., Dichtl, B., Georgiev, O. and Schaffner, W. (2012) Polyglutamine tracts as modulators of transcriptional activation from yeast to mammals. Biol. Chem. **393**, 63–70

3. Kim, D.H., Kim, G.S., Yun, C.H. and Lee, Y.C. (2008) Functional conservation of the glutamine-rich domains of yeast Gal11 and human SRC-1 in the transactivation of glucocorticoid receptor Tau 1 in *Saccharomyces cerevisiae*. Mol. Cell. Biol. **28**, 913–925

4. Hands, S., Sinadinos, C. and Wyttenbach, A. (2008) Polyglutamine gene function and dysfunction in the ageing brain. Biochim. Biophys. Acta **1779**, 507–521

5. Gusella, J.F. (1989) Location cloning strategy for characterizing genetic defects in Huntington's disease and Alzheimer's disease. FASEB J. **3**, 2036–2041

6. The Huntington's Disease Collaborative Research Group (1993) A novel gene containing a trinucleotide repeat that is expanded and unstable on Huntington's disease chromosomes. Cell **72**, 971–983

7. Andrade, M.A. and Bork, P. (1995) HEAT repeats in the Huntington's disease protein. Nat. Genet. **11**, 115–116

8. Faber, P.W., Barnes, G.T., Srinidhi, J., Chen, J., Gusella, J.F. and MacDonald, M.E. (1998) Huntingtin interacts with a family of WW domain proteins. Hum. Mol. Genet. **7**, 1463–1474

9. Cattaneo, E., Zuccato, C. and Tartari, M. (2005) Normal huntingtin function: an alternative approach to Huntington's disease. Nat. Rev. **6**, 919–930

10. DiFiglia, M., Sapp, E., Chase, K.O., Davies, S.W., Bates, G.P., Vonsattel, J.P. and Aronin, N. (1997) Aggregation of huntingtin in neuronal intranuclear inclusions and dystrophic neurites in brain. Science **277**, 1990–1993

11. Lindner, A.B., Madden, R., Demarez, A., Stewart, E.J. and Taddei, F. (2008) Asymmetric segregation of protein aggregates is associated with cellular aging and rejuvenation. Proc. Natl. Acad. Sci. U.S.A. **105**, 3076–3081

12. Davies, S.W., Turmaine, M., Cozens, B.A., DiFiglia, M., Sharp, A.H., Ross, C.A., Scherzinger, E., Wanker, E.E., Mangiarini, L. and Bates, G.P. (1997) Formation of neuronal intranuclear inclusions underlies the neurological dysfunction in mice transgenic for the HD mutation. Cell **90**, 537–548

13. Scherzinger, E., Sittler, A., Schweiger, K., Heiser, V., Lurz, R., Hasenbank, R., Bates, G.P., Lehrach, H. and Wanker, E.E. (1999) Self-assembly of polyglutamine-containing huntingtin

      fragments into amyloid-like fibrils: implications for Huntington's disease pathology. Proc. Natl. Acad. Sci. U.S.A. **96**, 4604–4609

14. Scherzinger, E., Lurz, R., Turmaine, M., Mangiarini, L., Hollenbach, B., Hasenbank, R., Bates, G.P., Davies, S.W., Lehrach, H. and Wanker, E.E. (1997) Huntingtin-encoded polyglutamine expansions form amyloid-like protein aggregates *in vitro* and *in vivo*. Cell **90**, 549–558

15. Sathasivam, K., Neueder, A., Gipson, T.A., Landles, C., Benjamin, A.C., Bondulich, M.K., Smith, D.L., Faull, R.L., Roos, R.A., Howland, D. et al. (2013) Aberrant splicing of HTT generates the pathogenic exon 1 protein in Huntington disease. Proc. Natl. Acad. Sci. U.S.A. **110**, 2366–2370

16. Waelter, S., Boeddrich, A., Lurz, R., Scherzinger, E., Lueder, G., Lehrach, H. and Wanker, E.E. (2001) Accumulation of mutant huntingtin fragments in aggresome-like inclusion bodies as a result of insufficient protein degradation. Mol. Biol. Cell **12**, 1393–1407

17. Sieradzan, K.A., Mechan, A.O., Jones, L., Wanker, E.E., Nukina, N. and Mann, D.M. (1999) Huntington's disease intranuclear inclusions contain truncated, ubiquitinated huntingtin protein. Exp. Neurol. **156**, 92–99

18. Sahl, S.J., Weiss, L.E., Duim, W.C., Frydman, J. and Moerner, W.E. (2012) Cellular inclusion bodies of mutant huntingtin exon 1 obscure small fibrillar aggregate species. Sci. Rep. **2**, 895

19. Pieri, L., Madiona, K., Bousset, L. and Melki, R. (2012) Fibrillar α-synuclein and huntingtin exon 1 assemblies are toxic to the cells. Biophys. J. **102**, 2894–2905

20. Harjes, P. and Wanker, E.E. (2003) The hunt for huntingtin function: interaction partners tell many different stories. Trends Biochem. Sci. **28**, 425–433

21. Olzscha, H., Schermann, S.M., Woerner, A.C., Pinkert, S., Hecht, M.H., Tartaglia, G.G., Vendruscolo, M., Hayer-Hartl, M., Hartl, F.U. and Vabulas, R.M. (2011) Amyloid-like aggregates sequester numerous metastable proteins with essential cellular functions. Cell **144**, 67–78

22. Ross, C.A. and Poirier, M.A. (2004) Protein aggregation and neurodegenerative disease. Nat. Med. **10**, S10–S17

23. Jarrett, J.T. and Lansbury, Jr, P.T. (1993) Seeding "one-dimensional crystallization" of amyloid: a pathogenic mechanism in Alzheimer's disease and scrapie? Cell **73**, 1055–1058

24. Wacker, J.L., Zareie, M.H., Fong, H., Sarikaya, M. and Muchowski, P.J. (2004) Hsp70 and Hsp40 attenuate formation of spherical and annular polyglutamine oligomers by partitioning monomer. Nat. Struct. Mol. Biol. **11**, 1215–1222

25. Olshina, M.A., Angley, L.M., Ramdzan, Y.M., Tang, J., Bailey, M.F., Hill, A.F. and Hatters, D.M. (2010) Tracking mutant huntingtin aggregation kinetics in cells reveals three major populations that include an invariant oligomer pool. J. Biol. Chem. **285**, 21807–21816

26. Kaganovich, D., Kopito, R. and Frydman, J. (2008) Misfolded proteins partition between two distinct quality control compartments. Nature **454**, 1088–1095

27. Wolfe, K.J., Ren, H.Y., Trepte, P. and Cyr, D.M. (2013) The Hsp70/90 cochaperone, Sti1, suppresses proteotoxicity by regulating spatial quality control of amyloid-like proteins. Mol. Biol. Cell **24**, 3588–3602

28. Martinez-Vicente, M., Talloczy, Z., Wong, E., Tang, G., Koga, H., Kaushik, S., de Vries, R., Arias, E., Harris, S., Sulzer, D. and Cuervo, A.M. (2010) Cargo recognition failure is responsible for inefficient autophagy in Huntington's disease. Nat. Neurosci. **13**, 567–576

29. Wang, J., Wang, C.E., Orr, A., Tydlacka, S., Li, S.H. and Li, X.J. (2008) Impaired ubiquitin-proteasome system activity in the synapses of Huntington's disease mice. J. Cell Biol. **180**, 1177–1189

30. Morfini, G.A., You, Y.M., Pollema, S.L., Kaminska, A., Liu, K., Yoshioka, K., Björkblom, B., Coffey, E.T., Bagnato, C. and Han, D. (2009) Pathogenic huntingtin inhibits fast axonal transport by activating JNK3 and phosphorylating kinesin. Nat. Neurosci. **12**, 864–871

31. Wyttenbach, A., Sauvageot, O., Carmichael, J., Diaz-Latoud, C., Arrigo, A.P. and Rubinsztein, D.C. (2002) Heat shock protein 27 prevents cellular polyglutamine toxicity and

suppresses the increase of reactive oxygen species caused by huntingtin. Hum. Mol. Genet. **11**, 1137–1151

32. Kadowaki, H., Nishitoh, H., Urano, F., Sadamitsu, C., Matsuzawa, A., Takeda, K., Masutani, H., Yodoi, J., Urano, Y., Nagano, T. and Ichijo, H. (2005) Amyloid β induces neuronal cell death through ROS-mediated ASK1 activation. Cell Death Diff. **12**, 19–24

33. Yang, W., Dunlap, J.R., Andrews, R.B. and Wetzel, R. (2002) Aggregated polyglutamine peptides delivered to nuclei are toxic to mammalian cells. Hum. Mol. Genet. **11**, 2905–2917

34. Huang, C.C., Faber, P.W., Persichetti, F., Mittal, V., Vonsattel, J.P., MacDonald, M.E. and Gusella, J.F. (1998) Amyloid formation by mutant huntingtin: threshold, progressivity and recruitment of normal polyglutamine proteins. Somat. Cell Mol. Genet. **24**, 217–233

35. Kitamura, A., Kubota, H., Pack, C.G., Matsumoto, G., Hirayama, S., Takahashi, Y., Kimura, H., Kinjo, M., Morimoto, R.I. and Nagata, K. (2006) Cytosolic chaperonin prevents polyglutamine toxicity with altering the aggregation state. Nat. Cell Biol. **8**, 1163–1170

36. Jana, N.R., Dikshit, P., Goswami, A., Kotliarova, S., Murata, S., Tanaka, K. and Nukina, N. (2005) Co-chaperone CHIP associates with expanded polyglutamine protein and promotes their degradation by proteasomes. J. Biol. Chem. **280**, 11635–11640

37. Bauer, P.O., Goswami, A., Wong, H.K., Okuno, M., Kurosawa, M., Yamada, M., Miyazaki, H., Matsumoto, G., Kino, Y., Nagai, Y. and Nukina, N. (201) Harnessing chaperone-mediated autophagy for the selective degradation of mutant huntingtin protein. Nat. Biotechnol. **28**, 256–263

38. Shoji-Kawata, S., Sumpter, R., Leveno, M., Campbell, G.R., Zou, Z., Kinch, L., Wilkins, A.D., Sun, Q., Pallauf, K. and MacDuff, D. (2013) Identification of a candidate therapeutic autophagy-inducing peptide. Nature **494**, 201–206

39. Jeong, H., Then, F., Melia, Jr, T.J., Mazzulli, J.R., Cui, L., Savas, J.N., Voisine, C., Paganetti, P., Tanese, N., Hart, A.C. and Yamamoto, A. (2009) Acetylation targets mutant huntingtin to autophagosomes for degradation. Cell **137**, 60–72

40. Sittler, A., Lurz, R., Lueder, G., Priller, J., Lehrach, H., Hayer-Hartl, M.K., Hartl, F.U. and Wanker, E.E. (2001) Geldanamycin activates a heat shock response and inhibits huntingtin aggregation in a cell culture model of Huntington's disease. Hum. Mol. Genet. **10**, 1307–1315

41. Wang, A.M., Miyata, Y., Klinedinst, S., Peng, H.M., Chua, J.P., Komiyama, T., Li, X., Morishima, Y., Merry, D.E. and Pratt, W.B. (2013) Activation of Hsp70 reduces neurotoxicity by promoting polyglutamine protein degradation. Nat. Chem. Biol. **9**, 112–118

42. Calamini, B., Silva, M.C., Madoux, F., Hutt, D.M., Khanna, S., Chalfant, M.A., Saldanha, S.A., Hodder, P., Tait, B.D., Garza, D. et al. (2012) Small-molecule proteostasis regulators for protein conformational diseases. Nat. Chem. Biol. **8**, 185–196

43. Sarkar, S., Perlstein, E.O., Imarisio, S., Pineau, S., Cordenier, A., Maglathlin, R.L., Webster, J.A., Lewis, T.A., O'Kane, C.J., Schreiber, S.L. and Rubinsztein, D.C. (2007) Small molecules enhance autophagy and reduce toxicity in Huntington's disease models. Nat. Chem. Biol. **3**, 331–338

44. Tsvetkov, A.S., Miller, J., Arrasate, M., Wong, J.S., Pleiss, M.A. and Finkbeiner, S. (2010) A small-molecule scaffold induces autophagy in primary neurons and protects against toxicity in a Huntington disease model. Proc. Natl. Acad. Sci. U.S.A. **107**, 16982–16987

45. Heiser, V., Scherzinger, E., Boeddrich, A., Nordhoff, E., Lurz, R., Schugardt, N., Lehrach, H. and Wanker, E.E. (2000) Inhibition of huntingtin fibrillogenesis by specific antibodies and small molecules: implications for Huntington's disease therapy. Proc. Natl. Acad. Sci. U.S.A. **97**, 6739–6744

46. Heiser, V., Engemann, S., Bröcker, W., Dunkel, I., Boeddrich, A., Waelter, S., Nordhoff, E., Lurz, R., Schugardt, N. and Rautenberg, S. (2002) Identification of benzothiazoles as potential polyglutamine aggregation inhibitors of Huntington's disease by using an automated filter retardation assay. Proc. Natl. Acad. Sci. U.S.A. **99**, 16400–16406

47. Ehrnhoefer, D.E., Duennwald, M., Markovic, P., Wacker, J.L., Engemann, S., Roark, M., Legleiter, J., Marsh, J.L., Thompson, L.M. and Lindquist, S. et al. (2006) Green tea

(–)-epigallocatechin-gallate modulates early events in huntingtin misfolding and reduces toxicity in Huntington's disease models. Hum. Mol. Genet. **15**, 2743–2751

48. Bilen, J. and Bonini, N.M. (2005) *Drosophila* as a model for human neurodegenerative disease. Annu. Rev. Genet. **39**, 153–171

49. Ehrnhoefer, D.E., Bieschke, J., Boeddrich, A., Herbst, M., Masino, L., Lurz, R., Engemann, S., Pastore, A. and Wanker, E.E. (2008) EGCG redirects amyloidogenic polypeptides into unstructured, off-pathway oligomers. Nat. Struct. Mol. Biol. **15**, 558–566

© The Authors Journal compilation © 2014 Biochemical Society
Essays Biochem. (2014) 56, 181–191: doi: 10.1042/BSE0560181

13

Prion disease and the 'protein-only hypothesis'

Jiyan Ma[1] and Fei Wang[1]

Center for Neurodegenerative Science, Van Andel Research Institute, Grand Rapids, MI 49503, U.S.A.

Abstract

Prion disease is the only naturally occurring infectious protein misfolding disorder. The chemical nature of the infectious agent has been debated for more than half a century. Early studies on scrapie suggested that the unusual infectious agent might propagate in the absence of nucleic acid. The 'protein-only hypothesis' provides a theoretical model to explain how a protein self-replicates without nucleic acid, which predicts that a prion, the proteinaceous infectious agent, propagates by converting its normal counterpart into the likeness of itself. Decades of studies have provided overwhelming evidence to support this hypothesis. The latest advances in generating infectious prions with bacterially expressed recombinant prion protein in the presence of cofactors not only provide convincing evidence supporting the 'protein-only hypothesis', but also indicate a role of cofactors in forming prion infectivity and encoding prion strains. In the present chapter, we review the literature regarding the chemical nature of the infectious agent, describe recent achievements in proving the 'protein-only hypothesis', and discuss the remaining questions in this research area.

Keywords:

infectious protein, prion infectivity, prion protein conversion, prion strain, 'protein-only hypothesis', recombinant prion, transmissible spongiform encephalopathy.

[1]*Correspondence may be addressed to either of these authors (email jiyan.ma@vai.org or fei.wang@vai.org).*

Introduction

TSEs (transmissible spongiform encephalopathies), also known as prion diseases, are a group of fatal neurodegenerative disorders that can be manifested as sporadic, inherited or acquired forms [1,2]. Prion disease affects a wide variety of mammals including kuru disease or vCJD (variant Creutzfeldt–Jacob disease) in humans, scrapie in sheep, BSE (bovine spongiform encephalopathy) in cattle and CWD (chronic wasting disease) in deer and elk [1,3]. It shares the characteristics of late-age onset, accumulation of misfolded protein aggregates in the central nervous system, and neurodegeneration with a large group of disorders including Alzheimer's and Parkinson's diseases. Despite the similarities, prion disease is the only naturally occurring infectious protein misfolding disorder that can be transmitted within and, on rare occasions, between species [4].

The infectious agent in TSEs has been intensely investigated and overwhelming evidence supports that a 'prion', a proteinaceous infectious particle, is responsible for the transmissibility. The 'protein-only hypothesis' predicts that a prion conveys its infectious structural information to its normally folded non-infectious counterpart, leading to the transmission of disease. The following sections summarize studies regarding the chemical nature of the infectious agent, describe the latest advances in generating infectious prions with bacterially expressed recPrP (recombinant prion protein), and discuss the potential role of cofactors in forming highly infectious prions and in enciphering the baffling prion strain phenomenon.

Exploring the chemical nature of the scrapie agent

Scrapie is the prototype of prion disease affecting sheep and goats, and was the most studied prion disease before rodents were introduced as disease models. Although scrapie was suspected as a contagious disease as early as the mid-18th Century, experimental evidence that scrapie could be transmitted to healthy sheep or goats by inoculating with brain homogenate from sick animals was not attained until the 1930s [5,6]. After establishing that scrapie is a transmissible disease, scientists started exploring the chemical nature of the infectious agent. A bacterium was first excluded because the agent was able to pass an antibacterial filter. A 'slow virus' was speculated because of the extraordinarily long incubation times of scrapie (>14 months in sheep and goats). Although extensive attempts failed to identify such a viral agent, those studies revealed unexpected properties of the agent that survives many common procedures used to inactivate viruses, including formalin treatment, boiling in water, extracting with organic solvents, digesting with nucleases, UV and ionizing radiations. These unusual properties led to alternative theories positing that the infectious agent could be a protein, a polysaccharide or a fragment of lipid membrane [7].

The 'protein-only hypothesis'

Despite the unusual characteristics, the mainstream thought remained that scrapie was caused by a novel viral agent containing nucleic acids (DNA or RNA) as the genetic information carrier. British scientists Tikvah Alper et al. [8] used ionizing radiation to determine the size of the scrapie agent based on the idea that the target size can be calculated from the dosage of electron beam used to inactivate the biological activity. Extrapolating from the exceptionally high electron dose required to inactivate scrapie infectivity, they concluded that the size of the scrapie agent was extraordinarily small, much smaller than bacteriophage, the smallest known virus at that time. More importantly, they found that scrapie infectivity remained after a high dosage of UV irradiation that would destroy nucleic acids, suggesting that the agent may replicate without nucleic acid [8]. On the basis of the unusual characteristics and the radiation results, Pattison and Jones [9] proposed that the scrapie agent could be a self-replicating protein, and Griffith [10], a mathematician without any biological science background, proposed three models to explain how a protein is capable of self-replicating in the absence of nucleic acid. The second model, currently known as the 'protein-only hypothesis', was derived from the following thermodynamic equations (eqns 1, 2 and 3) and assumptions.

Equations

$$a' \rightarrow a - \Delta F_1 \tag{1}$$
$$a + a \rightarrow a_2 + \Delta F_2 \tag{2}$$

Combining eqns (1) and (2), one can derive eqn (3):

$$a' + a' \rightarrow a_2 + \Delta F_2 - 2\Delta F_1 \tag{3}$$

Assumptions:

(i) a' is the normal cellular protein with a stable structure
(ii) a is in the reactive state bearing a different conformation from a'
(iii) ΔF_1 is so large that a'-to-a conversion hardly ever occurs
(iv) Without pre-existing a_2 (the hypothetical infectious protein structure), eqn (2) cannot take place even though the reaction is thermodynamically favourable.

However, when ΔF_2 is larger than $2\Delta F_1$ and pre-formed a_2 is present as a template, normal cellular protein a' could proceed to form new a_2 (eqn 3), completing the self-replication of a_2. Therefore if the scrapie agent is composed of protein and acts like a_2, this model readily explains how a proteinaceous agent, without nucleic acid, could self-replicate after being introduced into the healthy animals where normal cellular protein a' is present. Figure 1 illustrates a simplified thermodynamic diagram of a'-to-a_2 conversion.

This model describes the thermodynamic feasibility for an infectious proteinaceous agent to self-replicate via propagating its conformation. However, this putative infectious protein remained elusive for a long period of time.

Prions: proteinaceous infectious particles

In an effort to isolate the scrapie infectivity using differential sedimentation, detergent extraction and enzymatic digestion, Stanley Prusiner et al. [11] discovered that the infectivity in diseased hamster brain homogenates could be enriched in a fraction that was mostly composed of a partially protease-resistant protein with apparent molecular mass of 27–30 kDa. In 1982, Prusiner postulated that the agent is a 'prion', the "small proteinaceous infectious particles that are resistant

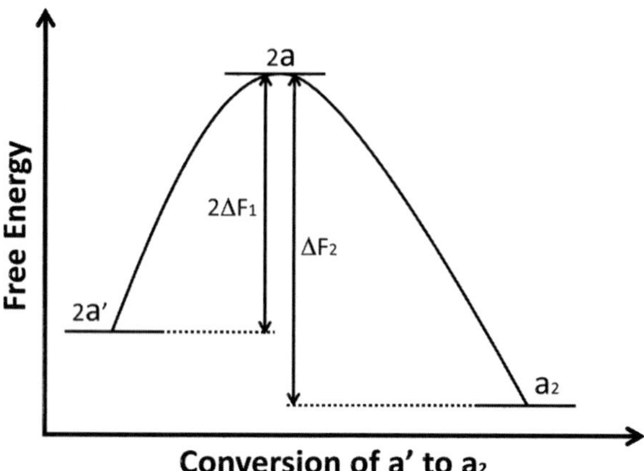

Figure 1. Conversion from a' to a_2

When ΔF_2 is larger than $2\Delta F_1$, the conversion from a' into a_2 is a thermodynamically favourable reaction. According to the 'protein-only hypothesis', in the presence of pre-existing a_2 template, the reaction can continue indefinitely, completing the self-replication of a_2 in the absence of nucleic acid. a', the stable normal cellular protein; a, the reactive state of a'; a_2, dimer formed from two units of a.

to inactivation by most procedures that modify nucleic acids" [11]. Purification of the PrP (prion protein) of 27–30 kDa, also known as PrP27–30, led to the identification of the PrP gene, *Prnp*, a single copy chromosomal gene that is highly conserved in mammals. The *Prnp* gene encodes PrP^C (normal cellular prion protein), which is primarily expressed in the central nervous system and, at much lower levels, in several peripheral tissues. The primary translation product of *Prnp* contains an N-terminal signal sequence targeting PrP to the secretory pathway, five octapeptide repeats, a highly conserved central hydrophobic domain, a globular C-terminal domain consisting of three α-helices and a short stretch of β-strands, and a signal sequence for adding a GPI (glycosylphosphatidylinositol) anchor (Figure 2). After removing N- and C-terminal signal sequences, adding N-linked sugars to two asparagine residues, and forming a single disulfide bond between two cysteine residues, the mature PrP^C localizes at the cell surface and attaches to the plasma membrane by its GPI anchor. Although PrP^C is expressed in both healthy and scrapie-affected animals, the scrapie-associated PrP27–30 can only be isolated from diseased brain homogenates after limited protease digestion. The disease-specific conformation of PrP is denoted as PrP^{Sc}, which has the same primary amino acid sequence as PrP^C, but differs drastically in protein conformation, resulting in distinct properties (Table 1). PrP^C is highly α-helical,

Table 1. Differences between PrP^C and PrP^{Sc}

PrP^C	PrP^{Sc}
Non-infectious	Infectious
Rich in α-helical content	Predominantly β-sheet
Soluble in mild detergents	Aggregated in mild detergents
Sensitive to protease digestion	Partially resistant to protease digestion

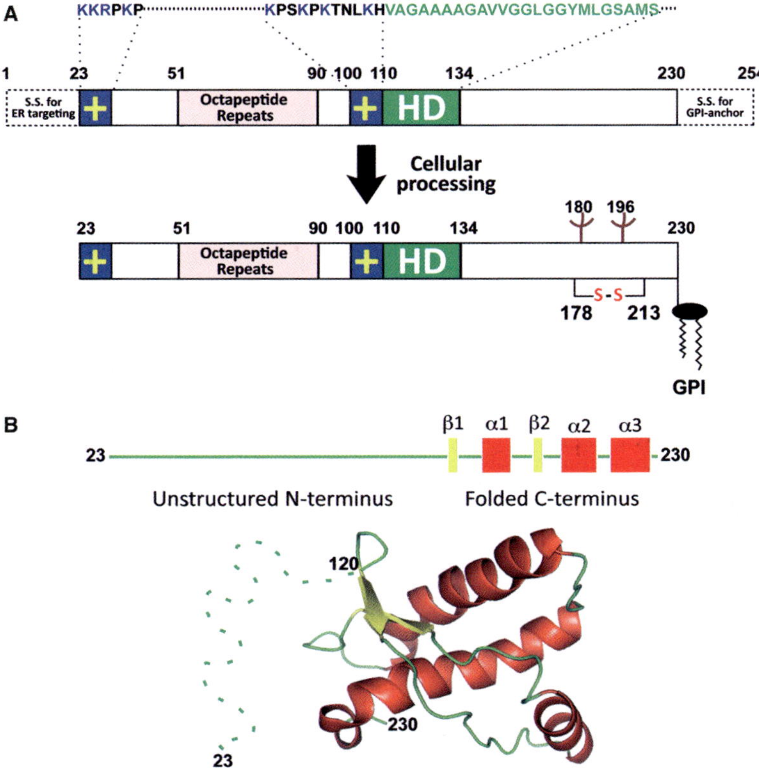

Figure 2. Schematic illustrations of mouse PrP

(**A**) Mouse PrP contains two positively charged (+) amino acid clusters (blue), five octapeptide repeats (pink) and a hydrophobic domain (green). S.S., signal sequence. After cellular processing, mature mouse PrP23–230 (mouse numbering) attaches to the cell membrane by a GPI anchor after N- and C-terminal signal sequences are removed, N-linked carbohydrates are added to Asn180 and Asn196, and a single disulfide bond forms between Cys178 and Cys213. (**B**) Mouse PrP is composed of an unstructured N-terminus and a globular C-terminus consisting of three α-helices and two short β-strands. The image of tertiary structure of mouse PrP120–230 (mouse numbering) (PDB code 1AG2) was generated in PyMOL. Dashed line is added to represent the unstructured N-terminus.

soluble in mild detergents and sensitive to protease digestion. In contrast, PrPSc is mainly β-sheet, highly aggregated and partially resistant to PK (proteinase-K) digestion.

Conversion of non-infectious PrPC into infectious PrPSc

After identifying the scrapie-infectivity-associated prion, Prusiner further proposed that the prion, composed entirely or principally of PrPSc, the misfolded isoform of normal PrPC, is the proteinaceous infectious agent and self-replication of PrPSc involving PrPC-to-PrPSc conversion induces prion diseases in hosts. The observation that PrP-knockout mice were resistant to prion infection strongly supports that PrP is essential for disease pathogenesis [12,13].

Given the aggregated nature of PrPSc, it is almost impossible to purify it to homogeneity to prove that PrPSc is the infectious agent. Based on the idea that PrPSc self-replication, the catalytic conversion of PrP^C into PrP^{Sc}, would produce an unlimited amount of newly formed PrP^{Sc}, a series of *in vitro* studies was carried out to correlate PrP^{Sc} with prion infectivity. According to the thermodynamic model [8], PrP^C with a stable structure needs to reach the reactive state, PrP*, before it converts into PrP^{Sc}. As PrP^{Sc} and PrP^C represent two distinct conformations of the same protein (Table 1), the reactive PrP* must represent an (at least partially unfolded) intermediate PrP species between the mainly α-helical PrP^C and the β-sheet-rich PrP^{Sc} (Figure 3). For PrP^C to reach this PrP* conformational state, exogenous energy is required to overcome the large energy barrier between PrP^C and PrP^{Sc}. Alternatively, other facilitating factors, such as denaturants or PrP-binding molecules, may lower the energy barrier and allow the conversion to occur.

The first cell-free conversion assay used a denaturant, GndHCl (guanidine hydrochloride), at low concentration to facilitate the PrP^{Sc}-seeded conversion [14]. Mixing partially purified PrP^{Sc} with purified ^{35}S-labelled PrP^C led to the formation of PK-resistant radioactive PrP species, which co-aggregated with unlabelled PrP^{Sc} seed. This cell-free conversion assay undoubtedly demonstrated the seeding capability of PrP^{Sc}, yet the low conversion efficiency resulted in an excessive amount of unlabelled PrP^{Sc} seed in the final product, making it difficult to assess the infectivity of newly generated radioactive PrP^{Sc}. To enhance the conversion efficiency, a new technique named PMCA (protein misfolding cyclic amplification) was developed, in which a mixture of a limited amount of crude diseased brain homogenate containing PrP^{Sc} and excess normal brain homogenate containing PrP^C was subjected to successive sonication and incubation cycles. After reaction, newly formed PrP^{Sc} can be detected by PK-digestion assay and used to seed a new round of PrP^C conversion, allowing indefinite propagation of PrP^{Sc} [15]. More importantly, after sufficient PMCA rounds that dilute out the original PrP^{Sc} seed from diseased brain homogenates, the newly formed PrP^{Sc} is capable of inducing *bona fide* prion disease in wild-type animals [16].

Compared with the low efficiency of the cell-free conversion assay, the ability of PMCA to efficiently propagate PrP^{Sc} and prion infectivity might be attributed to the following aspects. Sonication in PMCA is believed to fragment large PrP^{Sc} aggregates into smaller particles, increasing the PrP^{Sc}–PrP^C contacting surfaces and resulting in more efficient conversion. On the

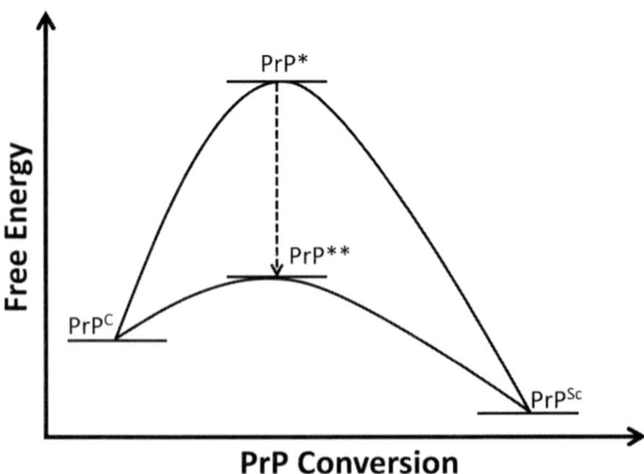

Figure 3. PrP conversion
To fulfil self-replication of PrP^{Sc}, the stable normal PrP^C needs to reach the reactive state, PrP* or PrP**, to further convert into PrP^{Sc}. Factors that lower the energy barrier would allow the reaction to go through the PrP** state, facilitating the PrP^C-to-PrP^{Sc} conversion.

other hand, sonication can certainly transfer energy to PrP^C helping it to reach the reactive PrP* state, or partially unfold PrP^C to facilitate the conversion. Therefore it is likely that with proper setups (in the form of power and duration of sonication, the incubation time and temperature), a certain amount of the reactive PrP intermediate, PrP*, could be generated from PrP^C, which is further converted into PrP^{Sc} under the catalytic influence of pre-existing PrP^{Sc} seed.

The concomitant propagation of PrP^{Sc} and the prion infectivity by PMCA strongly supports the 'protein-only hypothesis'. However, due to the use of crude brain homogenates in this assay, it is still difficult to conclusively pinpoint that PrP^{Sc} is the infectious agent. One can argue that other components in the brain homogenates, such as a small fragment of nucleic acid, may have been propagated during the PMCA, which might be the culprit in transmitting the disease. Notably, the 'virino hypothesis' postulates that the scrapie agent could be a nucleic acid–PrP^{Sc} complex. Although the nucleic acid carries the genetic information for transmitting the disease, PrP^{Sc} serves as the protective coat allowing the disease-causing nucleic acid to survive all the harsh treatments [17].

It is widely accepted that the most stringent proof for the 'protein-only hypothesis' would be the generation of infectious PrP^{Sc} from pure non-infectious PrP^C. Owing to its denaturation/refolding purification procedures and remarkably similar tertiary structure to PrP^C [18], purified bacterially expressed recPrP has been regarded as the purest available PrP species and is widely used in PrP conversion studies. Because scrapie-associated PrP27–30 forms short amyloid fibres after detergent extraction and protease digestion, it was reasoned that the *in vitro*-formed PrP amyloid fibrils might possess prion infectivity. Soluble, monomeric and mainly α-helical recPrP has been successfully converted into amyloid fibrils in the presence of denaturing chaotropic agents, such as GndHCl or urea [19,20]. Despite the similarities to PrP^{Sc} (in being highly aggregated, rich in β-sheet and with strong *in vitro* seeding capability), recPrP amyloid fibrils induced prion disease only in transgenic mice overexpressing PrP after a prolonged incubation period (an indication of minimal infectivity), but failed to cause disease in wild-type animals [21,22].

The minimal infectivity associated with recPrP amyloid fibrils may suggest that the *in vitro*-generated recPrP amyloid fibrils still have large structural differences from the infectious PrP^{Sc}. Alternatively, other non-PrP cofactors, which are not present in the pure recPrP amyloid fibril system, might be essential for generating the infectious PrP^{Sc} conformer. The latter possibility is consistent with a significant difference in PrP conversion efficiency between the cell-free and PMCA assays. These non-PrP cofactors in brain homogenates used in the PMCA reaction may interact with PrP^{Sc} and/or PrP^C to facilitate the conversion. Notably, polyanions, such as proteoglycans and nucleic acids have been shown to bind PrP, induce conformational changes in PrP and promote PrP conversion *in vitro* [23–25].

In addition to polyanions, lipids are also a plausible candidate for facilitating PrP conversion. The GPI-anchored PrP^C is in the vicinity of lipid membranes and PrP–lipid interactions have long been implicated in PrP^C-to-PrP^{Sc} conversion. PrP^C can be released from lipid membranes after PI-PLC (phosphoinositide-specific phospholipase C) cleavage of the GPI anchor. However, PI-PLC digestion failed to release PrP^{Sc} from lipid membranes, indicating an additional mode of interaction between PrP^{Sc} and lipid membranes. Moreover, it has been shown that a direct PrP–lipid interaction is required for PrP conversion in the presence of lipid membranes in a modified cell-free PrP conversion assay [7].

The PrP–lipid interaction has been verified by experiments showing that bacterially expressed recPrP binds to synthetic liposomes and the binding destabilizes the well-structured C-terminal domain of recPrP [26]. The recPrP–lipid interaction is initiated by the electrostatic binding between positively charged amino acid residues of recPrP and negatively charged anionic phospholipid headgroups, which is followed by the hydrophobic interactions between recPrP hydrophobic domain and lipid acyl chains. The lipid interaction converts α-helical structured recPrP into a β-sheet-rich, C-terminal PK-resistant conformation, both of which are biochemical hallmarks of PrP[Sc] [27]. These observations indicate that similar to denaturant treatment, PrP–lipid interactions are able to unfold recPrP to another stable conformational state.

The similar biochemical properties of lipid-bound recPrP to those of infectious PrP[Sc] led to the hypothesis that recPrP–lipid interactions may lead recPrP to reach the reactive PrP* state and thereby lower the energy barrier for the conversion into PrP[Sc] (Figure 3). This hypothesis was tested by PMCA using a substrate mixture of bacterially expressed recPrP plus two cofactors: a negatively charged phospholipid [POPG (1-palmitoyl-2-oleoyl-*sn*-glycero-3-phospho-(10-rac-glycerol)] and polyanions (total RNA isolated from normal mouse liver). Indeed, recPrP[Sc] generated by this approach not only possesses all the hallmarks of diseased brain-derived PrP[Sc] (aggregated, C-terminal PK-resistant, capable of seeding the conversion of PrP[C] in normal brain homogenate by PMCA and converting PrP[C] in cultured cells to create a chronic infected state), but also induces prion disease in wild-type mice after a short incubation period and with a relatively synchronized onset, indicating a high degree of specific prion infectivity [28]. When the total mouse liver RNA is replaced by synthetic poly(rA) (polyriboadenylic acid), the resulting recPrP[Sc] is equally infectious and causes prion disease in wild-type animals with a 100% attack rate. Since poly(rA) does not contain meaningful genetic information, the latter experiment reveals that the role of poly(rA) is to facilitate PrP conformational change instead of providing genetic information for the infectivity, and disproves the 'virino hypothesis' [29]. Generation of recPrP[Sc] *in vitro* with defined cofactors strongly supports that the pathogen in prion disease is a protein-conformation-based infectious agent [28–30].

Cofactors: possible roles in prion infectivity and prion strains

Thus far, it remains unclear whether cofactors are essential for the infectivity or just contribute as a chaperone to facilitate PrP to reach the infectious conformation. The most recent success in generating infectious recPrP[Sc] with only a single cofactor, synthetic PE (phosphatidylethanolamine), indicates that polyanions such as RNA are not essential for prion infectivity [31]. However, whether lipid is required for prion infectivity remains unanswered. Early ionizing radiation studies indicated a role of lipids in maintaining high prion infectivity [32]. Recent attempts to generate infectious prions with bacterially expressed recPrP showed that the infectivity of pure recPrP amyloid fibrils or recPrP[Sc] formed by PMCA [33,34] in the absence of any cofactor is very low, but the infectivity of recPrP[Sc] generated by PMCA in the presence of a lipid cofactor is much higher. These results suggest that lipid cofactors might be important for PrP to gain and/or maintain the highly infectious conformation.

A puzzling observation in prion disease is the presence of multiple strains. The 'protein-only hypothesis' explains the prion strain phenomenon by variations in PrP[Sc] conformation. However, the fact that a single protein can stably exist in multiple conformations (>20 prion strains in mouse) is difficult to reconcile with the thermodynamic rules of protein folding. If the stable infectious PrP^{Sc} conformation is maintained by forming a PrP^{Sc}–cofactor complex, it is not difficult to envision that different cofactors (e.g. phospholipids with different head-groups) or different PrP/cofactor ratios would result in multiple stable infectious PrP^{Sc} conformations. A recent study showed that propagating three prion strains to recPrP with PE as the sole cofactor led to the convergence of three strains to a single new strain, supporting a role of cofactors in modulating prion strain phenotype [35]. If cofactors indeed contribute to the formation of prion strains, it would bring the peculiar prion strain phenomenon back to the protein-folding paradigm.

Conclusions

After decades of intense research and heated debate, the latest studies provide unequivocal evidence supporting that a protein-conformation-based infectious agent is responsible for the transmissibility of prion disease (or TSEs). If cofactors are essential for prion infectivity, does it disprove the 'protein-only hypothesis'? If one interprets 'protein-only' in the strictest manner that no other factors are required in the propagation of the infectious PrP^{Sc} conformers, then the requirement of a cofactor, even as a chaperone, would be inconsistent with the hypothesis. However, it might be more plausible to interpret the 'protein-only hypothesis' as requiring that the genetic information of prion infectivity be carried only by protein conformation. In this case, even if cofactors are required for the infectivity, the information of infectivity is still governed by protein conformation, which is consistent with the 'protein-only hypothesis'. Further studies to elucidate the role(s) of cofactors in prion infectivity and the formation and evolution of diverse prion strains would lead to a better understanding of the enigmatic agent in prion diseases. Moreover, the generation of recombinant prions *in vitro* makes it possible to study the high-resolution three-dimensional structure of the infectious PrP^{Sc}, which would provide a molecular basis for explaining the puzzling biological observations and for developing diagnostic and therapeutic tools. The clean recombinant prion system also offers a valuable platform to investigate the molecular mechanism of prion propagation and to screen for compounds that inhibit prion propagation. These studies are not only important for us to combat the devastating prion diseases, but they may also shed light on the mechanism of recently discovered 'prion-like' propagation of misfolded proteins in a variety of more common neurodegenerative disorders [36].

Summary

- Prion diseases are a group of infectious illnesses affecting humans and animals.
- The infectious agent in prion disease has been proposed to be a prion, an infectious protein that is capable of self-propagating in the absence of nucleic acid.
- The 'protein-only hypothesis' posits that prions self-replicate by conveying the infectious protein conformation to its normally folded counterpart.
- Various PrP conversion studies have provided unequivocal evidence supporting the 'protein-only hypothesis'.

- Generating highly infectious recombinant prions with bacterially expressed recPrP in the presence of defined cofactors supports that a protein-conformation-based infectious agent is responsible for the infectivity in prion disease.
- Experiments suggest that cofactors may play a role in maintaining the highly infectious prion conformation and encoding various prion strains.

References

1. Prusiner, S.B. (1998) Prions. Proc. Natl. Acad. Sci. U.S.A. **95**, 13363–13383
2. Aguzzi, A., Baumann, F. and Bremer, J. (2008) The prion's elusive reason for being. Annu. Rev. Neurosci. **31**, 439–477
3. Sigurdson, C.J. and Aguzzi, A. (2007) Chronic wasting disease. Biochim. Biophys. Acta **1772**(6), 610–618
4. Kraus, A., Groveman, B.R. and Caughey, B. (2013) Prions and the potential transmissibility of protein misfolding diseases. Annu. Rev. Microbiol. **67**, 543–564
5. Curril, J. and Chelle, P.L. (1936) Is the disease of scrapie inoculable? Comptes Rendus Hebdomadaires Des Seances De L Academie Des Sciences **203**, 1552–1554
6. Cuille, J. and Chelle, P.L. (1939) Experimental transmission of trembling to the goat. C.R. Seances Acad. Sci. **208**, 1058–1160
7. Wang, F. and Ma, J. (2013) Role of lipid in forming an infectious prion? Acta Biochim. Biophys. Sin. (Shanghai). **45**, 485–493
8. Alper, T., Cramp, W.A., Haig, D.A. and Clarke, M.C. (1967) Does the agent of scrapie replicate without nucleic acid? Nature **214**, 764–766
9. Pattison, I.H. and Jones, K.M. (1967) The possible nature of the transmissible agent of scrapie. Vet Rec. **80**, 2–9
10. Griffith, J.S. (1967) Self-replication and scrapie. Nature **215**, 1043–1044
11. Prusiner, S.B. (1982) Novel proteinaceous infectious particles cause scrapie. Science **216**, 136–144
12. Bueler, H., Aguzzi, A., Sailer, A., Greiner, R.A., Autenried, P., Aguet, M. and Weissmann, C. (1993) Mice devoid of PrP are resistant to scrapie. Cell **73**, 1339–1347
13. Sailer, A., Bueler, H., Fischer, M., Aguzzi, A. and Weissmann, C. (1994) No propagation of prions in mice devoid of PrP. Cell **77**, 967–968
14. Kocisko, D.A., Come, J.H., Priola, S.A., Chesebro, B., Raymond, G.J., Lansbury, P.T. and Caughey, B. (1994) Cell-free formation of protease-resistant prion protein. Nature **370**, 471–474
15. Saborio, G.P., Permanne, B. and Soto, C. (2001) Sensitive detection of pathological prion protein by cyclic amplification of protein misfolding. Nature **411**, 810–813
16. Castilla, J., Saa, P., Hetz, C. and Soto, C. (2005) *In vitro* generation of infectious scrapie prions. Cell **121**, 195–206
17. Kimberlin, R.H. (1982) Scrapie agent: prions or virinos? Nature **297**, 107–108
18. Hornemann, S., Schorn, C. and Wuthrich, K. (2004) NMR structure of the bovine prion protein isolated from healthy calf brains. EMBO Rep. **5**, 1159–1164
19. Swietnicki, W., Petersen, R., Gambetti, P. and Surewicz, W.K. (1997) pH-dependent stability and conformation of the recombinant human prion protein PrP(90–231). J. Biol. Chem. **272**, 27517–27520
20. Baskakov, I.V., Legname, G., Baldwin, M.A., Prusiner, S.B. and Cohen, F.E. (2002) Pathway complexity of prion protein assembly into amyloid. J. Biol. Chem. **277**, 21140–21148
21. Legname, G., Baskakov, I.V., Nguyen, H.O., Riesner, D., Cohen, F.E., DeArmond, S.J. and Prusiner, S.B. (2004) Synthetic mammalian prions. Science **305**, 673–676

22. Colby, D.W., Wain, R., Baskakov, I.V., Legname, G., Palmer, C.G., Nguyen, H.O., Lemus, A., Cohen, F.E., DeArmond, S.J. and Prusiner, S.B. (2010) Protease-sensitive synthetic prions. PLoS Pathog. **6**, e1000736

23. Wong, C., Xiong, L.W., Horiuchi, M., Raymond, L., Wehrly, K., Chesebro, B. and Caughey, B. (2001) Sulfated glycans and elevated temperature stimulate PrP(Sc)-dependent cell-free formation of protease-resistant prion protein. EMBO J. **20**, 377–386

24. Deleault, N.R., Lucassen, R.W. and Supattapone, S. (2003) RNA molecules stimulate prion protein conversion. Nature **425**, 717–720

25. Deleault, N.R., Harris, B.T., Rees, J.R. and Supattapone, S. (2007) Formation of native prions from minimal components *in vitro*. Proc. Natl. Acad. Sci. U.S.A. **104**, 9741–9746

26. Morillas, M., Swietnicki, W., Gambetti, P. and Surewicz, W.K. (1999) Membrane environment alters the conformational structure of the recombinant human prion protein. J. Biol. Chem. **274**, 36859–36865

27. Wang, F., Yang, F., Hu, Y., Wang, X., Jin, C. and Ma, J. (2007) Lipid interaction converts prion protein to a PrPSc-like proteinase K-resistant conformation under physiological conditions. Biochemistry **46**, 7045–7053

28. Wang, F., Wang, X., Yuan, C.G. and Ma, J. (2010) Generating a prion with bacterially expressed recombinant prion protein. Science **327**, 1132–1135

29. Wang, F., Zhang, Z., Wang, X., Li, J., Zha, L., Yuan, C.G., Weissmann, C. and Ma, J. (2012) Genetic informational RNA is not required for recombinant prion infectivity. J. Virol. **86**, 1874–1876

30. Zhang, Z., Zhang, Y., Wang, F., Wang, X., Xu, Y., Yang, H., Yu, G., Yuan, C. and Ma, J. (2013) *De novo* generation of infectious prions with bacterially expressed recombinant prion protein. FASEB J. **27**, 4768–4775

31. Deleault, N.R., Piro, J.R., Walsh, D.J., Wang, F., Ma, J., Geoghegan, J.C. and Supattapone, S. (2012) Isolation of phosphatidylethanolamine as a solitary cofactor for prion formation in the absence of nucleic acids. Proc. Natl. Acad. Sci. U.S.A. **109**, 8546–8551

32. Alper, T., Haig, D.A. and Clarke, M.C. (1978) The scrapie agent: evidence against its dependence for replication on intrinsic nucleic acid. J. Gen. Virol. **41**, 503–516

33. Makarava, N., Kovacs, G.G., Bocharova, O., Savtchenko, R., Alexeeva, I., Budka, H., Rohwer, R.G. and Baskakov, I.V. (2010) Recombinant prion protein induces a new transmissible prion disease in wild-type animals. Acta Neuropathol. **119**, 177–187

34. Kim, J.I., Cali, I., Surewicz, K., Kong, Q., Raymond, G.J., Atarashi, R., Race, B., Qing, L., Gambetti, P., Caughey, B. and Surewicz, W.K. (2010) Mammalian prions generated from bacterially expressed prion protein in the absence of any mammalian cofactors. J. Biol. Chem. **285**, 14083–14087

35. Deleault, N.R., Walsh, D.J., Piro, J.R., Wang, F., Wang, X., Ma, J., Rees, J.R. and Supattapone, S. (2012) Cofactor molecules maintain infectious conformation and restrict strain properties in purified prions. Proc. Natl. Acad. Sci. U.S.A. **109**, E1938–E1946

36. Prusiner, S.B. (2012) Cell biology: a unifying role for prions in neurodegenerative diseases. Science **336**, 1511–1513

© The Authors Journal compilation © 2014 Biochemical Society
Essays Biochem. (2014) 56, 193–205: doi: 10.1042/BSE0560193

14

Amyloid diseases of yeast: prions are proteins acting as genes

Reed B. Wickner[1], Herman K. Edskes, David A. Bateman, Amy C. Kelly, Anton Gorkovskiy, Yaron Dayani and Albert Zhou

Laboratory of Biochemistry and Genetics, National Institute of Diabetes and Digestive and Kidney Diseases, National Institutes of Health, Bethesda, MD 20892–0830, U.S.A.

Abstract

The unusual genetic properties of the non-chromosomal genetic elements [URE3] and [PSI+] led to them being identified as prions (infectious proteins) of Ure2p and Sup35p respectively. Ure2p and Sup35p, and now several other proteins, can form amyloid, a linear ordered polymer of protein monomers, with a part of each molecule, the prion domain, forming the core of this β-sheet structure. Amyloid filaments passed to a new cell seed the conversion of the normal form of the protein into the same amyloid form. The cell's phenotype is affected, usually from the deficiency of the normal form of the protein. Solid-state NMR studies indicate that the yeast prion amyloids are in-register parallel β-sheet structures, in which each residue (e.g. Asn^{35}) forms a row along the filament long axis. The favourable interactions possible for aligned identical hydrophilic and hydrophobic residues are believed to be the mechanism for propagation of amyloid conformation. Thus, just as DNA mediates inheritance by templating its own sequence, these proteins act as genes by templating their conformation. Distinct isolates of a given prion have different biological properties, presumably determined by differences between the amyloid structures. Many lines of evidence indicate that the *Saccharomyces cerevisiae* prions are pathological disease agents, although the example of the [Het-s] prion of *Podospora anserina* shows that a prion can have beneficial aspects.

Keywords:

[PIN+], [PSI+], [URE3], in-register parallel β-sheet, solid-state NMR, Sup35p, Ure2p.

[1]*To whom correspondence should be addressed (email wickner@helix.nih.gov).*

Introduction

Infectious elements in yeast generally appear as non-chromosomal genetic elements. Most differences between mated strains segregate 2+ :2− in meiosis, the pattern of a difference in a single chromosomal gene. However, if one parent in a genetic cross carries one of the yeast viruses and the other does not, all of the meiotic progeny will have the virus, a pattern called 4+ :0 segregation. Yeast viruses (and prions) do not exit one cell into the environment and then enter another as is the case for human viruses or prions. [URE3] [1] and [PSI+] [2] are two long-known yeast non-chromosomal genetic elements whose basis was unknown. The similarity of the phenotype of [URE3] to that of mutants in the *ure2* chromosomal gene, and the fact that *URE2* is necessary for the propagation of [URE3] [3], first led us to suspect that [URE3] was actually a prion form of the Ure2 protein, an altered form of Ure2p with the ability to catalyse the conversion of the normal form into the same altered (inactive) form [4]. Ure2p is a regulator of nitrogen catabolism, turning off the genes encoding enzymes and transporters needed for using poor nitrogen sources if a good nitrogen source was present in the medium [5,6]. If [URE3] were indeed a prion, we reasoned that overproduction of Ure2p should increase the frequency with which the [URE3] non-chromosomal genetic element would arise, and this too proved to be true [4]. Various treatments can induce very frequent mutation of the mitochondrial DNA or curing of yeast viruses: growth in the presence of guanidine [7] or ethidium bromide [8], for example, induces mutation in mitochondrial DNA and its loss. But although these mitochondrial DNA mutations or loss are irreversible, curing a prion should be reversible, since the prion-forming protein is still being made in the cell and should be able (rarely) to again convert into the prion form. Thus, *reversible* curability (not curability itself) is expected to be a trait of a prion [4]. Indeed, [URE3] can be cured by growth in the presence of low concentrations of guanidine, but, unlike guanidine-induced mitochondrial DNA curing, that of [URE3] is reversible (at low frequency), again indicating it is a prion [4].

Interestingly, these three properties had already been shown for [PSI+] and the *SUP35* gene [9–11], and we concluded that [PSI+] was likewise a prion of Sup35p [4]. Sup35p is a subunit of the translation termination factor, a protein whose activity is, unlike that of Ure2p, essential for growth of *Saccharomyces cerevisiae* [12,13].

The prion concept first arose as a leading hypothesis in studies of the uniformly lethal mammalian TSEs (transmissible spongiform encephalopathies) [14–16], but proving it was difficult because of the long incubation times for even infected rodents. Although the yeast prion systems can be non-lethal (but see below), show phenotypes unrelated to the TSE diseases and involve proteins with no sequence relation to the mammalian prion protein PrP, the yeast systems provided an important model in which it was possible to actually prove that proteins could be infectious elements, and quickly explore the mechanisms involved.

Most yeast prions are amyloid forms of a normally soluble protein

Amyloid is a filamentous polymer of identical protein monomers that is characterized by a cross-β structure (see next section). Amyloids play a prominent role in human degenerative diseases such as Alzheimer's disease, Parkinson's disease and amyotrophic lateral sclerosis. These neurodegenerative diseases, each quite common, are caused by deposits of amyloid, each of a specific protein or peptide, which cause damage to the brain. Type 2 (late onset) diabetes mellitus is associated with (although probably not caused by) deposits of amylin, a peptide that, similar to insulin, is made in the islets of the pancreas. Senile amyloidosis is a very common disorder of the elderly due to deposition of amyloid filaments of transthyretin, a protein normally found in serum.

Perhaps with the many amyloidoses of humans it is not surprising that yeast has several amyloid diseases. A series of studies showed that Sup35p is aggregated in cells carrying the [PSI+] prion, that Ure2p is aggregated in [URE3] cells, and similarly for the other identified yeast prions (see Table 1) [17–19]. Recombinant Sup35p could form amyloid *in vitro* [20,21] and introduction of this amyloid into yeast cells makes them prion positive [22,23]. Similar results were later obtained for Ure2p and [URE3] [24,25]. Thus these amyloid filaments are infectious.

Prion variants

A single prion protein sequence can form amyloids of different detailed structure resulting in different biological properties. These are called 'prion variants'. Since prions are proteins acting

Table 1. Prions of *S. cerevisiae* and *P. anserina*

Prion	Protein	Normal function	Prion phenotype	Reference
[URE3]	Ure2p	Nitrogen regulation	Inappropriate derepression of nitrogen catabolism genes and slow growth	[4]
[PSI+]	Sup35p	Translation termination	Readthrough of translation stop codons	[4]
[PIN+]	Rnq1p	Unknown	Rare cross-seeding of [PSI+] or other prions	[79]
[SWI+]	Swi1p	Chromatin remodelling	Inability to utilize non-fermentable carbon source and slow growth	[80]
[OCT+]	Cyc8p	Transcription repression	Derepressed transcription and flocculence	[81]
[MOT+]	Mot3p	Repressor of genes for anaerobic growth	Inappropriate derepression of anaerobic growth genes	[82]
[ISP+]	Sfp1p	Transcription factor	Decreased translation readthrough	[83]
[MOD+]	Mod5p	tRNA isopentenyl transferase	Slow growth and resistance to azole anti-fungal drugs	[84]
[Het-s]	HET-s	Heterokaryon incompatibility	Heterokaryon incompatibility in *P. anserina* (a functional prion)	[63]
[BETA]	Prb1p	Vacuolar protease B	Normal sporulation and survival in stationary phase (a functional prion)	[85]

as genes, prion variants can be thought of as different alleles of the protein gene. Each prion variant is (relatively) stable and propagates as cells divide. Prion variants were long known in mammalian prions, and were found in yeast prions soon after their discovery [25–27]. In yeast, variants are commonly distinguished based on whether their phenotype is 'strong' or 'weak', whether the variant is stably propagated or readily lost, response to excess or deficiency of certain chaperones, and transmission efficiency across interspecies or intraspecies barriers. The existence of variants is critical in understanding many aspects of prions, including structural studies, interactions of prions with other cellular components and the biological role of prions for yeast.

Prion domains, their structure and biological implications

Only a part of each prion protein actually forms the amyloid structure, and this part is sufficient to transmit the prion trait [20,24,28,29]. These 'prion domains' have been the focus of structural studies. The prion domains of Ure2p and Sup35p are the N-terminal ~70 residues and ~124 residues respectively, although the size of the prion domain varies somewhat with prion variant (see below for discussion of prion variants). One particularly clear demonstration of the role of the prion domain is in Ure2p, whose C-terminal part is essential for its role in regulating nitrogen assimilation, and which has glutathione peroxidase activity [30]. Remarkably, this activity is unaffected by amyloid formation, showing that the C-terminal domain is unchanged by amyloid formation, including its homodimer status [30]. The definition of amyloid includes the cross-β structure, meaning that the filaments are rich in β-sheet, and that the β-strands run perpendicular to the long axis of the filament. Within this definition are several possible architectures, depending on the relation of the β-strands to each other:

(i)   Antiparallel β-sheets have adjacent β-strands running in opposite directions. This is the most common type of β-sheet in monomeric proteins.

(ii)   In parallel β-sheets, the peptide chains are oriented in the same direction. If a parallel β-sheet is in-register, each residue is aligned with the same residue in the molecule before and after it in the filament (see Figure 1). Each molecule occupies a single 4.7 Å (1 Å = 0.1 nm) layer along the long axis of the filament. In-register parallel β-sheets are the most common architecture of pathologic amyloids (reviewed in [31]), and current evidence supports this form for the infectious amyloids of the prion domains of Sup35p, Ure2p and Rnq1p [32–34].

(iii)   In a β-helix, each molecule occupies more than one layer along the long axis of the filament. Each molecule forms a helix of two or more turns (see Figure 1). This architecture has been observed in the [Het-s] prion of *Podospora anserina* [35,36].

The parallel in-register structure is maintained because of favourable interactions between identical amino acid side chains. Hydrophilic side chains can form a line of hydrogen bonds along the filament long axis and hydrophobic residues can favourably interact, but only if they are aligned. Aligned charged residues would repel each other, but there are very few charged residues in these prion domains. These favourable interactions stabilize the in-register

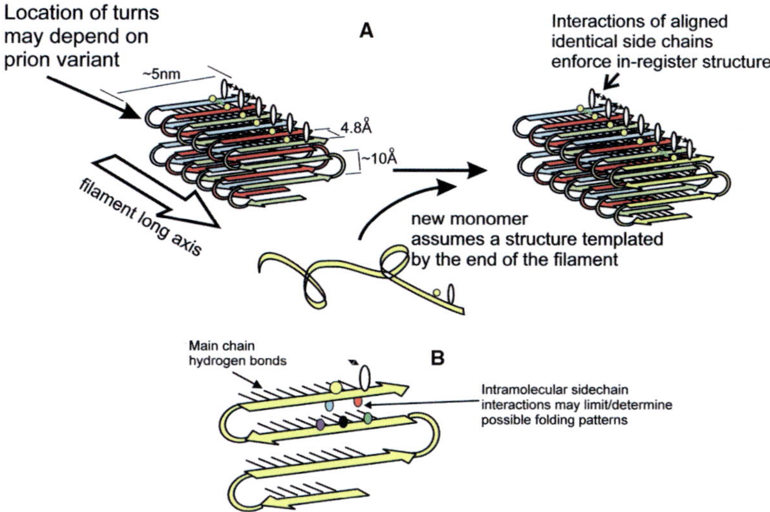

Figure 1. The in-register parallel architecture of yeast prion amyloid can explain templating of conformation

(**A**) The unstructured prion domain of molecules newly joining the end of the amyloid filament are directed to assume the same conformation as molecules already in the filament by the favourable interactions between identical side chains that can only occur if the molecules are in-register [77]. (**B**) Three interactions of an amino acid residue are shown. The black lines show the main chain hydrogen bonds of the β-sheet. The black double-headed arrow indicates the intermolecular side-chain interactions between identical residues (emphasized in **A**). Also shown are the interactions between non-identical side chains in the plane perpendicular to the long axis of the filaments. These interactions have been studied by X-ray crystallography of short peptides [78].

parallel structure and direct a new monomer joining the ends of the filaments to assume the same conformation as that of the other monomers in the filament. Like the hydrogen bonding of complementary bases in DNA allows templating of sequence, these interactions of identical side chains allow templating of conformation.

Biology of yeast prions

Prions arise stochastically, and not in response to specific environmental cues (an apparent exception will be discussed below). Thus, it would seem counterproductive to inactivate Ure2p at a random time, even though its normal function is to become inactive when good nitrogen sources are lacking in the medium, the appropriate time for this to happen. Similarly, allowing translational readthrough of all mRNAs by inactivation of Sup35p does not seem to be a useful way to regulate gene expression. Nonetheless, there have been suggestions that the [PSI+] prion, and even [URE3], are beneficial to yeast. A report that [PSI+] made cells resistant to heat or high ethanol concentrations [37] was not reproduced in a subsequent study [38], and the advantages of [PSI+] reported in that study were not reproduced (using the same strains) in a further study [39]. A report of specific induction of [PSI+] generation by certain unfavourable conditions [40] was, again, not reproducible [41], but even in the original report, [PSI+] was usually unfavourable for growth under the conditions reported to induce its appearance [40], suggesting that this is not an adaptive response.

Even deadly viruses are found in natural populations because infectious agents can spread and outstrip the damage they do to their hosts. An advantageous infectious agent would surely be nearly universal in its distribution because infectivity and benefit to the host would be working together, instead of in opposition. Thus an infectious agent that is rare in the wild must be detrimental to its host. To examine the issue of whether yeast prions are adaptive or detrimental, we surveyed 70 wild yeast strains, and found that none carried either [URE3] or [PSI+], although each of the known selfish DNA/RNA plasmids and viruses of yeast were found in varying proportions of the wild isolates [42]. This implied that these prions, even their mildest variants, must be detrimental to their hosts. Another study confirmed the rarity of [PSI+] in the wild, but did not examine [URE3] [43]. This study did report frequent phenotypes of wild strains that were affected by growth on guanidine, and inferred that these phenotypes were due to unknown prions [43]. We were able to quantify the detriment of acquiring a prion by comparing the frequency of the prions to that of 2 μm DNA, a selfish plasmid known to slow cell growth by 1–3% [44–46], but nevertheless found in over half of wild isolates [42]. We find that the mildest forms of the [PSI+], [URE3] and [PIN+] prions must have a >1% detrimental effect on growth and/or survival to account for their limited occurrence in the wild [41].

In trying to understand the overall effect of prion formation, one must consider the entire range of variants that can be formed. This range is as yet only beginning to be explored. In isolation of any prions, it is axiomatic that a lethal prion would not be recovered unless some special measures were taken to detect it. Sup35p is essential for growth, but the N-terminal prion domain is not essential. Low level expression of the essential C-terminal part of Sup35 lacking the prion domain allowed us to detect the formation of lethal [PSI+] prions [47]. Indeed, lethal and near-lethal variants of [PSI+] comprised more than half of total isolates, showing that [PSI+] generation is not generally a favourable event.

The method by which we isolated lethal [PSI+] variants implied that they were lethal because nearly all of the Sup35p joined the amyloid, leaving an insufficient amount for translation termination. This is not the mechanism of lethality of the TSE diseases, since the PrP protein is completely non-essential. Rather, the prion form of PrP has some toxic effect. Ure2p is likewise non-essential and, depending on the strain background, deletion of *URE2* may not even slow cell growth. Using such a strain, we found that many [URE3] isolates were extremely toxic, slowing cell growth dramatically [47]. Although the mechanism of [URE3] toxicity remains unclear, these results again show that acquisition of a yeast prion, like mutation of a chromosomal gene, is not generally a beneficial event.

The prion domains of Ure2p and Sup35p are perhaps misnamed as they have normal functions. The Sup35p prion domain is involved in the mRNA turnover process, interacting with poly(A)-binding protein and the poly(A)-degrading enzymes. In the absence of the Sup35p 'prion domain', turnover of all mRNAs is much slower [48]. The prion domain of Ure2p is necessary for the stability of Ure2p *in vivo*, and so plays an important role in the molecule [49]. Thus these domains are not conserved for the purpose of prion formation. In fact, the Ure2p elements of *Kluyveromyces lactis* or *Candida glabrata* that have an N-terminal 'prion domain'-like region cannot, in fact, form prions, even in their native hosts [50,51]. Prion-forming ability appears to be sporadically arising, rather than conserved.

Sequence comparisons of Ure2p and Sup35p show that the prion domains change much more rapidly than does the remainder of either molecule [52–56]. These accumulated changes result in barriers to transmission of the [URE3] and [PSI+] prion between species [52,55]. Even within the genus *Saccharomyces* there are barriers to transmission of [URE3] [57] and [PSI+] [58] based on sequence differences in the prion domains. There are even polymorphs in the Sup35p prion domain of wild *S. cerevisiae* isolates [54,59,60] that result in intraspecies barriers to transmission of [PSI+] [60]. Indeed, the rare wild isolates of [PSI+] are sensitive to these barriers [60]. Just as in humans, where polymorphism at residue 129 of PrP results in a barrier to prion transmission [61], it is likely that these Sup35p polymorphisms were selected because of the transmission barrier they provide [60]. This suggests that prion acquisition is unfavourable, not advantageous.

The above is not to contend that no prions can be beneficial, or that no yeast prions can be beneficial. We were the first to hail [62] a beneficial prion, the [Het-s] prion of the filamentous fungus *P. anserina*, which has a role in heterokaryon incompatibility, a normal function of filamentous fungi [63]. [Het-s] is striking in that it is present in 80% of wild strains of the appropriate chromosomal genotype, and forms only a single prion variant, as expected for a functional prion. This contrasts with the properties of those yeast prions investigated to date.

Prion clouds

Prions, similar to viruses and plasmids, are expected to be able to segregate during growth if they are mixed to begin with, and to mutate. Work on mammalian prions has suggested that prions exist as a 'cloud', a mixture of variants in one animal or cell [64,65], and classic experiments with mouse scrapie showed that prions can mutate (without change in the protein sequence) when subjected to selective pressure [66].

We found that [PSI+] transmission to different polymorphs of Sup35p depends strongly on the prion variant examined [60]. A given [PSI+] clone can be a mixture of variants with different patterns of transmission, and simple mitotic growth results in segregation of clones with different transmission patterns [67]. However, extensive growth of a clone with one pattern results in production of clones, some of which have different patterns, indicating that there is variant mutation occurring as well [67]. The details of the experimental procedure were such that the changes were occurring without selection or interference with amyloid propagation. Interestingly, either 'strong' [PSI+] or 'weak' [PSI+] can have any of the four transmission phenotypes. Thus yeast prions can exist as a cloud, a mixture of variants each of which is relatively stable, but that can interconvert over time under non-selective conditions. Further definition of the possible prion variant phenotypes and the mechanisms by which these phenotypes are produced will be an important area of future work.

Chaperones and prions

The involvement of chaperones, proteins that aid in the correct folding of other proteins, in prion phenomena began with Chernoff's identification of Hsp104 as a gene whose overproduction could cure [PSI+], although [PSI+] was not then known to be a prion [68]. Either overproduction or deficiency of Hsp104 cures [PSI+] [69]. Hsp104 working together with Hsp70 and Hsp40 chaperone families, break amyloid filaments producing new seeds, an essential step in prion propagation (reviewed by [70]). Other chaperones, co-chaperones and nucleotide exchange factors have also been found to play key roles in prion propagation (reviewed in [71]).

Btn2p, Cur1p and prion aggregate collection

A screen for proteins whose overproduction could cure the [URE3] prion produced two somewhat homologous proteins, Btn2p and Cur1p [72]. Deletion of both genes produced substantial effects on prion generation and increased prion stability, indicating that the normal levels of these proteins also affect prions [72]. In cells in the process of being cured of [URE3] by overproduced Btn2p, Ure2p and Btn2p were often co-localized in a single site, suggesting that sequestration of amyloid filaments might prevent one of the progeny cells from getting any seeds [72]. This was not observed in the case of curing of [URE3] by Cur1p. The involvement of the chaperone Hsp42 in aggregated protein sequestration was documented by Bukau and co-workers [73], and the interaction of Hsp42 with Btn2p (but not Cur1p) was shown by Malinovska et al. [74]. Several differences between Btn2p action and Cur1p action have been documented in spite of their sequence similarity. Mammalian cells have a centrosome-proximal structure at which aggregated proteins are collected [75]. In studying huntingtin aggregation in yeast, an aggresome-like structure was also identified [76]. Further work will be needed to completely define the actions of these systems, and their relation to each other.

Perspectives

In just under 20 years, the yeast prion field has reached a point where a great deal of information has accumulated and some of the central messages can be understood. However, there remain many very important areas that are largely unclear or controversial. The detailed structure of yeast prion variants has so far resisted all attempts at solution. What is the scope of prion variants, and how do they produce their many effects? The dramatic difference between a mild [PSI+] or [URE3] and a lethal form of the same prion suggests that there may be parallels in mammalian amyloidoses. Although Alzheimer's disease may be fatal, patients deceased from another cause are often found with extensive amyloidosis, but no brain damage. This is often taken as evidence that amyloid is not the toxic species, but it could well be that such patients have a mild amyloid variant, analogous to mild [PSI+] or mild [URE3] and a range of Aβ (amyloid β-peptide) structures have been defined [31].

The functions of Btn2p and Cur1p, as well as the role of yeast aggresomes in dealing with aggregated proteins of various sorts, remain to be elucidated. The many effects of elevated and depressed chaperones are far from understood. Yeast prions are largely pathogenic, but it remains possible that some functional yeast prions, such as [Het-s] of *P. anserina*, will be found. Certainly the non-amyloid prion [BETA], the active form of vacuolar protease B, is beneficial to the cell. With an increasing number of prions identified in *S. cerevisae*, it seems likely that many prions that are not simply homologues of those found in this yeast will be found in other organisms if appropriate searches are made. It is perhaps most striking that proteins can act as genes, not often, but enough to make it interesting.

Summary

- Certain yeast proteins can form self-propagating amyloid (a fibrous β-sheet-rich aggregate) that produces cellular defects, largely by inactivating the amyloid-forming protein.
- The self-propagation of the amyloids makes them infectious and heritable, so these proteins act as genes by templating their conformation, just as DNA templates its sequence.
- Chaperones play an important part in prion generation and propagation, and aggregate-collecting mechanisms also impinge on prion processes.

This work was supported by the Intramural Program of the National Institute of Diabetes and Digestive and Kidney Diseases.

References

1. Lacroute, F. (1971) Non-Mendelian mutation allowing ureidosuccinic acid uptake in yeast. J. Bacteriol. **106**, 519–522

2. Cox, B.S. (1965) PSI, a cytoplasmic suppressor of super-suppressor in yeast. Heredity **20**, 505–521

3. Aigle, M. and Lacroute, F. (1975) Genetical aspects of [URE3], a non-Mendelian, cytoplasmically inherited mutation in yeast. Molec. Gen. Genet. **136**, 327–335

4. Wickner, R.B. (1994) [URE3] as an altered *URE2* protein: evidence for a prion analog in *S. cerevisiae*. Science **264**, 566–569

5. Cooper, T.G. (2002) Transmitting the signal of excess nitrogen in *Saccharomyces cerevisiae* from the Tor proteins to th GATA factors: connecting the dots. FEMS Microbiol. Rev. **26**, 223–238

6. Magasanik, B. and Kaiser, C.A. (2002) Nitrogen regulation in *Saccharomyces cerevisiae*. Gene **290**, 1–18

7. Villa, L.L. and Juliani, M.H. (1980) Mechanism of rho⁻ induction in *Saccharomyces cerevisiae* by guanidine hydrochloride. Mutat. Res. **7**, 147–153

8. Goldring, E.S., Grossman, L.I., Krupnick, D., Cryer, D.R. and Marmur, J. (1970) The petite mutation in yeast: loss of mitochondrial DNA during induction of petites with ethidium bromide. J. Mol. Biol. **52**, 323–335

9. Lund, P.M. and Cox, B.S. (1981) Reversion analysis of [psi-] mutations in *Saccharomyces cerevisiae*. Genet. Res. **37**, 173–182

10. Chernoff, Y.O., Derkach, I.L. and Inge-Vechtomov, S.G. (1993) Multicopy SUP35 gene induces *de novo* appearance of psi-like factors in the yeast *Saccharomyces cerevisiae*. Curr. Genet. **24**, 268–270

11. Doel, S.M., McCready, S.J., Nierras, C.R. and Cox, B.S. (1994) The dominant *PNM2⁻* mutation which eliminates the [PSI] factor of *Saccharomyces cerevisiae* is the result of a missense mutation in the *SUP35* gene. Genetics **137**, 659–670

12. Stansfield, I. and Tuite, M.F. (1994) Polypeptide chain termination in *Saccharomyces cerevisiae*. Curr. Genet. **25**, 385–395

13. Frolova, L., LeGoff, X., Rasmussen, H.H., Cheperegin, S., Drugeon, G., Kress, M., Arman, I., Haenni, A.-L., Celis, J.E., Philippe, M. et al. (1994) A highly conserved eukaryotic protein family possessing properties of polypeptide chain release factor. Nature **372**, 701–703

14. Alper, T., Cramp, W.A., Haig, D.A. and Clarke, M.C. (1967) Does the agent of scrapie replicate without nucleic acid? Nature **214**, 764–766

15. Griffith, J.S. (1967) Self-replication and scrapie. Nature **215**, 1043–1044

16. Prusiner, S.B. (1982) Novel proteinaceous infectious particles cause scrapie. Science **216**, 136–144

17. Paushkin, S.V., Kushnirov, V.V., Smirnov, V.N. and Ter-Avanesyan, M.D. (1996) Propagation of the yeast prion-like [*psi*⁺] determinant is mediated by oligomerization of the *SUP35*-encoded polypeptide chain release factor. EMBO J. **15**, 3127–3134

18. Patino, M.M., Liu, J.-J., Glover, J.R. and Lindquist, S. (1996) Support for the prion hypothesis for inheritance of a phenotypic trait in yeast. Science **273**, 622–626

19. Edskes, H.K., Gray, V.T. and Wickner, R.B. (1999) The [URE3] prion is an aggregated form of Ure2p that can be cured by overexpression of Ure2p fragments. Proc. Natl. Acad. Sci. U.S.A. **96**, 1498–1503

20. King, C.-Y., Tittmann, P., Gross, H., Gebert, R., Aebi, M. and Wuthrich, K. (1997) Prion-inducing domain 2–114 of yeast Sup35 protein transforms *in vitro* into amyloid-like filaments. Proc. Natl. Acad. Sci. U.S.A. **94**, 6618–6622

21. Glover, J.R., Kowal, A.S., Shirmer, E.C., Patino, M.M., Liu, J.-J. and Lindquist, S. (1997) Self-seeded fibers formed by Sup35, the protein determinant of [*PSI* +], a heritable prion-like factor of *S. cerevisiae*. Cell **89**, 811–819

22. King, C.Y. and Diaz-Avalos, R. (2004) Protein-only transmission of three yeast prion strains. Nature **428**, 319–323

23. Tanaka, M., Chien, P., Naber, N., Cooke, R. and Weissman, J.S. (2004) Conformational variations in an infectious protein determine prion strain differences. Nature **428**, 323–328

24. Taylor, K.L., Cheng, N., Williams, R.W., Steven, A.C. and Wickner, R.B. (1999) Prion domain initiation of amyloid formation *in vitro* from native Ure2p. Science **283**, 1339–1343

25. Brachmann, A., Baxa, U. and Wickner, R.B. (2005) Prion generation *in vitro*: amyloid of Ure2p is infectious. EMBO J. **24**, 3082–3092

26. Derkatch, I.L., Chernoff, Y.O., Kushnirov, V.V., Inge-Vechtomov, S.G. and Liebman, S.W. (1996) Genesis and variability of [*PSI*] prion factors in *Saccharomyces cerevisiae*. Genetics **144**, 1375–1386

27. Schlumpberger, M., Prusiner, S.B. and Herskowitz, I. (2001) Induction of distinct [URE3] yeast prion strains. Mol. Cell. Biol. **21**, 7035–7046

28. TerAvanesyan, A., Dagkesamanskaya, A.R., Kushnirov, V.V. and Smirnov, V.N. (1994) The *SUP35* omnipotent suppressor gene is involved in the maintenance of the non-Mendelian determinant [psi +] in the yeast *Saccharomyces cerevisiae*. Genetics **137**, 671–676

29. Masison, D.C. and Wickner, R.B. (1995) Prion-inducing domain of yeast Ure2p and protease resistance of Ure2p in prion-containing cells. Science **270**, 93–95

30. Bai, M., Zhou, J.M. and Perrett, S. (2004) The yeast prion protein Ure2 shows glutathione peroxidase activity in both native and fibrillar forms. J. Biol. Chem. **279**, 50025–50030

31. Tycko, R. (2011) Solid-state NMR studies of amyloid fibril structure. Annu. Rev. Phys. Chem. **62**, 279–299

32. Shewmaker, F., Wickner, R.B. and Tycko, R. (2006) Amyloid of the prion domain of Sup35p has an in-register parallel β-sheet structure. Proc. Natl. Acad. Sci. U.S.A. **103**, 19754–19759

33. Baxa, U., Wickner, R.B., Steven, A.C., Anderson, D., Marekov, L., Yau, W.-M. and Tycko, R. (2007) Characterization of β-sheet structure in Ure2p1–89 yeast prion fibrils by solid state nuclear magnetic resonance. Biochemistry **46**, 13149–13162

34. Wickner, R.B., Dyda, F. and Tycko, R. (2008) Amyloid of Rnq1p, the basis of the [*PIN*⁺] prion, has a parallel in-register β-sheet structure. Proc. Natl. Acad. Sci. U.S.A. **105**, 2403–2408

35. Ritter, C., Maddelein, M.L., Siemer, A.B., Luhrs, T., Ernst, M., Meier, B.H., Saupe, S.J. and Riek, R. (2005) Correlation of structural elements and infectivity of the HET-s prion. Nature **435**, 844–848

36. Siemer, A.B., Arnold, A.A., Ritter, C., Westfeld, T., Ernst, M., Riek, R. and Meier, B.H. (2006) Observation of highly flexible residues in amyloid fibrils of the HET-s prion. J. Am. Chem. Soc. **128**, 13224–13228

37. Eaglestone, S.S., Cox, B.S. and Tuite, M.F. (1999) Translation termination efficiency can be regulated in *Saccharomyces cerevisiae* by environmental stress through a prion-mediated mechanism. EMBO J. **18**, 1974–1981

38. True, H.L. and Lindquist, S.L. (2000) A yeast prion provides a mechanism for genetic variation and phenotypic diversity. Nature **407**, 477–483

39. Namy, O., Galopier, A., Martini, C., Matsufuji, S., Fabret, C. and Rousset, C. (2008) Epigenetic control of polyamines by the prion [*PSI+*]. Nat. Cell. Biol. **10**, 1069–1075

40. Tyedmers, J., Madariaga, M.L. and Lindquist, S. (2008) Prion switching in response to environmental stress. PLoS Biol. **6**, e294

41. Kelly, A.C., Shewmaker, F.P., Kryndushkin, D. and Wickner, R.B. (2012) Sex, prions and plasmids in yeast. Proc. Natl. Acad. Sci. U.S.A. **109**, E2683–E2690

42. Nakayashiki, T., Kurtzman, C.P., Edskes, H.K. and Wickner, R.B. (2005) Yeast prions [URE3] and [*PSI+*] are diseases. Proc. Natl. Acad. Sci. U.S.A. **102**, 10575–10580

43. Halfmann, R., Jarosz, D.F., Jones, S.K., Chang, A., Lancster, A.K. and Lindquist, S. (2012) Prions are a common mechanism for phenotypic inheritance in wild yeasts. Nature **482**, 363–368

44. Futcher, A.B. and Cox, B.S. (1983) Maintenance of the 2 μm circle plasmid in populations of *Saccharomyces cerevisiae*. J. Bacteriol. **154**, 612–622

45. Mead, D.J., Gardner, D.C.J. and Oliver, S.G. (1986) The yeast 2 μ plasmid: strategies for the survival of a selfish DNA. Mol. Gen. Genet. **205**, 417–421

46. Futcher, B., Reid, E. and Hickey, D.A. (1988) Maintenance of the 2 μm circle plasmid of *Saccharomyces cerevisiae* by sexual transmission: an example of selfish DNA. Genetics **118**, 411–415

47. McGlinchey, R., Kryndushkin, D. and Wickner, R.B. (2011) Suicidal [PSI+] is a lethal yeast prion. Proc. Natl. Acad. Sci. U.S.A. **108**, 5337–5341

48. Hoshino, S., Imai, M., Kobayashi, T., Uchida, N. and Katada, T. (1999) The eukaryotic polypeptide chain releasing factor (eRF3/GSPT) carrying the translation termination signal to the 3′;-poly(A) tail of mRNA. J. Biol. Chem. **274**, 16677–16680

49. Shewmaker, F., Mull, L., Nakayashiki, T., Masison, D.C. and Wickner, R.B. (2007) Ure2p function is enhanced by its prion domain in *Saccharomyces cerevisiae*. Genetics **176**, 1557–1565

50. Safadi, R.A., Talarek, N., Jacques, N. and Aigle, M. (2011) Yeast prions: could they be exaptations? The *URE2*/[URE3] system in *Kluyveromyces lactis*. FEMS Yeast Res. **11**, 151–153

51. Edskes, H.K., Engel, A., McCann, L.M., Brachmann, A., Tsai, H.-F. and Wickner, R.B. (2011) Prion-forming ability of Ure2 of yeasts is not evolutionarily conserved. Genetics **188**, 81–90

52. Santoso, A., Chien, P., Osherovich, L.Z. and Weissman, J.S. (2000) Molecular basis of a yeast prion species barrier. Cell **100**, 277–288

53. Chernoff, Y.O., Galkin, A.P., Lewitin, E., Chernova, T.A., Newnam, G.P. and Belenkiy, S.M. (2000) Evolutionary conservation of prion-forming abilities of the yeast Sup35 protein. Mol. Microbiol. **35**, 865–876

54. Resende, C.G., Outeiro, T.F., Sands, L., Lindquist, S. and Tuite, M.F. (2003) Prion protein gene polymorphisms in *Saccharomyces cerevisiae*. Mol. Microbiol. **49**, 1005–1017

55. Edskes, H.K. and Wickner, R.B. (2002) Conservation of a portion of the *S. cerevisiae* Ure2p prion domain that interacts with the full-length protein. Proc. Natl. Acad. Sci. U.S.A. **99**, 16384–16391

56. Baudin-Baillieu, A., Fernandez-Bellot, E., Reine, F., Coissac, E. and Cullin, C. (2003) Conservation of the prion properties of Ure2p through evolution. Mol. Biol. Cell **14**, 3449–3458

57. Edskes, H.K., McCann, L.M., Hebert, A.M. and Wickner, R.B. (2009) Prion variants and species barriers among *Saccharomyces* Ure2 proteins. Genetics **181**, 1159–1167

58. Chen, B., Newnam, G.P. and Chernoff, Y.O. (2007) Prion species barrier between the closely related yeast proteins is detected despite coaggregation. Proc. Natl. Acad. Sci. U.S.A. **104**, 2791–2796

59. Jensen, M.A., True, H.L., Chernoff, Y.O. and Lindquist, S. (2001) Molecular population genetics and evolution of a prion-like protein in *Saccharomyces cerevisiae*. Genetics **159**, 527–535

60. Bateman, D.A. and Wickner, R.B. (2012) [PSI +] prion transmission barriers protect *Saccharomyces cerevisiae* from infection: intraspecies 'species barriers'. Genetics **190**, 569–579

61. Mead, S., Stumpf, M.P., Whitfield, J., Beck, J.A., Poulter, M., Campbell, T., Uphill, J.B., Goldstein, D., Alpers, M., Fisher, E.M. and Collinge, J. (2003) Balancing selection at the prion protein gene consistent with prehistoric kurulike epidemics. Science **300**, 640–643

62. Wickner, R.B. (1997) A new prion controls fungal cell fusion incompatibility. Proc. Natl. Acad. Sci. U.S.A. **94**, 10012–10014

63. Coustou, V., Deleu, C., Saupe, S. and Begueret, J. (1997) The protein product of the *het-s* heterokaryon incompatibility gene of the fungus *Podospora anserina* behaves as a prion analog. Proc. Natl. Acad. Sci. U.S.A. **94**, 9773–9778

64. Collinge, J. and Clarke, A.R. (2007) A general model of prion strains and their pathogenicity. Science **318**, 930–936

65. Li, J., Mahal, S.P., Demczyk, C.A. and Weissmann, C. (2011) Mutability of prions. EMBO Rep. **12**, 1243–1250

66. Kimberlin, R.H., Cole, S. and Walker, C.A. (1987) Temporary and permanent modifications to a single strain of mouse scrapie on transmission to rats and hamsters. J. Gen. Virol. **68**, 1875–1881

67. Bateman, D. and Wickner, R.B. (2013) The [PSI+] prion exists as a dynamic cloud of variants. PLoS Genet. **9**, e1003257

68. Chernoff, Y.O., Inge-Vechtomov, S.G., Derkach, I.L., Ptyushkina, M.V., Tarunina, O.V., Dagkesamanskaya, A.R. and Ter-Avanesyan, M.D. (1992) Dosage-dependent translational suppression in yeast *Saccharomyces cerevisiae*. Yeast **8**, 489–499

69. Chernoff, Y.O., Lindquist, S.L., Ono, B.-I., Inge-Vechtomov, S.G. and Liebman, S.W. (1995) Role of the chaperone protein Hsp104 in propagation of the yeast prion-like factor [psi⁺]. Science **268**, 880–884

70. Reidy, M. and Masison, D.C. (2011) Modulation and elimination of yeast prions by protein chaperones and co-chaperones. Prion **5**, 245–249

71. Liebman, S.W. and Chernoff, Y.O. (2012) Prions in yeast. Genetics **191**, 1041–1072

72. Kryndushkin, D., Shewmaker, F. and Wickner, R.B. (2008) Curing of the [URE3] prion by Btn2p, a Batten disease-related protein. EMBO J. **27**, 2725–2735

73. Specht, S., Miller, S.B. M., Mogk, A. and Bukau, B. (2011) Hsp42 is required for sequestration of protein aggregates into deposition sites in *Saccharomyces cerevisiae*. J. Cell. Biol. **195**, 617–629

74. Malinovska, L., Kroschwald, S., Munder, M.C., Richter, D. and Alberti, S. (2012) Molecular chaperones and stress-inducible protein-sorting factors coordinate the spaciotemporal distribution of protein aggregates. Mol. Biol. Cell **23**, 3041–3056

75. Kopito, R. (2000) Aggresomes, inclusion bodies and protein aggregation. Trends Cell Biol. **10**, 524–530

76. Wang, Y., Meriin, A.B., Zaarur, N., Romanova, N.V., Chernoff, Y.O., Costello, C.E. and Sherman, M.Y. (2009) Abnormal proteins can form aggresome in yeast: aggresome-targeting signals and components of the machinery. FASEB J. **23**, 451–463

77. Wickner, R.B., Edskes, H.K., Bateman, D.A., Kelly, A.C., Gorkovskiy, A., Dayani, Y. and Zhou, A. (2013) Amyloids and yeast prion biology. Biochemistry **52**, 1514 –1527

78. Nelson, R., Sawaya, M.R., Balbirnie, M., Madsen, A.O., Riekel, C., Grothe, R. and Eisenberg, D. (2005) Structure of the cross-β spine of amyloid-like fibrils. Nature **435**, 773–778

79. Derkatch, I.L., Bradley, M.E., Hong, J.Y. and Liebman, S.W. (2001) Prions affect the appearance of other prions: the story of *[PIN]*. Cell **106**, 171–182

80. Du, Z., Park, K.-W., Yu, H., Fan, Q. and Li, L. (2008) Newly identified prion linked to the chromatin-remodeling factor Swi1 in *Saccharomyces cerevisiae*. Nat. Genet. **40**, 460–465

81. Patel, B.K., Gavin-Smyth, J. and Liebman, S.W. (2009) The yeast global transcriptional co-repressor protein Cyc8 can propagate as a prion. Nat. Cell Biol. **11**, 344–349

82. Alberti, S., Halfmann, R., King, O., Kapila, A. and Lindquist, S. (2009) A systematic survey identifies prions and illuminates sequence features of prionogenic proteins. Cell **137**, 146–158

83. Rogoza, T., Goginashvili, A., Rodionova, S., Ivanov, M., Viktorovskaya, O., Rubel, A., Volkov, K. and Mironova, L. (2010) Non-mendelian determinant [ISP+] in yeast is a nuclear-residing prion form of the global transcriptional regulator Sfp1. Proc. Natl. Acad. Sci. U.S.A. **107**, 10573–10577

84. Suzuki, G., Shimazu, N. and Tanaka, M. (2012) A yeast prion, Mod5, promotes acquired drug resistance and cell survival under environmental stress. Science **336**, 355–359

85. Roberts, B.T. and Wickner, R.B. (2003) A class of prions that propagate via covalent auto-activation. Genes Dev. **17**, 2083–2087

© The Authors Journal compilation © 2014 Biochemical Society
Essays Biochem. (2014) 56, 207–219: doi: 10.1042/BSE0560207

15

Functional amyloid: widespread in Nature, diverse in purpose

Chi L.L. Pham*, Ann H. Kwan[†] and Margaret Sunde*[†1]

**Discipline of Pharmacology, School of Medical Sciences, University of Sydney, NSW 2006, Australia*
†School of Molecular Bioscience, University of Sydney, NSW 2006, Australia

Abstract

Amyloids are insoluble fibrillar protein deposits with an underlying cross-β structure initially discovered in the context of human diseases. However, it is now clear that the same fibrillar structure is used by many organisms, from bacteria to humans, in order to achieve a diverse range of biological functions. These functions include structure and protection (e.g. curli and chorion proteins, and insect and spider silk proteins), aiding interface transitions and cell–cell recognition (e.g. chaplins, rodlins and hydrophobins), protein control and storage (e.g. Microcin E492, modulins and PMEL), and epigenetic inheritance and memory [e.g. Sup35, Ure2p, HET-s and CPEB (cytoplasmic polyadenylation element-binding protein)]. As more examples of functional amyloid come to light, the list of roles associated with functional amyloids has continued to expand. More recently, amyloids have also been implicated in signal transduction [e.g. RIP1/RIP3 (receptor-interacting protein)] and perhaps in host defence [e.g. aDrs (anionic dermaseptin) peptide]. The present chapter discusses in detail functional amyloids that are used in Nature by micro-organisms, non-mammalian animals and mammals, including the biological roles that they play, their molecular composition and how they assemble, as well as the coping strategies that organisms have evolved to avoid the potential toxicity of functional amyloid.

Keywords:
amyloid, biofilm, chorion protein, curli, fibril, hydrophobin, self-assembly, surface adhesion.

[1]*To whom correspondence should be addressed (email margaret.sunde@sydney.edu.au).*

Introduction

The amyloid structure has traditionally been associated with misfolded and partially folded proteins in the context of pathology and diseases. However, recent studies have identified amyloid structures serving important functional roles in organisms ranging from bacteria to insects to mammals [1]. In some organisms, the unique structural traits of the cross-β structural core have been exploited by Nature to serve a multitude of biological roles not merely restricted to the provision of a structural framework. Indeed, functional amyloids serving roles as diverse as surface protection and modification, mediation of host interactions, pigment biosynthesis, haemostatic control, hormone storage and release and signal transduction have been discovered [1]. Despite the many roles served by functional amyloid, such structures are a double-edged sword as large, self-assembling and insoluble protein aggregates can be extremely toxic and detrimental to an organism. Therefore the assembly process of functional amyloid must be tightly regulated both spatially and temporally to harness its utility. To this end, Nature has evolved many molecular, structural and cellular adaptations and coping mechanisms [2]. This chapter focuses on the functional amyloids that are employed in Nature by life forms as diverse as simple micro-organisms, to higher order non-mammalian animals and mammals, including humans.

Functional amyloids with a structural purpose

Many microbes have evolved a diverse suite of proteins that are suited to self-assembly into the cross-β amyloid fold under a range of conditions, to provide a robust fibrillar protein scaffold that can present additional functional characteristics including stability, amphipathicity, adhesion and toxicity. Amyloid fibrils play a key role in the formation and stability of bacterial biofilms. Many different proteins have been identified as the amyloid-forming component of bacterial fibrils [3–26] (Table 1). Bacteria including *Escherichia coli*, *Salmonella*, *Citrobacter* and *Shewanella* produce curli fimbriae with amyloid characteristics and these protein fibrils form a major part of the extracellular matrix in biofilms formed by these bacteria, in association with exopolysaccharides [3] (Figure 1A). The amyloid fibrils increase biofilm stability and resistance to protease degradation and as such, these amyloids contribute to host invasion and colonization. Curli fibril assembly involves six members of the curli protein family, with CsgA and CsgB making up the fibrils and CsgD-G responsible for expression, secretion and assembly [4]. In *Pseudomonas fluorescens*, fibrils composed of the protein FapC contribute to biofilm formation and stability [2] and in *Mycobaterium tuberculosis* the protein Mtp is involved in pili formation [3]. In the natural environment, screening with amyloid-specific dyes has identified material with amyloid character in Proteobacteria, Bacteriodetes, Choroflexi and Actinobacteria, while amyloids have also been detected in flocs associated with water treatment processes [3].

Although the most well-known and studied functional amyloids tend to be from micro-organisms, amyloid structures playing beneficial roles are also known to exist in higher order organisms, ranging from insects to spiders to fish to mammals [1]. In these higher organisms, the roles served by functional amyloids are even more diverse (Table 1), even though the

Table 1. Functional amyloids are found in a wide variety of organisms ranging from simple bacteria to humans

Species	Protein	Function	Reference(s)
Bacteria			
E. coli	Curli	Biofilm formation and host invasion	[3–5]
Salmonella spp.	Curli	Biofilm formation and host invasion	[3–5]
S. coelicolor	Chaplin	Modulation of water surface tension	[5,6]
Pseudomonas spp.	FapC	Biofilm formation	[2,5]
Xanthomonas spp. and other plant pathogens	HpaG	Plant pathogen virulence factor	[5]
K. pneumonia	Microcin E492 (Mcc)	Storage and regulation of toxicity	[5,7]
Bacillus subtilis	TasA	Biofilm formation	[2,5]
Streptococcus mutans	P1	Adhesion and host interaction	[8]
S. aureus	Modulin	Toxin and biofilm stabilization	[9]
M. tuberculosis	Mtp	Pili formation	[10]
Unicellular eukaryotes			
Plasmodium falciparum	MSP2	Erythrocyte invasion*	[11]
Fungi			
Podospora anserina	HET-s	Regulation of heterokaryon formation	[5,12]
S. cerevisiae	Ure2p	Regulation of nitrogen catabolism	[12]
S. cerevisiae	Sup35p	Regulation of stop-codon readthrough	[12]
S. cerevisiae	Nsp1	Control of nucleocytoplasmic mixing at nuclear pore	[5]
Candida albicans	Fungal adhesin	Cell adhesion	[3]
S. cerevisiae	Fungal adhesin	Cell adhesion	[3]
Most filamentous fungi	Hydrophobin	Coat formation and modulation of adhesion and surface tension	[13]
Plants			
Hevea brasiliensis	REF	Biosynthesis of natural rubber	[14]

(Continued)

Table 1. Functional amyloids are found in a wide variety of organisms ranging from simple bacteria to humans   (*Continued*)

Species	Protein	Function	Reference(s)
Animalia (excluding mammals)			
Insects and fish	Chorion protein	Structural and protection	[5,15–17]
Nephila clavipes	Spidroin	Structural	[18]
A. diadematus	Spidroin	Structural	[18]
C. flava	Silk protein	Structural	[19]
M. signata	Silk protein (MalXB)	Structural	[20]
A. californica	CPEB	Memory storage	[21]
P. dacnicolor	aDrs	Host defence*	[22]
Mammals			
Homo sapiens	Pmel17	Melanin synthesis	[23]
H. sapiens	Peptide hormone	Storage and controlled release	[24]
H. sapiens	RIP1/RIP3	Regulators of necroptosis	[25]
Mus musculus and probably other mammals	CRES and cst8	Sperm maturation and maintenance of the luminal milieu	[26]

*Function is putative or it is unclear if the amyloid has a function *in vivo*

provision of a stable and robust structural framework remains as the underlying theme. One such example is the chorion proteins. Silkmoth chorion is a proteinaceous layer with remarkable mechanical and physicochemical properties and which represents the major component (over 90% by weight) of the eggshell [17] (Figure 1C). This layer is composed of ~200 proteins and serves to protect the oocyte and the developing embryo from a range of potential environmental hazards, as well as to enable physiological functions, such as fertilization and respiratory gas exchange. Chorion proteins can be divided into two classes, known as A and B, on the basis of sequence alignment. Members of both protein classes are composed of three domains: the highly conserved central domain and two relatively variable flanking regions. Characteristic tandem repeats of hexapeptides are present in all three domains and the repeats in the central domain have been shown to be the basis for the amyloidogenic properties of silkmoth chorion [15,16]. Using electron microscopy, amyloid-specific dye binding experiments, X-ray diffraction and infra-red spectroscopy, peptide analogue representatives covering parts and the entirety of the central domain from both class A and B proteins have been shown to self-assemble into amyloid-like fibrils *in vitro*, with similar structural characteristics to those observed on native silkmoth chorion. Similarly, the chorion of the annual killifish *Austrofundulus limnaeus* has been shown to be composed of amyloid proteins which

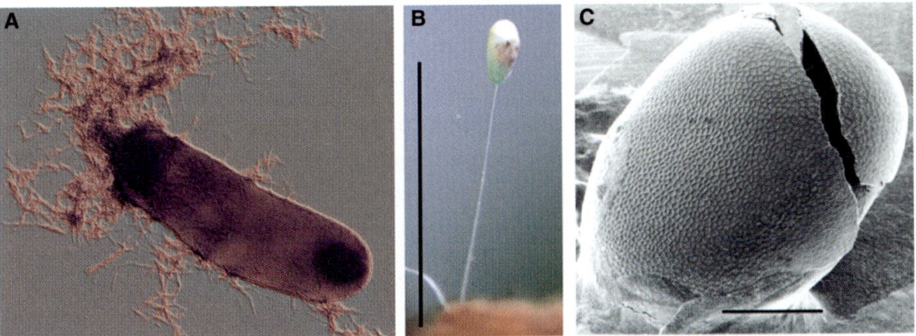

Figure 1. Examples of micro-organisms that utilize amyloid fibrils for functional purposes
(**A**) *E. coli* expressing curli amyloid fibrils (reproduced with permission from http://labs.mcdb. lsa.umich.edu/labs/chapman/). (**B**) An egg suspended on the egg-stalk silk of the green lacewing fly, *Chrysopa carnea*. Scale bar, 50 mm. Reproduced with permission from [34], Lintz, E.S. and Scheibel, T.R. (2013) Dragline, egg stalk and byssus: a comparison of outstanding protein fibers and their potential for developing new materials. Adv. Funct. Mater. **23**, 4467–4482. (**C**) The chorion of the silkmoth *Bombyx mori*. Scale bar, 400 µm. Reproduced with permission from http://biophysics.biol.uoa.gr/LepChorionDB/Manual.php.

allow the embryos to survive the drying ephemeral ponds which form and dry out on a seasonal basis, where all living fish are killed [27]. It has been proposed that the amyloidogenic properties of the egg proteins allow for increased intermolecular contacts and interactions to form upon dehydration, which could serve to decrease water permeability of the egg envelope during the dry season.

The superior mechanical properties and the insoluble nature of the stacked β-sheets found in amyloid fibres have also been exploited by insects and spiders for silk production. A number of insect and spider silks with many morphological and structural similarities to disease amyloids have been identified, including the egg-stalk silk from the green lacewing fly *Chrysopa flava* (Figure 1B) and *Mallada signata* [19,20] and the dragline silk from the spiders *Nephila edulis* and *Araneus diadematus* [18]. As for the chorion proteins, the major protein components in dragline silk, MaSp1/2 (major ampullate spidroin 1/2) and ADF-3/4 (*Araneus diadematus* fibroin-3/4) from the two spider species, are characterized by short repeat motifs in the sequence. Remarkably, the proteins are stored at a concentration of up to 50% (w/v) in the spider gland in the form of liquid crystals, and thread assembly is initiated as the local environment along the gland duct lumen changes to favour formation of hydrogen bonds and β-pleated structures. In many ways, the silk-spinning process mimics amyloid formation in disease states on a molecular level with engineered ADF-4-based protein fragments shown to self-assemble into nanofibrils *in vitro* [18].

Functional amyloids that enable interface transitions and cell–cell recognition

Many microbial amyloids are amphipathic structures that mediate interactions across air–liquid interfaces. The fibrillar rodlet layers observed on the filamentous soil bacteria *Streptomyces* and on the aerial surfaces of filamentous fungi have an amyloid substructure that presents a hydrophobic face towards the air and a hydrophilic face in contact with cell wall components [28] (Figures 2A and 2B). These rodlet layers allow the vegetative hyphae to breach the air–liquid interface and to complete sporulation. The *Streptomyces coelicolor* rodlet layer is comprised of two types of proteins, the chaplins and the rodlins, whereas the amyloid fibrils on fungal spores are composed of hydrophobin proteins [6,13]. The presence of the hydrophobic outer coating on fungal spores provided by the amphipathic amyloid monolayer allows for resistance to wetting and effective dispersal of spores in air (Figures 3A–3D). Fungal repellent proteins may also adopt amyloid structures and be involved in aerial hyphae formation and attachment to host cells (Figures 3E and 3F) [29].

Microbial amyloid also plays a key role in mediating attachment of the organisms to surfaces. The Mtp fibres produced by *M. tuberculosis* bind laminin, a human extracellular matrix protein, and improve cellular adhesion and internalization [10] (Figure 2C). Curli fibrils have also been shown to bind to host extracellular matrix proteins such as fibronectin and laminin [7]. The amyloid rodlet structures composed of hydrophobins produced by plant pathogenic fungi, e.g. MPG1 from *Magnaporthe grisea*, the causative agent of rice blast, facilitate adherence to waxy leaf surfaces [30]. Deletion of the hydrophobin layer reduces infectivity. Adhesins from *Candida albicans* are involved in host tissue adhesion [3]. The MSP2 protein on the surface of the malaria parasite *Plasmodium falciparum*, which has been proposed as a candidate for an antimalarial vaccine, has been shown to form an amyloid structure *in vitro* [11]. However, the conformation and function of this protein on the surface of the parasite is not yet known. In addition, these functional amyloids may mediate particular interactions with the host immune system. The presence of a functional amyloid monolayer composed of the hydrophobin RodA on the surface of the spores of the human pathogenic fungus *Aspergillus fumiga-*

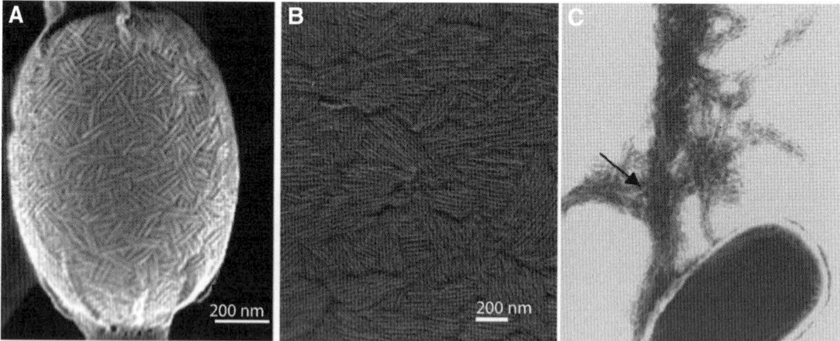

Figure 2. Microbial amyloid fibrils as monolayer spore coatings and bacterial pili
(**A**) Chaplin rodlets on the surface of a wild-type *S. coelicolor* M600 spore. Adapted with permission from [35], Di Berardo, C., Capstick, D.S., Bibb, M.J., Findlay, K.C., Buttner, M.J. and Elliot, M.A. (2008) Function and redundancy of the chaplin cell surface proteins in aerial hypha formation, rodlet assembly, and viability in *Streptomyces coelicolor*. J. Bacteriol. **190**, 5879–5889. (**B**) Hydrophobin rodlets on the surface of *A. fumigatus* spore, provided by Professor Jean-Paul Latgé (*Aspergillus* Unit, Paris, France). (**C**) Mtp pili production by *M. tuberculosis* clinical isolate CDC1551 at magnification ×45000. Reproduced with permission from [10], Alteri, C.J., Xicohtencatl-Cortes, J., Hess, S., Caballero-Olin, G., Giron, J.A. and Friedman, R.L. (2007) *Mycobacterium tuberculosis* produces pili during human infection. Proc. Natl. Acad. Sci. U.S.A. **104**, 5145–5150, Copyright 2007 National Academy of Sciences, U.S.A.

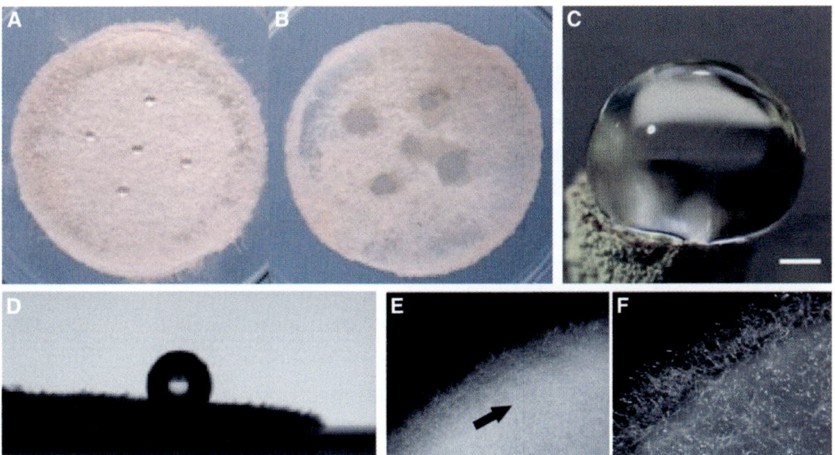

Figure 3. Functional amyloids that modulate interface transitions
(**A**) Water droplets resting on the hydrophobic surface of the mycelium of wild-type *Neurospora crassa* and (**B**) water droplets soaking into the mycelium of a knockout strain lacking the hydrophobin EAS, image produced by Professor Ross Beever (deceased; previously at Landcare Research Auckland). (**C**) A water droplet attached to the super-hydrophobic surface of the lichen *Cladonia chlorophaea*. Scale bar, 200 nm. Reproduced with permission from [36], Hamlett, C.A.E., Shirtcliffe, N.J., Pyatt, F.B., Newton, M.I., McHale, G. and Koch, K. (2011) Passive water control at the surface of a superhydrophobic lichen. Planta **234**, 1267–1274. (**D**) A water droplet resting on the hydrophobic surface of a fungal colony of *Penicillium expansum*. Adapted with permission from [37], Siqueira, V. and Lima, N. (2012) Surface hydrophobicity of culture and water biofilm of *Penicillium* spp. Curr. Microbiol. **64**, 93–99. (**E**) Formation of aerial hyphae by wild-type *Ustilago maydis* colonies and (**F**) aerial hyphae produced by *U. maydis* lacking the repellent gene *rep1*. Reproduced with permission from [38], Teertstra, W.R., Deelstra, H.J., Vranes, M., Bohlmann, R., Kahmann, R., Kamper, J. and Wosten, H.A.B. (2006) Repellents have functionally replaced hydrophobins in mediating attachment to a hydrophobic surface and in formation of hydrophobic aerial hyphae in *Ustilago maydis*. Microbiology **152**, 3607–3612.

tus prevents immune recognition by the infected host [31]. Curli fibres produced by *E. coli* are recognized by Toll-like receptors, but also serve to protect bacteria through stabilization of biofilms and promote adherence to host cells and surfaces [7].

Functional amyloids as protein control or storage systems

Many functional amyloids are important for facilitating self- and non-self interactions between the organism and its environment, especially when toxicity or pathogenesis is involved. The switch between amyloid and non-amyloid forms may be used to control function, especially when one of the forms is cytotoxic. The amyloid fibrils utilized by microorganisms can represent a non-toxic repository of proteins or a structural form with distinct properties. For example, Microcin E492 is a bactericidal peptide expressed by *Klebsiella pneumonia* which in monomeric and oligomeric forms is able to form cytotoxic pores in bacteria, but which can also form inert fibrils. The amyloid form appears to represent a safe storage form of the peptide [7]. The phenol soluble modulins are virulence factors produced by *Staphylococcus aureus* that exhibit anti-microbial activity against niche-occupying bacteria in a soluble form and which have now also been shown to form amyloid fibrils that stabilize the *S. aureus* biofilms [9]. In the frog *Pachymedusa dacnicolor*, a secreted peptide known as aDrs (anionic dermaseptin) proposed to be involved in host defence has been shown to assemble into amyloid-like fibrils in a pH-dependent manner [22]. This peptide exists in two forms, with the leucine residue at the second position existing as an L- or D-isomer. Interestingly, both forms of the peptide can assemble into amyloid fibres, but with different assembly kinetics, morphologies and superstructural architectures. It has therefore been suggested that the L/D-isomerization may act as a stereochemical switch to control amyloid assembly with biological consequence.

PMEL is a transmembrane glycoprotein, synthesized in the endoplasmic reticulum and then trafficked through to the Golgi and the trans-Golgi network before reaching the early endosome/stage I premelanosomes [23]. Amyloid fibrils, composed of a fragment of the protein PMEL, play a specialized role in storage in mammalian melanocytes. Melanins are tyrosine-based polymers found in the melanosomes, the membrane-bound organelles of melanocytes and the retinal pigment epithelial cells. The function of melanin is to protect the skin and eyes from UV radiation and oxidative damage. The biosynthesis of melanin involves the action of the enzyme tyrosinase, which converts tyrosine into L-dopa. This readily oxidizes to form the reactive intermediate indole-5,6-quinone that subsequently polymerizes to form melanin. Formation of melanin is accelerated in the presence of PMEL fibrils within the melanosomes and both cytotoxic intermediates and mature melanin bind to the fibrils and remain sequestered within the melanosomes [23,32] (Figure 4).

A number of proteolytic processing events occur within the trans-Golgi network and the early endosome to ultimately release the N-terminal Mα fragments from the C-terminal-membrane-associated Mβ fragment of PMEL [23]. Some short fibrillar material consisting of Mα fragments can be observed in stage I melanosomes. Further self-association of the Mα fragment into amyloid fibrils occurs in the lumen of stage II melanosomes. Amyloid fibrils formed by PMEL subsequently assemble into fibril matrices that act as a scaffold to enable the formation of melanin during stages III and IV of melanosome development, giving a characteristic black pigment [23] (Figure 4). In promoting melanin biosynthesis, PMEL amyloid fibrils sequester the indole-5,6-quinone reactive intermediates from the cellular milieu, thus preventing oxidative damage and cytotoxicity [23,32]. The deposition of melanin on to the PMEL amyloid fibril matrix also serves to concentrate melanin for storage and cellular transport [23].

It is known that secretory granules in mammals are composed of highly concentrated and densely packed protein aggregates that have a distinct structural organization. Maji et al. [24] demonstrated that many peptides and protein hormones of the endocrine system are stored as amyloid fibrils within secretory granules. The fibrils formed here are less toxic than amyloid fibrils associated with diseases and may be inert upon storage within membrane-enclosed granules. Furthermore, these fibrils are able to release biologically active monomeric hormone, a prerequisite for granule secretion. However, it must be noted that not all amyloids formed by endocrine hormones are functional and beneficial. Amyloid fibrils formed from the amylin peptide, which is produced in the β-cells of pancreatic islets, are a well-studied example of disease amyloid associated with Type II diabetes.

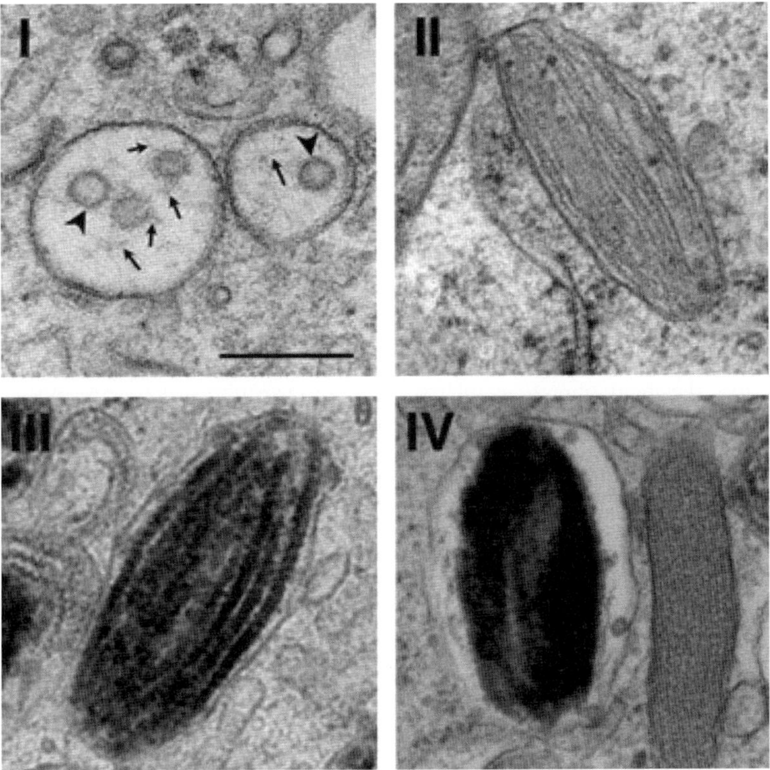

Figure 4. The four stages of melanosome maturation accompanied by PMEL amyloid formation

The arrows in stage I indicate the presence of short PMEL fibrils that further associate and assemble into fibril matrices during stage II. The fibril matrices act as a scaffold to promote melanin pigment formation in stages III and IV. Scale bar, 200 nm. Images obtained with permission from [39], Hurbain, I., Geerts, W.J., Boudier, T., Marco, S., Verkleij, A.J., Marks, M.S. and Raposo, G. (2008) Electron tomography of early melanosomes: implications for melanogenesis and the generation of fibrillar amyloid sheets. Proc. Natl. Acad. Sci. U.S.A. **105**, 19726–19731, Copyright 2008 National Academy of Sciences, U.S.A.

Other biological functions associated with amyloid fibrils

Apart from structural and protective roles, functional amyloids have been suggested to serve roles in functions as diverse as signal transduction, epigenetic inheritance, memory formation and host defence. In some cases, the biological role of the amyloid remains to be elucidated, as in the case of a reproductive-specific cystatin protein, cst8, which can form amyloid fibrils *in vitro* and may play a role in sperm maturation or maintenance of the luminal environment of the epididymis [26].

Functional amyloid structures formed in higher organisms have been implicated in the protein–protein interactions that underlie programmed necrosis (known as necroptosis), which serves as an alternative cell death pathway to apoptosis [25]. RIP1 (receptor-interacting protein 1) and RIP3 are important mammalian regulators of necroptosis. Following inhibition of caspase 8 activity within the DISC (death-inducing signalling complex), the apoptosis pathway is inhibited and necroptosis is induced by the assembly of the necrosome, where RIP1 and RIP3 interact with each other to form the core of necrosome [33]. The interaction of RIP1 and RIP3 occurs through their RHIM (RIP homotypic interaction motif) domains. Recently, RIP1/RIP3 complexes have been shown to form amyloid fibrils and the amyloid core is located within the RHIM domain. Mutations within the core RHIM domain of RIP1 or RIP3 disrupt formation of the RIP1/RIP3 complexes, inhibit amyloid assembly and cause defects in kinase activation and induction of necroptosis. Both RIP1 and RIP3 kinase activities are required for necroptosis and thus, the formation of amyloidal RIP1/RIP3 complexes is essential for signal transduction in necroptosis [25].

In yeast, the ability of proteins such as Sup35 and Ure2p to switch between soluble and aggregated amyloid forms gives rise to an epigenetic non-Mendelian type of inheritance when the cytoplasmic amyloid is passed to progeny during cell division. The infectious 'prion' nature of the amyloid aggregates induces conversion of soluble protein into the amyloid form and inheritance of the phenotype. The amyloid HET-s prion system in *Podospora anserina* regulates heterokaryon incompatibility between genetically similar fungi [12]. Similarly, the N-terminal domain of a neuron-specific isoform of CPEB (cytoplasmic polyadenylation element-binding protein) in *Aplysia californica*, a Californian sea slug, has been shown to confer a self-perpetuating change in state on the glucocorticoid receptor, a hallmark of the infectious yeast prions. In addition, the prion form of full-length CPEB has an enhanced ability to alter the translation rate of local mRNA at selective neuron junctions, leading to the suggestion that this functional amyloid may help to maintain perpetuating changes associated with memory storage [21].

Conclusions

The widespread nature and diversity of purpose of natural functional amyloid systems is rapidly coming to light. From providing a stable and proteolysis-resistant structural scaffold (e.g. biofilm formation and protection of chorion), altering surface properties (amphipathic hydrophobin monolayers), facilitating cell adhesion (Mtp pili) and protein–protein interactions (RIP kinases), to providing safe storage forms of proteins (endocrine hormones) and cytotoxic species (PMEL amyloid), amyloid underlies a range of biological systems.

In contrast with disease-associated amyloid, where the aggregation of protein into amyloid fibrils is a consequence of proteins adopting a non-native and non-functional form, the formation of functional amyloid involves the association and interaction of natively folded proteins and must be stringently controlled and regulated. Such regulation is essential to avoid the unwanted accumulation of protein aggregates that interfere with the normal functioning of cellular processes. Thus research into the molecular details of how organisms control and regulate the biogenesis of functional amyloid should not only lead to an in-depth understanding of diverse cellular processes, but may also provide insights into therapeutic strategies for the prevention and treatment of amyloid diseases [1]. Furthermore, one of the exciting outcomes emerging from functional amyloid research over the last decade is the discovery that some functional amyloids possess unique physiochemical properties that can be exploited for use in drug delivery, surface coating and other areas of nanobiotechnology.

Summary

- Amyloids play important and varied functional roles in organisms as diverse as bacteria and humans.
- The stable cross-β-fibril structure provides a structural scaffold upon which functionality such as amphipathicity, adhesion and toxicity is displayed.
- Many bacterial amyloid fibrils act to stabilize biofilms.
- Functional amyloids provide a protective coating surrounding fungal spores and silkmoth embryos.
- Many functional amyloid fibrils mediate interactions across hydrophobic–hydrophilic interfaces and facilitate surface adhesion.
- Functional amyloid coatings play a role in mediating recognition by the host immune system.
- Functional amyloids have also been implicated as toxins or as a storage form for sequestration of toxins.
- Some peptide hormones may be stabilized and stored in an amyloid form.
- Prion forms of functional amyloid play a role in epigenetic inheritance and memory.

References

1. Fowler, D.M., Koulov, A.V., Balch, W.E. and Kelly, J.W. (2007) Functional amyloid: from bacteria to humans. Trends Biochem. Sci. **32**, 217–224
2. Otzen, D. (2010) Functional amyloid: turning swords into plowshares. Prion **4**, 256–264
3. Blanco, L.P., Evans, M.L., Smith, D.R., Badtke, M.P. and Chapman, M.R. (2012) Diversity, biogenesis and function of microbial amyloids. Trends Microbiol. **20**, 66–73
4. Chapman, M.R., Robinson, L.S., Pinkner, J.S., Roth, R., Heuser, J., Hammar, M., Normark, S. and Hultgren, S.J. (2002) Role of *Escherichia coli* curli operons in directing amyloid fiber formation. Science **295**, 851–855
5. Shewmaker, F., McGlinchey, R.P. and Wickner, R.B. (2011) Structural insights into functional and pathological amyloid. J. Biol. Chem. **286**, 16533–16540
6. Sawyer, E.B., Claessen, D., Gras, S.L. and Perrett, S. (2012) Exploiting amyloid: how and why bacteria use cross-β fibrils. Biochem. Soc. Trans. **40**, 728–734
7. DePas, W.H. and Chapman, M.R. (2012) Microbial manipulation of the amyloid fold. Res. Microbiol. **163**, 592–606
8. Oli, M.W., Otoo, H.N., Crowley, P.J., Heim, K.P., Nascimento, M.M., Ramsook, C.B., Lipke, P.N. and Brady, L.J. (2012) Functional amyloid formation by *Streptococcus mutans*. Microbiology **158**, 2903–2916
9. Schwartz, K. and Boles, B.R. (2013) Microbial amyloids: functions and interactions within the host. Curr. Opin. Microbiol. **16**, 93–99
10. Alteri, C.J., Xicohtencatl-Cortes, J., Hess, S., Caballero-Olin, G., Giron, J.A. and Friedman, R.L. (2007) *Mycobacterium tuberculosis* produces pili during human infection. Proc. Natl. Acad. Sci. U.S.A. **104**, 5145–5150
11. Adda, C.G., Murphy, V.J., Sunde, M., Waddington, L.J., Schloegel, J., Talbo, G.H., Vingas, K., Kienzle, V., Masciantonio, R., Howlett, G.J. et al. (2009) *Plasmodium falciparum* merozoite surface protein 2 is unstructured and forms amyloid-like fibrils. Mol. Biochem. Parasitol. **166**, 159–171
12. Wickner, R.B., Edskes, H.K., Bateman, D.A., Kelly, A.C., Gorkovskiy, A., Dayani, Y. and Zhou, A. (2013) Amyloids and yeast prion biology. Biochemistry **52**, 1514–1527

13. Sunde, M., Kwan, A.H., Templeton, M.D., Beever, R.E. and Mackay, J.P. (2008) Structural analysis of hydrophobins. Micron **39**, 773–784

14. Berthelot, K., Lecomte, S., Estevez, Y., Coulary-Salin, B., Bentaleb, A., Cullin, C., Deffieux, A. and Peruch, F. (2012) Rubber elongation factor (REF), a major allergen component in *Hevea brasiliensis* latex has amyloid properties. PLoS ONE **7**, e48065

15. Iconomidou, V.A., Chryssikos, G.D., Gionis, V., Galanis, A.S., Cordopatis, P., Hoenger, A. and Hamodrakas, S.J. (2006) Amyloid fibril formation propensity is inherent into the hexapeptide tandemly repeating sequence of the central domain of silkmoth chorion proteins of the A-family. J. Struct. Biol. **156**, 480–488

16. Iconomidou, V.A., Chryssikos, G.D., Gionis, V., Vriend, G., Hoenger, A. and Hamodrakas, S.J. (2001) Amyloid-like fibrils from an 18-residue peptide analogue of a part of the central domain of the B-family of silkmoth chorion proteins. FEBS Lett. **499**, 268–273

17. Iconomidou, V.A., Vriend, G. and Hamodrakas, S.J. (2000) Amyloids protect the silkmoth oocyte and embryo. FEBS Lett. **479**, 141–145

18. Kenney, J.M., Knight, D., Wise, M.J. and Vollrath, F. (2002) Amyloidogenic nature of spider silk. Eur. J. Biochem. **269**, 4159–4163

19. Parker, K.D. and Rudall, K.M. (1957) The silk of the egg-stalk of the green lace-wing fly: structure of the silk of *Chrysopa* egg-stalks. Nature **179**, 905–906

20. Weisman, S., Okada, S., Mudie, S.T., Huson, M.G., Trueman, H.E., Sriskantha, A., Haritos, V.S. and Sutherland, T.D. (2009) Fifty years later: the sequence, structure and function of lacewing cross-β silk. J. Struct. Biol. **168**, 467–475

21. Si, K., Lindquist, S. and Kandel, E.R. (2003) A neuronal isoform of the *Aplysia* CPEB has prion-like properties. Cell **115**, 879–891

22. Gossler-Schofberger, R., Hesser, G., Reif, M.M., Friedmann, J., Duscher, B., Toca-Herrera, J.L., Oostenbrink, C. and Jilek, A. (2012) A stereochemical switch in the aDrs model system, a candidate for a functional amyloid. Arch. Biochem. Biophys. **522**, 100–106

23. Watt, B., van Niel, G., Raposo, G. and Marks, M.S. (2013) PMEL: a pigment cell-specific model for functional amyloid formation. Pigment Cell Melanoma Res. **26**, 300–315

24. Maji, S.K., Perrin, M.H., Sawaya, M.R., Jessberger, S., Vadodaria, K., Rissman, R.A., Singru, P.S., Nilsson, K.P., Simon, R., Schubert, D. et al. (2009) Functional amyloids as natural storage of peptide hormones in pituitary secretory granules. Science **325**, 328–332

25. Li, J., McQuade, T., Siemer, A.B., Napetschnig, J., Moriwaki, K., Hsiao, Y.S., Damko, E., Moquin, D., Walz, T., McDermott, A. et al. (2012) The RIP1/RIP3 necrosome forms a functional amyloid signaling complex required for programmed necrosis. Cell **150**, 339–350

26. Whelly, S., Johnson, S., Powell, J., Borchardt, C., Hastert, M.C. and Cornwall, G.A. (2012) Nonpathological extracellular amyloid is present during normal epididymal sperm maturation. PLoS ONE **7**, e36394

27. Podrabsky, J.E., Carpenter, J.F. and Hand, S.C. (2001) Survival of water stress in annual fish embryos: dehydration avoidance and egg envelope amyloid fibers. Am. J. Physiol. Regul. Integr. Comp. Physiol. **280**, R123–131

28. Gebbink, M.F., Claessen, D., Bouma, B., Dijkhuizen, L. and Wosten, H.A. (2005) Amyloids: a functional coat for microorganisms. Nat. Rev. Microbiol. **3**, 333–341

29. Teertstra, W.R., van der Velden, G.J., de Jong, J.F., Kruijtzer, J.A., Liskamp, R.M., Kroon-Batenburg, L.M., Muller, W.H., Gebbink, M.F. and Wosten, H.A. (2009) The filament-specific Rep1-1 repellent of the phytopathogen *Ustilago maydis* forms functional surface-active amyloid-like fibrils. J. Biol. Chem. **284**, 9153–9159

30. Talbot, N.J., Kershaw, M.J., Wakley, G.E., De Vries, O., Wessels, J. and Hamer, J.E. (1996) MPG1 encodes a fungal hydrophobin involved in surface interactions during infection-related development of *Magnaporthe grisea*. Plant Cell **8**, 985–999

31. Aimanianda, V., Bayry, J., Bozza, S., Kniemeyer, O., Perruccio, K., Elluru, S.R., Clavaud, C., Paris, S., Brakhage, A.A., Kaveri, S.V. et al. (2009) Surface hydrophobin prevents immune recognition of airborne fungal spores. Nature **460**, 1117–1121

32. Fowler, D.M., Koulov, A.V., Alory-Jost, C., Marks, M.S., Balch, W.E. and Kelly, J.W. (2006) Functional amyloid formation within mammalian tissue. PLoS Biol. **4**, e6

33. Wu, W., Liu, P. and Li, J. (2012) Necroptosis: an emerging form of programmed cell death. Crit. Rev. Oncol. Hematol. **82**, 249–258

34. Lintz, E.S. and Scheibel, T.R. (2013) Dragline, egg stalk and byssus: a comparison of outstanding protein fibers and their potential for developing new materials. Adv. Funct. Mater. **23**, 4467–4482

35. Di Berardo, C., Capstick, D.S., Bibb, M.J., Findlay, K.C., Buttner, M.J. and Elliot, M.A. (2008) Function and redundancy of the chaplin cell surface proteins in aerial hypha formation, rodlet assembly, and viability in *Streptomyces coelicolor*. J. Bacteriol. **190**, 5879–5889

36. Hamlett, C.A.E., Shirtcliffe, N.J., Pyatt, F.B., Newton, M.I., McHale, G. and Koch, K. (2011) Passive water control at the surface of a superhydrophobic lichen. Planta **234**, 1267–1274

37. Siqueira, V. and Lima, N. (2012) Surface hydrophobicity of culture and water biofilm of *Penicillium* spp. Curr. Microbiol. **64**, 93–99

38. Teertstra, W.R., Deelstra, H.J., Vranes, M., Bohlmann, R., Kahmann, R., Kamper, J. and Wosten, H.A.B. (2006) Repellents have functionally replaced hydrophobins in mediating attachment to a hydrophobic surface and in formation of hydrophobic aerial hyphae in *Ustilago maydis*. Microbiology **152**, 3607–3612

39. Hurbain, I., Geerts, W.J., Boudier, T., Marco, S., Verkleij, A.J., Marks, M.S. and Raposo, G. (2008) Electron tomography of early melanosomes: implications for melanogenesis and the generation of fibrillar amyloid sheets. Proc. Natl. Acad. Sci. U.S.A. **105**, 19726–19731

INDEX

H

I

K

L

M

N

O

P